CONTENTS

Introduction	iii
1. The Mediterranean Diet	1
2. Foods to Avoid and to Eat	3
3. Benefits of the Mediterranean Diet	7
4. Getting Started with the Mediterranean Diet	10
5. Meal Preparation	14
6. Mediterranean Recipes	252
Afterword	485

INTRODUCTION

The Mediterranean Diet is a diet developed in the United States in the 1980s and inspired by Italy's and Greece's eating habits in the 1960s. Its main aspects include proportionally excessive intake of olive oil, nuts and seeds, unprocessed cereals, fruits, veggies, moderate to high fish consumption, and regular drinking of dairy products (mostly as cheese and yogurt). Olive oil has been known as a potential health factor in reducing mortality from all causes and the risk of chronic diseases.

There are many opposing views on the Mediterranean Diet, and there are controversies over some sources saying it is not that great since there are numerous other diets that have a similar style. However, the Mediterranean Diet is an excellent way of living and has been proven to produce great results. It is an excellent way of maintaining health and living a long, healthy life. It is undoubtedly a great diet plan to follow as it can create long-term effects in keeping one's heart healthy and their body functioning at optimum levels.

The Mediterranean Diet is one of the very first and most popular diets in the world today, as it has changed the way people view dieting and adhering to a strict diet plan. Be as it may, there is a lot more to it than merely following a strict diet plan and sticking to it will undoubtedly be enough to keep one fit and healthy.

It is a lifestyle more than a mere diet. It's safe to say the Mediterranean Diet is both a brain-friendly and body-friendly diet because it preserves and keeps them balanced in their respective ways. The dietary pattern is associated with reductions of all-cause mortality in observational studies. There is also some indication that the Mediterranean Diet decreases the risk of heart failure and early death; that is why the American Medical Association and the

(AHA) American Heart Association suggest this diet. Therefore, as long as you follow this Mediterranean Diet and continue to enrich your lifestyle with the balanced meal options it provides, you are assured of leading a safe and wonderful life without the fear of diseases.

Chapter One

THE MEDITERRANEAN DIET

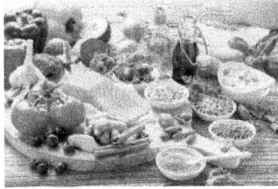

*T*he Mediterranean Diet refers to the traditional eating habits and lifestyles of people living around the Mediterranean Sea – Italy, Spain, France, Greece, and some North African countries. The Mediterranean Diet has become very popular in recent times, as people from these regions have better health and suffer from fewer ailments, such as cancer and cardio-vascular issues. Food plays a key role in this.

Research has uncovered the many benefits of this diet. According to the results of a 2013 study, many overweight and diabetic patients showed a surprising improvement in their cardiovascular health after doing the Mediter-ranean Diet for 5 years. The study was conducted among 7000 people in Spain. There was a marked 30% reduction in cardiovascular disease in this high-risk group.

The report took the world by storm after the New England Journal of Medicine published the findings. Several studies have indicated its many health benefits; the Mediterranean Diet may stabilize the level of blood sugar, prevent Alzheimer's disease, reduce the risk of heart disease and stroke, improve brain health, ease anxiety and depression, promote weight loss, and even lower the risk of certain types of cancer.

The diet differs from country to country, and even within the regions of these countries because of cultural, ethnic, agricultural, religious, and economic differences. So, there is no one standard Mediterranean Diet. However, there are several common factors.

The Mediterranean Diet food pyramid is a nutrition guide to help people eat the right foods in the correct quantities and the prescribed frequency as per the traditional eating habits of people from the Mediterranean coast countries. The pyramid was developed by the World Health Organization, Harvard School of Public Health, and the old ways Preservation Trust in 1993.

There are 6 food layers in the pyramid with physical activity at the base, which is an important element to maintain a healthy life. Just above it is the first food layer, consisting of whole grains, bread, beans, pasta, and nuts. It is the strongest layer having foods that are recommended by the Mediterranean Diet. Next comes fruits and vegetables. As you move up the pyramid, you will find foods that must be eaten less and less, with the topmost layer consisting of foods that should be avoided or restricted.

The Mediterranean Diet food pyramid is easy to understand and it provides an easy way to follow the eating plan.

The Food Layers: Whole Grains, Bread, Beans – The lowest and the widest layer with foods that are strongly recommended. Your meals should be made of mostly these items. Eat whole-wheat bread, whole-wheat pita, whole-grain roll and bun, whole-grain cereal, whole-wheat pasta, and brown rice. 4 to 6 servings a day will give you plenty of nutrition.

Fruits, Vegetables – Almost as important as the lowest layer. Eat non-starchy vegetables daily like asparagus, broccoli, beets, tomatoes, carrots, cucumber, cabbage, cauliflower, turnips 4 to 8 servings daily. Take 2 to 4 servings of fruits every day. Choose seasonal fresh fruits.

Olive oil – Cook your meals preferably in extra-virgin olive oil. Daily consumption. Healthy for the body, it lowers the low-density lipoprotein cholesterol (LDL) and total cholesterol level. Up to 2 tablespoons of olive oil is allowed. The diet also allows for canola oil.

Poultry, cheese, yogurt – The diet should include cheese, yogurt, eggs, chicken, and other poultry products, but in moderation. Maximum 2-3 times a week. Low-fat dairy is best. Soymilk, cheese, or yogurt is better.

Meats, sweets – This is the topmost layer consisting of foods that are best avoided. Red meats can be eaten once or twice a week maximum, sweets only once a month. Remember, the Mediterranean diet is plant-based. There is very little room for meat, especially red meat. If you cannot live without it, then take red meat in small portions. Choose lean cuts. Have sweets only to celebrate – for instance, you can have a couple of sweets after following the diet for a month.

Chapter Two

FOODS TO AVOID AND TO EAT

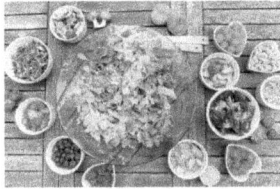

oods to Avoid if on the Mediterranean Diet

The premise of the Mediterranean diet is simple; you need to get the body burning fat rather than glucose for energy. However, the Mediterranean diet isn't a diet where carbohydrates are completely avoided. You can eat vegetables, and even a couple of fruits, virtually without limit. The key, however, is knowing which ones are permitted and which ones must be avoided.

A guiding principle to the Mediterranean Diet is that green vegetables can be consumed, while you want to avoid foods you intuitively know are starchy or sugary. So, let's start with grains. The bottom line when it comes to bread, pasta, rice, corn, oats, barley, and the like is that you can't eat these foods at all. That might be off-putting for a lot of people, but you should be aware that many substitutes are available that use almond or coconut flour in place of wheat, so you can follow a Mediterranean diet and still enjoy some bread and those type of foods. However, many people find they lose their cravings for these kinds of foods after they have been on the Ketogenic diet for some time.

Another large class of food to avoid includes most fruits. Although fruit is known for having a relatively low glycemic index, it's not low enough to avoid having the body rely on sugar for energy. Also, the fact is fruit contains fructose, which is a very potent sugar as far as carbohydrates are involved. The advantage of fruit over fruit juice is that fruit also contains a lot of fiber, which slows down digestion a bit, and it's not concentrated like fruit juice. So, the impact isn't as bad; however, if you are going on a Ketogenic diet, most fruit must be avoided.

The goal of the Mediterranean Diet is to consume minimal carbohydrates so that they only make up between 5-10% of your total calories. To accomplish this, you should avoid the following products and foods (unless they are made out of a substitute like almond flour and explicitly labeled as Mediterranean Diet friendly):

- Bread
- Pasta
- Rice
- Quinoa
- Potatoes
- Muesli
- Lentils
- Couscous
- Sweet potatoes
- Bananas and plantains
- Most round fruits including oranges, apples, peaches, nectarines, and kiwis
- Soda
- Fruit juice
- Donuts and pastries
- Bagels
- Chocolate
- Sugar-containing condiments like ketchup, maple syrup
- Pudding, jelly, and jam
- Green peas
- Legumes
- Beans
- Cashews and pistachios
- French fries
- Milkshakes
- Sugary lattes and other fancy drinks from Starbucks and other coffee outlets
- Mixed alcoholic drinks that contain any syrups or sugary flavored additives
- Sports drinks
- Milk
- Cottage cheese
- Table sugar
- Brown sugar
- Powdered sugar
- Oatmeal, porridge, wheat-based cereals
- Honey
- Barbecue sauce
- Agave
- Cake and cookies

- Potato chips
- Crackers
- Ice-cream and sherbet
- Beer
- Be careful of packaged foods that may contain more carbs than you think and avoid omega-6 based 'vegetable oils' like corn oil, canola oil, etc.

What Can You Eat if on the Mediterranean Diet?

The Mediterranean diet is based on a diet containing fresh, whole foods that contain low amounts of carbohydrates. You can freely consume the following foods while following a Mediterranean diet.

- Fresh meat including beef, chicken, lamb, pork, and turkey (consume skin-on poultry)
- Bacon
- Fatty fish like salmon, mackerel, anchovies, and sardines
- Any other fish and seafood as long as it's not breaded
- Hot dogs and sausage (but check carb content)
- Butter, ghee, and heavy cream
- Cream cheese
- Coconut milk (get full fat, watch carbs)
- Olive oil and avocado oil
- Cheese of any kind (but do not use low-fat varieties, get regular cheese)
- Eggs
- Full fat mayo
- Processed meat (but check for carbs, as they are sometimes added)
- Cabbage
- Cauliflower
- Broccoli
- Zucchini
- Cucumber
- Asparagus
- Celery
- Bell peppers
- Chili peppers
- Carrots, parsnip, and onions (but in moderation)
- Leafy greens (spinach, arugula, kale, mustard greens, collard greens)
- Eggplant
- Olives
- Avocados
- Lettuce
- Green onions and leeks

- Mushrooms (in moderation)
- Nuts (any except cashews and pistachios, but in moderation)
- Blueberries, strawberries, raspberries, and blackberries (in moderation)
- Tomatoes
- Pork rinds
- Water
- Unsweetened tea (can use artificial sweeteners but in small amounts)
- Coffee (if you use sweetener, use artificial sweetener in small amounts)
- Hard alcoholic drinks (but no sugars or syrups in mixed drinks)
- Wine (if not a sugary variety; can drink merlot, cabernet sauvignon, Malbec, Chianti, Zinfandel, etc. or dry white wines)
- Bone broth (can add butter)

Chapter Three

BENEFITS OF THE MEDITERRANEAN DIET

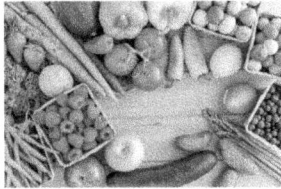

*W*e've also heard about the Mediterranean Diet's advantages. It can help fight obesity and provide our cardiovascular health with fascinating advantages. These aspects are why it has been called one of the best known and most detailed diets.

Often our lifestyle, quicker and with less time to devote not only to the kitchen but also to ourselves, causes us to eat inappropriately and with excessive amounts of fats and chemical components that could impact our health.

The Mediterranean Diet means a diverse and balanced contribution of natural and conventional items from this region bathed by the Mediterranean Sea, in addition to a particular lifestyle. Fruits, fruits, legumes, cereals, olive oil as a source of fat, fish, and eggs, and poultry are essential in more moderate amounts.

The Mediterranean diet, as the Mediterranean Diet Foundation site says, is a significant cultural heritage that is much more than just a nutritious, rich, and balanced template. Will you know the benefits of dieting in the Mediterranean? Continue reading. We're telling you everything about it!

The importance of this diet has made it recognized by the United Nations Educational, Scientific and Cultural Organization (UNESCO) as an Intangible Heritage of Mankind. It also has a traditional and customary character because it includes cultural and folkloric influences.

The Mediterranean Diet is a type of diet involving both the use of healthy ingredients and healthy preparation methods. Because of its inherent characteristics, it is not only a high-flavored diet but also rich in benefits for our health. That's why we're going to talk about its benefits.

Benefits of the Mediterranean Diet

1. Fight the so-called bad cholesterol

The abundant consumption of seafood, fish, and vegetables, as opposed to the moderate intake of red meat, is one of the main benefits of the Mediterranean diet. This is linked to a decrease in cholesterol.

1. It is beneficial for the heart

Due to the presence of unsaturated fatty acids in combination with nitrates and dietary nitrates, the Mediterranean diet helps to reduce the risk of cardiovascular diseases. Nuts, fish oil, olives, and avocado contain such fatty acids.

1. Prevent stroke

Strokes, better known as stroke, are one of the most common clinical conditions today. The Mediterranean diet significantly reduces the risk of suffering this as it is rich in olive oil and nuts that prevent stroke. This is in line with the findings of the Center for Human Nutrition and Aging Research at Tufts University in the USA and researchers at the Carlos III Health Institute

1. Avoid stomach problems

Combined with polyphenols (antioxidant substances) in apples and red wine, green vegetable nitrates function as a gastric defender. It avoids stomach problems such as ulcers and helps to alleviate them if they have them already.

1. Control of diabetes

Thanks to the low-fat diet and sweetened desserts, the Mediterranean diet helps control Type 2 diabetes.

1. Decreases the risk of Alzheimer's and dementia

In the Mediterranean diet, eggs are an important element. Due to an optimum state of the blood vessels, these food brain functions are improved. Hence, the risk of mental deterioration in people following this diet is rising.

1. Help against obesity

Adequate food intake, reasonable carbohydrate consumption, carbohydrates, and pasteurized or soft drinks, as well as the inclusion of vegetables, "healthy" fats, and proteins, enables both weight loss and ideal weight main-tenance.

1. Help prevent Parkinson's disease

The foods on this diet have great antioxidant power, which prevents cell deterioration and reduces the chance of suffering from Parkinson's disease.

1. Protect the bones

Adequate intake of calcium-rich products helps to strengthen the bones, which helps prevent fractures and bone conditions.

1. Provides agility

The nutritious foods from this diet favor firmness and muscle strength, which becomes more physical fitness, regardless of age.

1. Anti-aging

The abundance of antioxidants and calcium, as well as the reduction in the likelihood of suffering from different conditions, suggest better physical health and, with it, a healthy, long, and productive life.

Chapter Four

GETTING STARTED WITH THE MEDITERRANEAN DIET

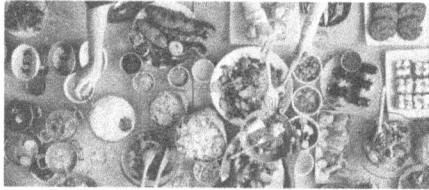

Your goals

Before you get started with this diet, spend some time, and come up with the goals you wish to achieve. Your goals will determine your level of motivation whenever you decide to follow a diet. Perhaps you want to lose weight, or maybe want to improve your overall health. Regardless of your goals, it is quintessential that you know what you wish to achieve from the diet. If you don't have any goals, it becomes difficult to stay on track in the long run.

Pick a date

Once you know your goal, you should work on setting a timeline. Select a date you want to start this diet. Don't be in a rush, and don't think that you can get started with this diet right this instance. It takes a while to prepare your mind and body for the diet you wish to follow. The Mediterranean diet doesn't require any drastic dietary changes. However, if your diet is rich in processed foods and sugars, your body will take time to adjust to the new diet. Therefore, pick a date and ensure you start your diet on that particular date. Don't make any excuses, and don't try to put it off until a later date. If you keep telling yourself that you can start this diet tomorrow, then tomorrow will never come. Take a calendar, mark the date, and get started.

Take the first step

Once you have made up your mind about this diet, then it is time to get started. Don't get scared – instead, think of it as a stepping-stone towards better health. If you get scared, remind yourself of the goals you wish to achieve from this diet. It will make it easier to keep going.

Clean your pantry

Before you start this diet, you should clean your pantry. Go through the

Mediterranean diet shopping list given in the next section and make a list of all the ingredients you will require. Once you have this list, it's time to go shopping for groceries. Simultaneously, you're also supposed to get rid of any other items that don't fit the Mediterranean diet eating protocols. So, it is time to get rid of all processed foods, unhealthy carbs, and sugary treats. Think of it as spring-cleaning for your kitchen. It is quintessential that you do this because if you're surrounded by temptations all the time, the chances of giving in to your urges to eat unhealthy foods will increase. Out of sight, out of mind, is the best approach when it comes to junk food.

Make the transition

Once you follow the steps mentioned up until now, it is time to make the transition. As mentioned in the previous point, if your diet is predominantly rich in processed foods and sugars, it might be a little tricky to shift to any other diet. You might not know this, but a diet rich in sugars is quite addictive to your body. Therefore, there are two ways in which you can change your diet. You can either go cold turkey or make a slow transition to the new diet. Slowly start eliminating all unhealthy foods from your diet while incorporating Mediterranean diet-friendly foods. This way, you are conditioning your mind and body to get used to the new diet. Give yourself at least two to three weeks before you come to any conclusions about this diet.

Support system

You must have a support system in place if you want to stick to this diet in the long run. Let go of the "I will just wing it" attitude. There will be days when you have little to no motivation. This is where your support system comes into the picture. Whenever you feel like you don't have the motivation to keep going, you can depend on your support system. Your support system can include your partner, loved ones, friends, or anyone else you want. Talk to them about your reasons for following the diet and tell them what you wish to achieve. By doing this, you are making yourself accountable to someone else. This, in turn, increases your motivation to stick to this diet. Also, you can always go online and get in touch with those who are following the same diet as you.

Be patient

A common mistake a lot of dieters make is that they are always in a hurry. Making any sort of dietary change is not easy, and it takes time. Not just time, but consistency as well. Don't think that you'll be able to shed all those extra pounds overnight. After all, you didn't gain all that extra weight within a day or two. Therefore, you can't expect yourself to get rid of it quickly. Whenever you make a dietary change, you might notice certain fluctuations in your energy levels. This happens because your body is trying to get used to the new diet. So, don't be upset with yourself if you can't exercise as vigorously as you used to. Within two to three weeks, your energy levels will stabilize, your body will get used to the new diet, and you will be able to exercise the way you want. Until then, be patient and don't weigh yourself daily. It might be quite tempting to see whether you've lost any weight lately, but it is not practical. There will be days when the scale doesn't fluctuate like you want to. Instead, make it a point to weigh yourself every week as it will help keep track of your progress.

Shopping List

Use this basic shopping list whenever you shop for groceries. Ensure that you stock your pantry with all these ingredients and get rid of any other item which is not suitable for your diet.

Your shopping list must include:

- Veggies like kale, garlic, spinach, arugula, onions, carrots
- Fruits like grapes, oranges, apples, and bananas
- Berries like blueberries, strawberries, raspberries
- Frozen veggies
- Grains like whole-grain pasta, whole-grain bread
- Legumes like beans, lentils, chickpeas
- Nuts like walnuts, cashews, almonds
- Seeds like pumpkin seeds and sunflower seeds
- Condiments like turmeric, cinnamon, salt, pepper
- Shrimp and shellfish
- Fish like mackerel, trout, tuna, salmon, and sardines
- Cheese
- Yogurt and Greek yogurt
- Potatoes and sweet potatoes
- Chicken
- Eggs
- Olives
- Olive oil and avocado oil

If you buy healthy and adequate ingredients, you will most certainly eat the right foods and you will stay on your diet.

Tricks and Tips That Will Make Things Easier

- Make sure you always have olive oil at hand. You have to forget about using butter if you are on the Mediterranean diet, but you can replace it with extra virgin olive oil.
- Give up consuming sodas and replace them with some red wine. Cut out the sweet drinks from your diet and try one glass of red wine instead.
- Replace white rice with brown rice. The Mediterranean diet allows you to continue to eat rice but make sure you replace the white rice with brown rice. Consume whole grains like buckwheat, corn, and quinoa.
- Your snacks should mainly contain fruits. Consume more citrus,

melons, berries, or grapes. You can also try seeds as a
Mediterranean diet snack, but fruits would be a better option.

- Exercise a lot and drink plenty of water. This is the main principle
to follow if you are on a Mediterranean diet. It will help you look
better and feel amazing. That's a fact!

- Another great idea to keep in mind when you are on such a diet is
to make a great shopping list. It will help you buy the right
ingredients. Choose organic products if you can, but only if they
suit your budget.

- You must keep your body hydrated. Regardless of the dietary
changes you make, the one thing you must always concentrate on is
proper hydration. When your body is hydrated, all the toxins
present within will be flushed out. Not just this, but it also helps
improve the health of your skin. You must consume at least eight
glasses of water daily. Also, when you're transitioning to this diet or
making any dietary changes, hunger pangs are quite common. To
keep hunger pangs at bay, ensure that your body is thoroughly
hydrated.

Chapter Five

MEAL PREPARATION

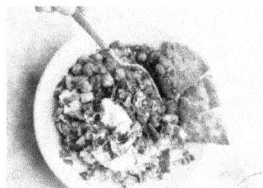

*I*f you haven't heard of the term "meal prep" before now, it's a beautiful day to learn something that will save you time, stress, and inches on your waistline. Meal prep, short for meal preparation, is a habit that was developed mostly by the bodybuilding community to accurately track your macronutrients. If you work a nine to five job like most of us, you know the struggle of feeding yourself a healthy dinner after work when you're tired, hungry, and just want to go home. When western society started getting more and more fast-paced, we developed fast-food restaurants that could serve you from your car. While we all love to indulge in a little junk food now and then, fast-food restaurants are marketed more towards routine family use than a one-off indulgence. If you have kids, you're probably even more familiar with this struggle. Some of the members of the fitness community had finally had enough, and so they developed a way to cook healthy homemade meals every single week without busting the bank, sacrificing time in the gym, or sacrificing time with your loved ones.

The basic idea behind meal prep is that each weekend, you manage your free time around cooking and preparing all your meals for the upcoming week. While most meal preppers do their grocery shopping and cooking on Sundays, to keep their meals the freshest, you can choose to cook on a Saturday if that works better with your schedule. Meal prep each week uses one large grocery list of bulk ingredients to get all the supplies you need to make four dinners and four lunches of your choice. This may make you think that you'll have to do a bit of mental math quadrupling the serving size, but all you must do is simply multiply each ingredient by four.

Although you don't have to meal prep more than one meal with four portions each week, if you're already in the kitchen, you most likely have cooking time to work on something else. Many bodybuilders even prep their breakfasts and on-the-go snacks during the weekend to save time and make sure they know what they're eating. For the average person, meal prepping four dinners alone will already free up a ton of time during the week, which can be used for a gym session, perhaps, or more time relaxing with the family.

When you cook for meal prep, you're going to be creating one meal in four portions – which can take up a lot of dishes. Investing in some good pots, pans, and skillets will help you work more efficiently in the kitchen, and matching Tupperware is something a good meal prepper can never resist. Once you've cooked your entire four-portion meal in one batch, you can separate individual matching portions that you will eat throughout the week. Most cooked vegetables and meats can last for up to five days in the refrigerator, but you can feel free to freeze your entrees as well if you need the space. Uncooked vegetables normally have only three to four days, that's why you're only reaching about four days in advance. If you want to keep your meals fresher for longer, you can always look for glass Tupperware with locking seals that can keep freshness in for longer.

Each week, you can do repeat this process with new recipes and new ingredients. However, it's worth it to note that if you're someone who likes consistency, meal prepping might be a bit of an adjustment. Meal prep tends to make only one identical dinner meal and one identical lunch meal each week – which means that eaters who like to have a different dinner each night might have their work cut out for them. One of the easiest ways to combat this is by simply making dinner and lunch that can be interchanged whenever necessary to create variety. Once you've learned how to meal prep, you will save yourself enough time in the evenings to relax, practice some self-care, and extend your dinner hours to have a fun conversation with friends and family. Now, meal preparation isn't just a cool technique to save you time and money – meal prep at its very core was designed to help you conveniently manage your weight loss, which is exactly what you need to succeed.

BREAKFAST

1. Cheesy Olives Bread
Preparation Time: 1 hour and 40 minutes
Cooking Time: 30 minutes
Servings: 10
Ingredients:

- 4 cups whole-wheat flour
- 3 tbsps. oregano, chopped
- 2 tsps. dry yeast
- ¼ cup olive oil
- 1 ½ cups black olives, pitted and sliced

- 1 cup of water
- ½ cup feta cheese, crumbled

Directions:
In a bowl, mix the flour with the water, the yeast, and the oil. Stir and knead your dough very well.

Put the dough in a bowl, cover with plastic wrap, and keep in a warm place for 1 hour.

Divide the dough into 2 bowls and stretch each ball well. Add the rest of the ingredients to each ball and tuck them inside. Knead the dough well again.

Flatten the balls a bit and leave them aside for 40 minutes more.

Transfer the balls to a baking sheet lined with parchment paper, make a small slit in each, and bake at 425°F for 30 minutes.

Serve the bread as a Mediterranean breakfast.

Nutrition: Calories 251, Fat: 7.3g, Fiber: 2.1g, Carbs: 39.7g, Protein: 6.7g

2. Sweet Potato Tart

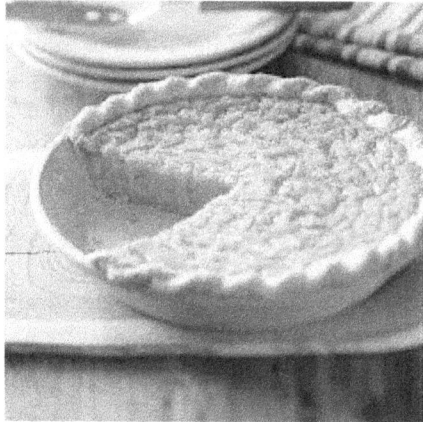

Preparation Time: 10 minutes
Cooking Time: 1 hour and 10 minutes
Servings: 8
Ingredients:

- 2 pounds sweet potatoes, peeled and cubed
- ¼ cup olive oil + a drizzle
- 7 oz. feta cheese, crumbled
- 1 yellow onion, chopped
- 2 eggs, whisked
- ¼ cup almond milk
- 1 tbsp. herbs de Provence

- A pinch of salt and black pepper
- 6 phyllo sheets
- 1 tbsp. parmesan, grated

Directions:

In a bowl, combine the potatoes with half of the oil, salt, and pepper, toss, spread on a baking sheet lined with parchment paper, and roast at 400°F for 25 minutes.

Meanwhile, heat a pan with half of the remaining oil over medium heat, add the onion, and sauté for 5 minutes.

In a bowl, combine the eggs with the milk, feta, herbs, salt, pepper, onion, sweet potatoes, and the rest of the oil and toss.

Arrange the phyllo sheets in a tart pan and brush them with a drizzle of oil.

Add the sweet potato mix and spread it well into the pan.

Sprinkle the parmesan on top and bake covered with tin foil at 350°F for 20 minutes.

Remove the tin foil, bake the tart for 20 minutes more, cool it down, slice, and serve for breakfast.

Nutrition: Calories 476, Fat: 16.8g, Fiber: 10.2g, Carbs: 68.8g, Protein: 13.9g

3. Stuffed Pita Breads

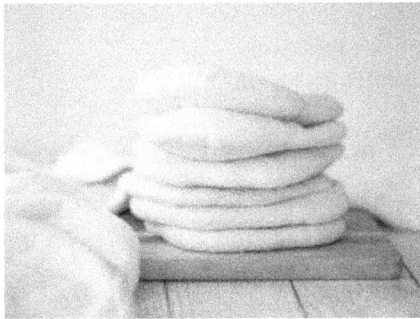

Preparation Time: 5 minutes
Cooking Time: 15 minutes
Servings: 4
Ingredients:

- 1 ½ tbsp olive oil
- 1 tomato, cubed
- 1 garlic clove, minced
- 1 red onion, chopped
- ¼ cup parsley, chopped

- 15 oz. canned fava beans, drained and rinsed
- ¼ cup lemon juice
- Salt and black pepper to the taste
- 4 whole-wheat pita bread pockets

Directions:
Heat a pan with the oil over medium heat, add the onion, stir, and sauté for 5 minutes.
Add the rest of the ingredients, stir, and cook for 10 minutes more
Stuff the pita pockets with this mix and serve for breakfast.
Nutrition: Calories 382, Fat: 1.8g, Fiber: 27.6g, Carbs: 66g, Protein: 28.5g
4. Blueberries Quinoa

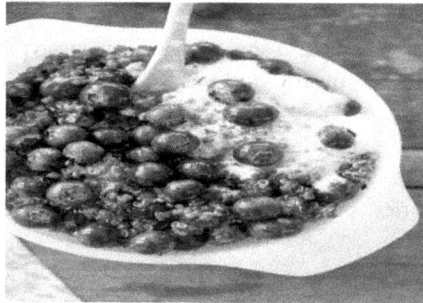

Preparation Time: 5 minutes
Cooking Time: 0 minutes
Servings: 4
Ingredients:

- 2 cups almond milk
- 2 cups quinoa, already cooked
- ½ tsp cinnamon powder
- 1 tbsp. honey
- 1 cup blueberries
- ¼ cup walnuts, chopped

Directions:
In a bowl, mix the quinoa with the milk and the rest of the ingredients, toss, divide into smaller bowls and serve for breakfast.
Nutrition: Calories 284, Fat: 14.3g, Fiber: 3.2g, Carbs: 15.4g, Protein: 4.4g
5. Endives, Fennel and Orange Salad

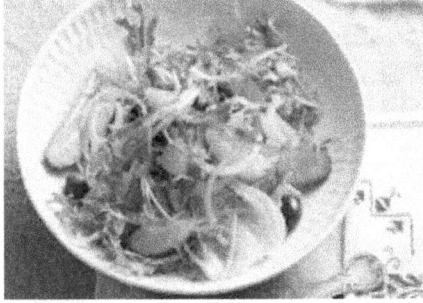

Preparation Time: 5 minutes
Cooking Time: 0 minutes
Servings: 4
Ingredients:

- 1 tbsp. balsamic vinegar
- 2 garlic cloves, minced
- 1 tsp. Dijon mustard
- 2 tbsps. olive oil
- 1 tbsp. lemon juice
- Sea salt and black pepper to taste
- ½ cup black olives, pitted and chopped
- 1 tbsp. parsley, chopped
- 7 cups baby spinach
- 2 endives, shredded
- 3 medium navel oranges, peeled and cut into segments
- 2 bulbs fennel, shredded

Directions:
In a salad bowl, combine the spinach with the endives, oranges, fennel, and the rest of the ingredients, toss and serve for breakfast.

Nutrition: Calories 97, Fat: 9.1g, Fiber: 1.8g, Carbs: 3.7g, Protein: 1.9g
6. Raspberries and Yogurt Smoothie

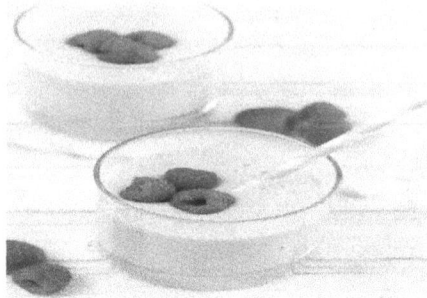

Preparation Time: 5 minutes
Cooking Time: 0 minutes
Servings: 2
Ingredients:

- 2 cups raspberries
- ½ cup Greek yogurt
- ½ cup almond milk
- ½ tsp vanilla extract

Directions:
In your blender, combine the raspberries with the milk, vanilla, and the yogurt, pulse well, divide into 2 glasses and serve for breakfast.
   Nutrition: Calories 245, Fat: 9.5g, Fiber: 2.3g, Carbs: 5.6g, Protein: 1.6g
7. Homemade Muesli
Preparation Time: 15 minutes
Cooking Time: 20 minutes
Servings: 8
Ingredients:

- 3 ½ cups rolled oats
- ½ cup wheat bran
- ½ tsp kosher salt
- ½ tsp ground cinnamon
- ½ cup sliced almonds
- ¼ cup raw pecans, coarsely chopped
- ¼ cup raw pepitas (shelled pumpkin seeds)
- ½ cup unsweetened coconut flakes
- ¼ cup dried apricots, coarsely chopped
- ¼ cup dried cherries

Directions:

Take a medium bowl and combine the oats, wheat bran, salt, and cinnamon. Stir well.

Place the mixture onto a baking sheet.

Next place the almonds, pecans, and pepitas onto another baking sheet and toss.

Pop both trays into the oven and heat to 350°F.

Bake for 10-12 minutes.

Remove from the oven and pop to one side.

Leave the nuts to cool but take the one with the oats, sprinkle with the coconut, and pop back into the oven for 5 minutes more.

Remove and leave to cool.

Find a large bowl and combine the contents of both trays then stir well to combine.

Throw in the apricots and cherries and stir well.

Pop into an airtight container until required.

Nutrition: Calories 250, Fat: 10g, Carbs: 36g, Protein: 7g

8. Tangerine and Pomegranate Breakfast Fruit Salad

Preparation Time: 15 minutes

Cooking Time: 20 minutes

Servings: 5

Ingredients:

For the grains:

- 1 cup pearl or hulled barley
- 3 cups of water
- 3 tbsps. olive oil, divided
- ½ tsp kosher salt

For the fruit:

- ½ large pineapple, peeled and cut into 1 ½" chunks
- 6 tangerines
- 1 ¼ cups pomegranate seeds
- 1 small bunch of fresh mint

For the dressing:

- ⅓ cup honey
- Juice and finely grated zest of 1 lemon
- Juice and finely grated zest of 2 limes
- ½ tsp kosher salt
- ¼ cup olive oil
- ¼ cup toasted hazelnut oil (olive oil is fine too)

Directions:

Place the grain into a strainer and rinse well.

Grab 2 baking sheets, line with paper, and add the grain. Spread well to cover then leave to dry.

Next, place the water into a saucepan and pop over medium heat.

Place a skillet over medium heat, add 2 tbsps. of the oil then add the barley. Toast for 2 minutes.

Add the water and salt and bring to a boil.

Reduce to simmer and cook for 40 minutes until most of the liquid has been absorbed.

Turn off the heat and leave to stand for 10 minutes to steam cook the rest.

Meanwhile, grab a medium bowl and add the honey, juices, zest, and salt, and stir well.

Add the olive oil then nut oil and stir again. Pop until the fridge until needed.

Remove the lid from the barley then place it onto another prepared baking sheet and leave to cool.

Drizzle with oil and leave to cool completely then pop into the fridge.

When ready to serve, divide the grains, pineapple, orange, pomegranate, and mint between the bowls.

Drizzle with the dressing then serve and enjoy.

Nutrition: Calories 400, Fat: 23g, Carbs: 50g, Protein: 3g

9. Hummus and Tomato Breakfast Pittas

Preparation Time: 5 minutes

Cooking Time: 10 minutes

Servings: 4

Ingredients:

- 4 large eggs, at room temperature
- Salt, to taste
- 2 whole-wheat pita bread with pockets, cut in half
- ½cup hummus
- 1 medium cucumber, thinly sliced into rounds
- 2 medium tomatoes, large dice
- A handful of fresh parsley leaves, coarsely chopped
- Freshly ground black pepper
- Hot sauce (optional)

Directions:

Grab a large saucepan, fill with water, and pop over medium heat until it boils.

Add the eggs and cook for 7 minutes.

Immediately drain the water and place the eggs under cool water until they cool down. Pop to one side until you can handle them comfortably.

Peel the eggs and cut them into ¼" slices, sprinkle with salt, and pop to one side.

Grab a pitta pocket and spread with hummus, fill with cucumber and tomato, season well then add an egg. Sprinkle with parsley and hot sauce then serve and enjoy.

Nutrition: Calories 377, Fat: 31g, Carbs: 17g, Protein: 11g

10.　Baked Ricotta & Pears

Preparation Time: 15 minutes

Cooking Time: 30 minutes

Servings: 4

Ingredients:

- ¼ cup White whole wheat flour
- 1 tbsp. Sugar
- ¼ tsp Nutmeg
- Ricotta cheese
- 16 oz. container whole-milk
- 2Large eggs
- 1Diced pear
- 2 tbsp. Water
- 1 tsp. Vanilla extract
- 1 tbsp. Honey
- Also Needed: 4 - 6 oz. ramekins

Directions:

Warm the oven to 400°F.

Lightly spritz the ramekins with a cooking oil spray.

Whisk the flour, nutmeg, sugar, vanilla, eggs, and ricotta together in a large mixing container.

Spoon the fixings into the dishes. Bake them for 20 to 25 minutes or until they're firm and set. Transfer them to the countertop and wait for them to cool.

In a saucepan, using the medium temperature setting, toss the cored and diced pear into the water for about ten minutes until it's slightly softened.

Take the pan from the burner and stir in the honey.

Serve the ricotta ramekins with the warm pear when it's ready.

Nutrition: Calories 312, Protein: 17g, Fat: 17g

11.　Egg White Scramble with Cherry Tomatoes & Spinach

Preparation Time: 5 minutes

Cooking Time: 8-10 minutes

Servings: 4

Ingredients:

- 1 tbsp. Olive oil

- 1 whole Egg
- 10 Egg whites
- ¼ tsp. Black pepper
- ½ tsp. Salt
- 1 garlic clove, minced
- 2 cups cherry tomatoes, halved
- 2 cups packed fresh baby spinach
- ½ cup Light cream or Half & Half
- ¼ cup finely grated parmesan cheese

Directions:
Whisk the eggs, pepper, salt, and milk.

Prepare a skillet using the med-high temperature setting.

Toss in the garlic when the pan is hot to sauté for approximately 30 seconds.

Pour in the tomatoes and spinach and continue to sauté it for one additional minute. The tomatoes should be softened, and the spinach wilted.

Add the egg mixture into the pan using the medium heat setting. Fold the egg gently as it cooks for about two to three minutes.

Remove from the burner, and sprinkle with a sprinkle of cheese.

Nutrition: Calories 142, Protein: 15g, Fat: 2g

12.   Blueberry, Hazelnut, and Lemon Breakfast Grain Salad
Preparation Time: 5 minutes
Cooking Time: 10 minutes
Servings: 8
Ingredients:

- 1 cup steel-cut oats
- 1 cup dry golden quinoa
- ½ cup dry millet
- 3 tbsps. olive oil, divided
- ¾ tsp salt
- 1 x 1" piece fresh ginger, peeled and cut into coins
- 2 large lemons, zest and juice
- ½ cup maple syrup
- 1 cup Greek yogurt
- ¼ tsp nutmeg
- 2 cups hazelnuts, roughly chopped and toasted
- 2 cups blueberries or mixed berries
- 4 ½ cups water

Directions:
Grab a mesh strainer and add the oats, quinoa, and millet. Wash well then pop to one side.

Find a 3-quart saucepan, add a tbsp of the oil, and pop over medium heat.

Add the grains and cook for 2-3 minutes to toast.

Pour in the water, salt, ginger coins, and lemon zest.

Bring to the boil then cover and turn down the heat. Leave to simmer for 20 minutes.

Turn off the heat and leave to sit for five minutes.

Fluff with a fork, remove the ginger then leave to cool for at least an hour.

Grab a large bowl and add the grains.

Take a medium bowl and add the remaining olive oil, lemon juice, maple syrup, yogurt, and nutmeg. Whisk well to combine.

Pour this over the grains and stir well.

Add the hazelnuts and blueberries, stir again then pop into the fridge overnight.

Serve and enjoy.

Nutrition: Calories 363, Fat: 11g, Carbs: 60g, Protein: 7g

13. Feta & Quinoa Egg Muffins

Preparation Time: 20 minutes

Cooking Time: 45-50 minutes

Servings: 12

Ingredients:

- 1 cup cooked quinoa
- 2 cups baby spinach, chopped
- ½ cup Kalamata olives
- 1 cup tomatoes
- ½ cup white onion
- 1 tbsp. fresh oregano
- ½ tsp. salt
- 2 tsp.+ more for coating pans olive oil
- 8 eggs
- 1 cup crumbled feta cheese
- Also Needed: 12-cup muffin tin

Directions:

Heat the oven to reach 350° F.

Lightly grease the muffin tray cups with a spritz of cooking oil.

Prepare a skillet using the medium temperature setting and add the oil. When it's hot, toss in the onions to sauté for two minutes.

Dump the tomatoes into the skillet and sauté for one minute. Fold in the spinach and continue cooking until the leaves have wilted (1 min.).

Transfer the pot to the countertop and add the oregano and olives. Set it aside.

Crack the eggs into a mixing bowl, using an immersion stick blender to mix them thoroughly. Add the cooked veggies in with the rest of the fixings.

Stir until it's combined and scoop the mixture into the greased muffin cups.

Set the timer to bake the muffins for 30 minutes until browned, and the muffins are set.

Cool for about ten minutes.

Nutrition: Calories 113, Protein: 7g, Fat: 7g

14.   5-Minute Heirloom Tomato & Cucumber Toast

Preparation Time: 10 minutes

Cooking Time: 6-10 minutes

Servings: 1

Ingredients:

- 1 small Heirloom tomato
- 1 Persian cucumber
- 1 tsp. Olive oil
- 1 pinch Oregano
- Kosher salt and pepper as desired
- 2 tsp. Low-fat whipped cream cheese
- 2 pieces Trader Joe's Whole Grain Crispbread or your choice
- 1 tsp. Balsamic glaze

Directions:

Dice the cucumber and tomato. Combine all the fixings except for the cream cheese.

Smear the cheese on the bread and add the mixture (step 1).

Top it off with the balsamic glaze and serve.

Nutrition: Calories: 177, Protein: 3g, Fat: 8g

15.   Garbanzo Bean Salad

Preparation Time: 10 minutes

Cooking Time: 0 minutes

Servings: 4

Ingredients:

- 1 ½ cups cucumber, cubed
- 15 oz. canned garbanzo beans, drained and rinsed
- 3 oz. black olives, pitted and sliced
- 1 tomato, chopped
- ¼ cup red onion, chopped
- 5 cups salad greens
- A pinch of salt and black pepper
- ½ cup feta cheese, crumbled
- 3 tbsps. olive oil
- 1 tbsp. lemon juice
- ¼ cup parsley, chopped

Directions:

In a salad bowl, combine the garbanzo beans with the cucumber, tomato, and the rest of the ingredients except the cheese and toss.

Divide the mix into small bowls, sprinkle the cheese on top, and serve for breakfast.

Nutrition: Calories 268, Fat: 16g, Fiber: 7g, Carbs: 24g, Protein: 9g

16. **Brown Rice Salad**

Preparation Time: 10 minutes

Cooking Time: 0 minutes

Servings: 4

Ingredients:

- 9 oz. brown rice, cooked
- 7 cups baby arugula
- 15 oz. canned garbanzo beans, drained and rinsed
- 4 oz. feta cheese, crumbled
- ¾ cup basil, chopped
- A pinch of salt and black pepper
- 2 tbsps. lemon juice
- ¼ tsp lemon zest, grated
- ¼ cup olive oil

Directions:

In a salad bowl, combine the brown rice with the arugula, the beans, and the rest of the ingredients, toss and serve cold for breakfast.

Nutrition: Calories 473, Fat: 22g, Fiber: 7g, Carbs: 53g, Protein: 13g

17. **Greek Yogurt with Walnuts and Honey**

Preparation Time: 5 Minutes

Cooking Time: 0 minutes

Servings: 4

Ingredients:

- 4 cups Greek yogurt, fat-free, plain or vanilla
- ½ cup California walnuts, toasted, chopped
- 3 tbsps. honey or agave nectar
- Fresh fruit, chopped or granola, low-fat (both optional)

Directions:

Spoon yogurt into 4 individual cups.

Sprinkle 2 tbsps. of walnuts over each and drizzle 2 tsps. of honey over each.

Top with fruit or granola, whichever is preferred.

Nutrition: Calories 300, Fat: 10g, Fiber: 1g, Carbs: 25g, Protein: 29g

18. **Tahini Pine Nuts Toast**

Preparation Time: 5 minutes
Cooking Time: 0 minutes
Servings: 2
Ingredients:

- 2 whole-wheat bread slices, toasted
- 1 tsp. water
- 1 tbsp. tahini paste
- 2 tsps. feta cheese, crumbled
- Juice of ½ lemon
- 2 tsps. pine nuts
- A pinch of black pepper

Directions:
In a bowl, mix the tahini with the water and the lemon juice, whisk well, and spread over the toasted bread slices.

Top each serving with the remaining ingredients and serve for breakfast.

Nutrition: Calories 142, Fat: 7.6g, Fiber: 2.7g, Carbs: 13.7g, Protein: 5.8g

19. Feta - Avocado & Mashed Chickpea Toast
Preparation Time: 10 minutes
Cooking Time: 15 minutes
Servings: 4
Ingredients:

- 15 oz. can Chickpeas
- 2 oz. - ½ cup Diced feta cheese
- 1 Pitted avocado

Fresh juice:

- 2 tsp. Lemon (or 1 tbsp. orange)
- ½ tsp. Black pepper
- 2 tsp. Honey
- 4 slices Multigrain toast

Directions:
Toast the bread. Drain the chickpeas in a colander. Scoop the avocado flesh into the bowl.

Use a large fork/potato masher to mash them until the mix is spreadable.

Pour in the lemon juice, pepper, and feta.

Combine and divide onto the four slices of toast.

Drizzle using the honey and serve.

Nutrition: Calories: 337, Protein: 13g, Fat: 13g

20. Feta Frittata

Preparation Time: 15 minutes
Cooking Time: 25 minutes
Servings: 2
Ingredients:

- 1 small clove Garlic
- 1 Green onion
- 2 Large eggs
- ½ cup Egg substitute
- 4 tbsp. Crumbled feta cheese - divided
- ⅓ cup Plum tomato
- 4 thin Avocado slices
- 2 tbsp. Reduced-fat sour cream
- Also Needed: 6-inch skillet

Directions:

Thinly slice/mince the onion, garlic, and tomato. Peel the avocado before slicing.

Heat the pan using the medium temperature setting and spritz it with cooking oil.

Whisk the egg substitute, eggs, and the feta cheese.

Add the egg mixture into the pan. Cover and simmer for four to six minutes.

Sprinkle it using the rest of the feta cheese and tomato. Cover and continue cooking until the eggs are set or about two to three more minutes.

Wait for about five minutes before cutting it into halves.

Serve with the avocado and sour cream.

Nutrition: Calories: 203, Fat: 12 g, Protein: 17g

21.   Fruit Bulgur Breakfast Bowls
Preparation Time: 15 minutes
Cooking Time: 20 minutes
Servings: 6
Ingredients:

- 2 cups 2% milk
- 1½ cups Uncooked bulgur
- 1 cup Water
- ½ tsp. Cinnamon
- 2 cups Frozen/fresh pitted dark sweet cherries
- 8 Dried/fresh chopped figs
- ½ cup Chopped almonds

Directions:

Combine the cinnamon, water, milk, and bulgur.

Stir once and bring to a boil. Put a top on the pot. Reduce the temperature setting to medium low.

Continue cooking until the liquid is absorbed (approx.10 min.).

Extinguish the flame, but leave the pan on the stove and stir in the cherries (frozen or thawed), almonds, and figs.

Stir well to thaw the cherries and hydrate the figs. Stir in the mint, and scoop into Servings bowls.

Serve with warm milk or serve it chilled to your liking.

Nutrition: Calories: 301, Fat: 6g, Protein: 9g

22.   Ham & Egg Cups
Preparation Time: 15 minutes
Cooking Time: 30 minutes
Servings: 8
Ingredients:

- 8 thin slices Cooked ham - deli-style
- ¼ cups/1 oz Mozzarella cheese
- 8 Eggs
- 8 tsp. Basil (Optional)
- Black pepper to taste
- 6/as desired Grape or cherry tomatoes
- Also Needed: 8-count Muffin tin

Directions:

Program the oven setting to 350° F. Coat the muffin tin cups with the spray.

Press the ham slice into the bottom and add the cheese to each of the prepared cups. Break an egg into the cup and sprinkle with the pepper. Add the pesto, if using. Slice the tomatoes into halves and place them on each of the cups.

Bake them for 18 to 20 minutes. The egg whites should be set, like a regular poached egg.

Leave them in the cups for three to five minutes. Then, carefully take the cups out of the tin and serve.

Nutrition: Calories: 145, Protein: 11g, Fat: 10g

23.   Spinach and Artichoke Frittata
Preparation Time: 15 minutes
Cooking Time: 20 minutes
Servings: 4-6
Ingredients:

- 10 large free-range eggs
- ½ cup sour cream
- 1 tbsp. Dijon mustard

- 1 tsp. salt
- ¼ tsp freshly ground black pepper
- 1 cup grated Parmesan cheese, divided
- 2 tbsps. olive oil
- 14 oz. marinated artichoke hearts, drained, patted dry, and quartered
- 5 oz. baby spinach
- 2 cloves garlic, minced

Directions:
Preheat your oven to 400°F.

Grab a large bowl and add the eggs, sour cream, mustard, salt, pepper, and ½ of the parmesan. Whisk to combine.

Pop a skillet over medium heat and add the oil.

Add the artichokes and cook for 5 minutes until soft.

Add the spinach and garlic, toss and cook for a further 2 minutes.

Spread over the skillet then pour in the egg until the veggies are covered.

Top with the remaining parmesan then cook for 2-3 minutes until the edges start to set.

Pop into the oven and cook for 12-15 minutes until cooked to perfection.

Remove from the oven, leave to cool for 5 minutes then serve and enjoy.

Nutrition: Calories: 185, Fat: 13g, Carbs: 7g, Protein: 11g

24.   Avocado and Egg Breakfast Pizza
Preparation Time: 15 minutes
Cooking Time: 20 minutes
Servings: 4
Ingredients:

- 1 large Hass avocado
- 1 tbsp. finely chopped cilantro
- 1 ½ tsp lime juice
- ⅛ tsp salt
- ½ lb. pizza dough, homemade or store-bought
- 4 large eggs
- 1 tbsp. vegetable oil
- Hot sauce, for Servings (optional)

Directions:
Grab a medium bowl and add the avocado, cilantro, lime juice, and salt. Mash well until smooth.

Take the pizza dough and divide it into 4 equal pieces.

Using a dusting of flour and a rolling pin, roll out into a circle approx. 6" wide.

Grab a skillet then lightly oil.

Place the dough into the skillet and cook for a few minutes on each side until fluffy.

Repeat with the remaining dough.

Divide the avocado mixture between the pizzas and spread to cover.

Add more oil to the pan then cook the eggs until cooked exactly as you like them.

Remove from the pan and pop onto the pizzas.

Serve and enjoy.

Nutrition: Calories: 400, Fat: 23g, Carbs: 50g, Protein: 3g

25.   Spinach Feta Breakfast Wraps

Preparation Time: 15 minutes

Cooking Time: 20 minutes

Servings: 4

Ingredients:

- 10 large free-range eggs
- ½ lb. baby spinach
- 4 large whole-wheat tortillas
- ½ pint cherry or grape tomatoes, halved
- 4 oz. feta cheese, crumbled
- Butter or olive oil, to taste
- Salt and pepper, to taste

Directions:

Grab a large bowl and add the eggs. Whisk well.

Pop a skillet over medium heat and add enough butter or oil to cover the bottom of the pan.

Add the eggs and cook to perfection.

Remove from the pan and leave to cool slightly.

Add a touch more oil or butter to the pan and add the spinach, cooking until wilted.

Pop your tortilla wraps into the microwave for a few seconds until warm.

Place the wrap onto a flat surface then top with eggs, spinach, tomato, and feta.

Wrap then repeat with the remaining tortillas.

Serve and enjoy.

Nutrition: Calories: 1061, Fat: 68g, Carbs: 77g, Protein: 55g

26.   Summer Vegetables with Eggs

Preparation Time: 5 minutes

Cooking Time: 30 minutes

Servings: 2

Ingredients:

- 1 tbsp. olive oil

- 1 small yellow onion, halved and thinly sliced
- 1 clove garlic, minced
- 2 medium summer squash or zucchini
- 2 medium tomatoes, chopped
- ½ tsp fresh thyme
- 1 tsp. ground Spanish piquillo pepper or Spanish paprika
- 1 medium red bell pepper
- Salt and pepper, to taste
- 2 large free-range eggs

Directions:

Pop a skillet over medium heat then add the olive oil.

Add the onion and cook for five minutes until soft.

Throw in the garlic and cook for a further minute.

Add the squash or zucchini and cook for 10 minutes until it begins to get soft.

Add the tomatoes, thyme, and paprika and leave to cook for 20 minutes until thick.

Meanwhile, roast your pepper by popping onto a fork and holding over a naked flame for a minute or two until the skin begins to blacken and burn.

Leave to cool slightly then remove the core and seeds and chop into 1" chunks.

Take the skillet from the heat and add the roasted peppers and salt and pepper. Leave to cool.

Place another skillet over medium heat, add the oil then cook your eggs exactly as you like them.

Serve everything together and enjoy.

Nutrition: Calories: 212, Fat: 13g, Carbs: 17g, Protein: 10g

27.   Crispy White Beans with Greens and Poached Egg

Preparation Time: 15 minutes

Cooking Time: 20 minutes

Servings: 4

Ingredients:

- 3 tbsps. olive oil, divided
- 1 x 15 oz. can cannellini beans, drained and rinsed
- 1 tsp. kosher salt, divided
- 2 tsps. za'atar, divided
- 10 oz. Swiss chard, stems removed and leaves thinly sliced
- 2 cloves garlic, minced
- ¼ tsp red pepper flakes, plus more for Servings
- 1 tbsp. freshly squeezed lemon juice
- 4 large eggs, poached

Directions:
Place a large skillet over medium heat and add 2 tbsps. of oil.
Throw in the beans and cook for 2-4 minutes until starting to brown.
Add ½ tsp of salt and 1 tsp. of the za'atar and stir well.
Continue to cook the beans for 3-5 minutes more until blistering.
Add the remaining oil then throw in the chard, remaining salt, remaining za'atar garlic, and red pepper flakes. Stir well and cook for five minutes.
Remove from the heat, add the lemon juice and stir well.
Serve topped with a poached egg and more red pepper flakes.
Nutrition: Calories: 187, Fat: 15g, Carbs: 6g, Protein: 8g

28.   Caprese Avocado Toast
Preparation Time: 5 minutes
Cooking Time: 10 minutes
Servings: 2
Ingredients:

- 2 slices hearty sandwich bread
- 1 medium avocado, halved and pit removed
- 8 grape tomatoes, halved
- 12 bite-sized mozzarella balls
- 4 large fresh basil leaves, torn
- 2 tbsps. balsamic glaze

Directions:
Toast the bread however you like.
Meanwhile, mash the avocado well.
When the toast is done, spread the avocado over the top.
Add tomatoes, mozzarella and basil, drizzle with the balsamic glaze then serve and enjoy.
Nutrition: Calories: 187, Fat: 15g, Carbs: 6g, Protein: 8g

29.   'Huevos' Rancheros
Preparation Time: 10 minutes
Cooking Time: 15 minutes
Servings: 6
Ingredients:

- Salsa, ex. 16 oz. jar Old El Paso
- 6 Eggs
- 6-inch Flour tortillas/soft tacos
- ¾ cup Shredded cheese
- Also Needed: 10-inch skillet

Directions:
Heat the salsa until it's bubbly. Gently crack the eggs into the skillet.

Place a top on the pot and simmer using the med-low temperature setting for six to seven minutes. The eggs should be thoroughly cooked.

Warm the tortillas and serve using a sprinkle of cheese.

Spoon one egg onto each of the salsa filled tortillas and serve.

Nutrition: Calories: 240, Protein: 11g, Fat: 12g

30.   Marinara Eggs with Parsley - Gluten-Free

Preparation Time: 10 minutes

Cooking Time: 20 minutes

Servings: 6

Ingredients:

- 1 tbsp. Olive oil
- 6 large Eggs
- ½ or 1 cup Medium onion
- 2 cloves or 1 tsp. Garlic
- 2 cans of 14.5 oz. diced tomatoes, undrained, no-salt-added
- ½ cup Chopped Italian fresh flat-leaf parsley
- Optional: Crusty Italian bread with grated parmesan or Romano cheese

Directions:

Heat a skillet using the med-high temperature setting. Add the oil.

Dice and toss the onions into the skillet. Sauté them for about five minutes. Stir occasionally and fold in the minced garlic, continuing to stir it for another minute.

Pour in the tomatoes with the juices into the pan and let it simmer until bubbling or for two to three minutes. Crack an egg into a coffee mug.

Once the tomatoes are boiling, lower the heat to medium. Use the spoon to make six indentions in the tomato mixture.

Add the egg to one of the slots and continue until you've used all of the eggs.

Place a top on the pot and cook for six to seven minutes or until done.

Garnish them with the parsley and serve with bread and grated cheese to your liking.

Nutrition: Calories: 122, Fat: 7g, Protein: 7g

31.   Nutty Orange Polenta

Preparation Time: 10 minutes

Cooking Time: 15 minutes

Servings: 6

Ingredients:

- 2 18-oz. tubes Plain polenta
- 2 ¼ - 2 ½ cups 2% milk, divided
- 2 Oranges

- ½ cup Pecans
- ¼ cup 2% Plain Greek yogurt
- 8 tsp. Honey

Directions:

Slice the polenta into rounds and place in a microwavable dish to heat for 45 seconds.

Prepare a pot using the medium heat setting and add the polenta. Mash it until it's roughly mashed.

In a microwavable dish, pour in the milk and heat it for one minute.

Pour two cups of warm milk into the pot with the polenta and whisk it thoroughly.

Add in milk a few tbsps. at a time until it's the way you like it. Let the mixture cook slowly for about five minutes. Take the pan off the burner.

Peel and chop the onions and pecans.

Serve and garnish them with the oranges, pecans, honey, and yogurt before Servings.

Nutrition: Calories: 234, Fat: 7g, Protein: 3g

32.   Peanut Butter & Banana Greek Yogurt Bowl

Preparation Time: 5 minutes

Cooking Time: 5 minutes

Servings: 4

Ingredients:

- 2 medium bananas
- ¼ cup Flaxseed meal
- 1 tsp. Nutmeg
- ¼ cup Peanut butter
- 4 cups Vanilla Greek yogurt

Directions:

Peel and slice the bananas. Divide the yogurt into four Servings dishes. Top each one with sliced bananas.

Microwave the peanut butter for 30 to 40 seconds until it's thoroughly melted. Drizzle the sauce over the banana slices and lightly dust them using the flaxseed meal and nutmeg to serve.

Nutrition: Calories: 370, Fat: 10.6g, Protein: 22.7g

33.   Poached Eggs

Preparation Time: 10 minutes

Cooking Time: 10 minutes

Servings: 2

Ingredients:

- ½ tsp. Salt

- 1 tsp. Champagne vinegar
- 2 Fresh eggs

Directions:
Prepare a cooking pot with cold water. Wait for it to boil using the medium temperature setting. Stir in the salt and vinegar.

Break each of the eggs into a ramekin. Place it close to the water and slide it out of the dish. Simmer until set.

Use a slotted spoon to lift it from the pan to help prevent sticking. Continue cooking until the yolk is runny and the white is cooked or about six minutes.

Prepare a container with ice water. Place the eggs into the bowl of ice water (It slows and stops the cooking process.)

Put them in paper towels to remove the water and serve.

Nutrition: Calories 72, Fat: 5g, Protein: 6.3g

34.   Portobello Pesto Egg Omelet - Gluten-Free
Preparation Time: 10 minutes
Cooking Time: 25 minutes
Servings: 1
Ingredients:

- 1 tsp. Olive oil
- 1 Portobello mushroom cap
- ¼ cup Red onion
- 4 Egg whites
- 1 tsp. Water
- Black pepper & salt to taste
- 1 tsp. Prepared pesto
- ¼ cup Shredded low-fat mozzarella cheese

Directions:
Pour and warm the oil in a skillet using the medium temperature setting.

Chop and add the onions and mushrooms to sauté for about three to five minutes or until they're softened.

Crack the eggs into a bowl and whisk in the salt, pepper, and water. Dump the eggs on top of the onions and mushrooms.

Continue cooking for about five minutes, stirring occasionally. Sprinkle it using the cheese and top it off with some pesto.

Fold the omelet in half and continue cooking for about two to three more minutes before Servings.

Nutrition: Calories: 259, Fat: 12g, Protein: 28g

35.   Prosciutto - Lettuce - Tomato & Avocado Sandwiches
Preparation Time: 5 minutes
Cooking Time: 10-12 minutes

Servings: 4
Ingredients:

- 2 oz./8 thin slices Prosciutto
- 1 Ripe avocado cut in half
- 4 full leaves Romaine lettuce
- 1 Large ripe tomato
- 8 Whole grain or whole wheat bread slices
- ¼ tsp. Black pepper and kosher salt

Directions:
Tear the lettuce leaves into eight pieces (total). Slice the tomato into eight rounds. Toast the bread and place it on a plate.

Scoop out the avocado flesh from the skin and toss it to a mixing bowl. Lightly dust it using the pepper and salt. Whisk or gently mash the avocado until it's creamy. Spread over the bread.

Make one sandwich. Take a slice of avocado toast; top it with a lettuce leaf, a prosciutto slice, and a tomato slice. Top with another slice of lettuce tomato and continue.

Repeat the process until all ingredients are depleted.

Nutrition: Calories 240, Fat: 9g, Protein: 12g

36.   Pumpkin Pancakes
Preparation Time: 15 minutes
Cooking Time: 40 minutes
Servings: 6
Ingredients:

- 1 ½ cup of milk
- 1Egg
- 2 tbsp. Vegetable oil
- 1 cup Pumpkin puree
- 2 tbsp. Vinegar
- 1 tsp. Baking soda
- 1 tsp. Ground allspice
- 2 cups All-purpose flour
- 3 tbsp. Brown sugar
- 2 tsp. Baking powder
- ½ tsp. Salt
- ½ tsp. Ground ginger
- 1 tsp. Cinnamon

Directions:
Whisk the egg, oil, vinegar, pumpkin, and the milk in a mixing bowl.
Mix the baking powder, salt, ginger, cinnamon, allspice, baking soda,

brown sugar, and the flour in another container.

Stir the fixings in one bowl to combine.

Warm a frying pan or oiled griddle using the med-high heat setting.

Pour the batter into the griddle and brown. Serve them hot.

Nutrition: Calories 278, Fat: 7.2g, Protein: 7.9g

37.   Scrambled Eggs with Roasted Peppers & Goat Cheese - Gluten-Free

Preparation Time: 5 minutes

Cooking Time: 15 minutes

Servings: 4

Ingredients:

- 1 ½ tsp. Olive oil
- 1 medium pepper / 1 cup Bell peppers
- 2 cloves /1 tsp. Garlic
- 6 Large eggs
- ¼ tsp. Sea salt
- 2 tbsp. Water
- 2 oz. / ½ cup Crumbled goat cheese
- 2 tbsp Chopped fresh mint

Directions:

Prepare a skillet using the med-high temperature setting on the stovetop. Add the oil. Once it's hot, toss in the peppers and sauté for five minutes.

Mince and stir in the garlic. Continue cooking for one minute.

Beat the water, eggs, and salt in a mixing container.

Reduce the temperature setting to medium low.

Empty the egg mixture over top of the peppers. Simmer it for one to two minutes until they're set on the bottom.

Sprinkle with the goat cheese and continue cooking for one to two more minutes. Stir until they are soft set.

Garnish with loosely packed fresh mint and serve.

Nutrition: Calories 201, Fat: 15g, Protein: 15g

38.   Spinach Omelet

Preparation Time: 15 minutes

Cooking Time: 25-30 minutes

Servings: 4

Ingredients:

- 3 tbsp. Olive oil
- 1 Small onion
- 1 Garlic clove
- 4 Large tomatoes
- 8 Eggs

- ¼ tsp. Black pepper
- 1 tsp. Fine sea salt
- 2 oz. Feta cheese
- 1 tbsp. Flat-leaf parsley

Directions:
Core and chop the tomatoes, parsley, and onion.
Set the oven to reach 400°F.
Pour the oil into an oven-proof skillet using the high heat temperature setting. Stir in the onions and sauté them until softened (5-7 min.).
Pour in the tomatoes, garlic, salt, and pepper.
Sauté the mixture for five more minutes and add the whisked eggs.
Stir and cook them for three to five minutes. When the bottom is set, put the skillet into the hot oven. Continue cooking for five additional minutes.
Transfer to the countertop and top it off with the parsley and feta. Serve the omelet warm.
Nutrition: Calories 295, Fat: 14g, Protein: 15g
39.   Yogurt Parfait with Roasted Grapes & Greek - Gluten-Free
Preparation Time: 15 minutes
Cooking Time: 30 minutes
Servings: 4
Ingredients:

- 4 cups of 1 ½ lbs. Seedless grapes
- 1 tbsp. Olive oil
- 2 cups of 2% Greek yogurt, plain
- 4 tsp. Honey
- ½ cup Chopped walnuts

Directions:
Set the oven temperature to 450° F with the pan inside.
Rinse the grapes and discard the stems. Dab them using a towel and toss them with the oil.
Bake them for about 20 to 23 minutes until they are slightly shriveled. Stir about halfway through the cooking process.
Take the pan from the oven. Cool for five minutes.
Meanwhile, assemble the parfaits by adding the yogurt to the glass.
Once the grapes are cooled, garnish the yogurt using a tsp of honey, 2 tbsp. of the walnuts, and a portion of the grapes.
Prepare all four Servings and serve or place in the fridge for later.
Nutrition: Calories 300, Fat: 17g, Protein: 7g
40.   Zucchini Egg White Frittata
Preparation Time: 15 minutes
Cooking Time: 25 minutes

Servings: 1
Ingredients:

- 1 tsp. Olive oil
- 1 tbsp. Minced shallot
- 1 clove Minced garlic
- 1 small Zucchini
- 4 Egg whites
- Black pepper and kosher salt as desired
- ½ tsp. Freshly chopped thyme

Directions:
Slice or shave the zucchini into strips. Chop the thyme.

Warm a skillet using the medium temperature setting and pour in the oil.

Mince and add the garlic and shallot to the skillet and sauté them for about five minutes. Stir in the zucchini. Continue cooking for about five minutes, stirring occasionally.

Whisk the salt, thyme, and egg whites together and mix into the zucchini mixture.

Continue cooking the mixture undisturbed for about two minutes using the low-temperature heat setting.

Flip the frittata and continue cooking one more minute.

Serve with a shake of salt and pepper to your desired taste.

Nutrition: Calories 137, Fat: 5g, Protein: 16.5g

41. Avocado Chickpea Pizza
Preparation Time: 20 minutes
Cooking Time: 20 minutes
Servings: 2
Ingredients:

- 1 ¼ cups chickpea flour
- A pinch of salt and black pepper
- 1 ¼ cups water
- 2 tbsps. olive oil
- 1 tsp. onion powder
- 1 tsp. garlic, minced
- 1 tomato, sliced
- 1 avocado, peeled, pitted, and sliced
- 2 oz. gouda, sliced
- ¼ cup tomato sauce
- 2 tbsps. green onions, chopped

Directions:
In a bowl, mix the chickpea flour with salt, pepper, water, the oil, onion

powder and the garlic, stir well until you obtain a dough, knead a bit, put in a bowl, cover and leave aside for 20 minutes.

Transfer the dough to a working surface, shape a bit circle, transfer it to a baking sheet lined with parchment paper and bake at 425 ° F for 10 minutes.

Spread the tomato sauce over the pizza, also spread the rest of the ingredients and bake at 400 ° F for 10 minutes more.

Cut and serve for breakfast.

Nutrition: Calories 416, Fat: 24.5g, Fiber: 9.6g, Carbs: 36.6g, Protein: 15.4g

42.   **Cheesy Yogurt**
Preparation Time: 4 hours and 5 minutes
Cooking Time: 0 minutes
Servings: 4
Ingredients:

- 1 cup Greek yogurt
- 1 tbsp. honey
- ½ cup feta cheese, crumbled

Directions:
In a blender, combine the yogurt with the honey and the cheese and pulse well.

Divide into bowls and freeze for 4 hours before Servings for breakfast.

Nutrition: Calories 161, Fat: 10g, Fiber: 0g, Carbs: 11.8g, Protein: 6.6g

43.   **Lentils and Cheddar Frittata**
Preparation Time: 10 minutes
Cooking Time: 15 minutes
Servings: 4
Ingredients:

- 1 red onion, chopped
- 2 tbsps. olive oil
- 1 cup sweet potatoes, boiled and chopped
- ¾ cup ham, chopped
- 4 eggs, whisked
- ¾ cup lentils, cooked
- 2 tbsps. Greek yogurt
- Salt and black pepper to the taste
- ½ cup cherry tomatoes, halved
- ¾ cup cheddar cheese, grated

Directions:
Heat up a pan with the oil over medium heat, add the onion, stir, and sauté for 2 minutes.

Add the rest of the ingredients except the eggs and the cheese, toss and cook for 3 minutes more.

Add the eggs, sprinkle the cheese on top, cover the pan and cook for 10 minutes more.

Slice the frittata, divide between plates, and serve.

Nutrition: Calories 274, Fat :17.3g, Fiber: 3.5g, Carbs: 8.9g, Protein: 11.4g

44. Seeds and Lentils Oats
Preparation Time: 10 minutes
Cooking Time: 50 minutes
Servings: 4
Ingredients:

- ½ cup red lentils
- ¼ cup pumpkin seeds, toasted
- 2 tsps. olive oil
- ¼ cup rolled oats
- ¼ cup coconut flesh, shredded
- 1 tbsp. honey
- 1 tbsp. orange zest, grated
- 1 cup Greek yogurt
- 1 cup blackberries

Directions:
Spread the lentils on a baking sheet lined with parchment paper, introduce in the oven and roast at 370°F for 30 minutes.

Add the rest of the ingredients except the yogurt and the berries, toss and bake at 370 ° F for 20 minutes more.

Transfer this to a bowl, add the rest of the ingredients, toss, divide into smaller bowls and serve for breakfast.

Nutrition: Calories 204, Fat: 7.1g, Fiber: 10.4g, Carbs: 27.6g, Protein: 9.5g

45. Tuna and Cheese Bake
Preparation Time: 5 minutes
Cooking Time: 15 minutes
Servings: 4
Ingredients:

- 10 oz. canned tuna, drained and flaked
- 4 eggs, whisked
- ½ cup feta cheese, shredded
- 1 tbsp. chives, chopped
- 1 tbsp. parsley, chopped
- Salt and black pepper to the taste
- 3 tsps. olive oil

Directions:

Grease a baking dish with the oil, add the tuna and the rest of the ingredients except the cheese, toss and bake at 370°F for 15 minutes.

Sprinkle the cheese on top, leave the mix aside for 5 minutes, slice and serve for breakfast.

Nutrition: Calories 283, Fat: 14.2g, Fiber: 5.6g, Carbs: 12.1g, Protein: 6.4g

46.   Tuna Sandwich
Preparation Time: 5 minutes
Cooking Time: 0 minutes
Servings: 2
Ingredients:

- 6 oz. canned tuna, drained and flaked
- 1 avocado, peeled, pitted, and mashed
- 4 whole wheat bread slices
- A pinch of salt and black pepper
- 1 cup baby spinach
- 1 tbsp. feta cheese, crumbled

Directions:

In a bowl, mix the tuna with the cheese, salt and pepper and stir well.

Spread the mashed avocado on the bread slices, divide the tuna mix on 2 of them, divide the spinach as well, top with the other 2 slices and serve for breakfast.

Nutrition: Calories 283, Fat: 11.2g, Fiber: 3.4g, Carbs: 9.8g, Protein: 4.5g

47.   Yogurt Figs Mix
Preparation Time: 5 minutes
Cooking Time: 5 minutes
Servings: 4
Ingredients:

- 8 oz. figs, chopped
- 2 cups Greek yogurt
- 1 tbsp. honey
- 1 tsp. cinnamon powder
- 1 tbsp. almonds, chopped
- 1 tbsp. walnuts, chopped
- ¼ cup pistachios, chopped

Directions:

Heat up a pan over medium heat, add the figs and the rest of the ingredients except the yogurt, stir and cook for 5 minutes.

Divide the yogurt into bowls, divide the figs mix on top, toss gently and serve.

Nutrition: Calories 198, Fat: 4.2g, Fiber: 6.3g, Carbs: 42.1g, Protein: 3.4g

48. Mango and Spinach Bowls

Preparation Time: 5 minutes

Cooking Time: 0 minutes

Servings: 4

Ingredients:

- 1 cup baby arugula
- 1 cup baby spinach, chopped
- 1 mango, peeled and cubed
- 1 cup strawberries, halved
- 1 tbsp. hemp seeds
- 1 cucumber, sliced
- 1 tbsp. lime juice
- 1 tbsp. tahini paste
- 1 tbsp. water

Directions:

In a salad bowl, mix the arugula with the rest of the ingredients except the tahini and the water and toss.

In a small bowl, combine the tahini with the water, whisk well, add to the salad, toss, divide into small bowls and serve for breakfast.

Nutrition: Calories 211, Fat: 4.5g, Fiber: 6.5g, Carbs: 10.2g, Protein: 3.5g

49. Oregano Quinoa and Spinach Muffins

Preparation Time: 10 minutes

Cooking Time: 35 minutes

Servings: 6

Ingredients:

- 1 cup quinoa
- 2 cups water
- 1 cup spinach, torn
- 2 spring onions, chopped
- 2 eggs, whisked
- ¼ cup parmesan cheese, grated
- ½ tsp garlic powder
- Sea salt and black pepper to the taste
- 2 tsps. oregano, dried
- Cooking spray

Directions:

Put the water in a pan, heat up over medium heat, add the quinoa, bring to a simmer, cook for 10 minutes, take off the heat, fluff with a fork and transfer to a bowl.

Add the rest of the ingredients except the cooking spray and stir well.

Grease a muffin tin with the cooking spray, divide the quinoa and spinach mix, introduce in the oven at 350°F and bake for 25 minutes.

Serve the muffins warm for breakfast.

Nutrition: Calories 267, Fat: 11.2g, Fiber: 2.3g, Carbs: 8.5g, Protein: 4.5g

50.   Apricots Couscous
Preparation Time: 15 minutes
Cooking Time: 4 minutes
Servings: 4
Ingredients:

- 3 cups almond milk
- 1 tsp. cinnamon powder
- 1 cup apricots, chopped
- 1 cup couscous, uncooked
- 3 tsps. honey
- 4 tsps. avocado oil

Directions:

Heat up a pan with the milk over medium heat, add the cinnamon and the rest of the ingredients, toss, and simmer for 4 minutes.

Divide the mix into bowls, leave aside for 15 minutes and serve for breakfast,

Nutrition: Calories 617, Fat: 44g, Fiber: 7.1g, Carbs: 52.3g, Protein: 10.2g

51.   Tapioca Pudding
Preparation Time: 30 minutes
Cooking Time: 15 minutes
Servings: 3
Ingredients:

- ¼ cup pearl tapioca
- ¼ cup maple syrup
- 2 cups almond milk
- ½ cup coconut flesh, shredded
- 1 and ½ tsp lemon juice

Directions:

In a pan, combine the milk with the tapioca and the rest of the ingredients, bring to a simmer over medium heat, and cook for 15 minutes.

Divide the mix into bowls, cool it down and serve for breakfast.

Nutrition: Calories 361, Fat: 28.5g, Fiber: 2.7g, Carbs: 28.3g, Protein: 2.8g

52.   Banana and Quinoa Casserole
Preparation Time: 10 minutes
Cooking Time: 1 hour and 20 minutes

Servings: 8
Ingredients:

- 3 cups bananas, peeled and mashed
- ¼ cup pure maple syrup
- ¼ cup molasses
- 1 tbsp. cinnamon powder
- 2 tsps. vanilla extract
- 1 tsp. cloves, ground
- 1 tsp. ginger, ground
- ½ tsp allspice, ground
- 1 cup quinoa
- ¼ cup almonds, chopped
- 2 ½ cups almond milk

Directions:
In a baking dish, combine the bananas with the maple syrup, molasses, and the rest of the ingredients, toss and bake at 350°F for 1 hour and 20 minutes.
Divide the mix between plates and serve for breakfast.
Nutrition: Calories 213, Fat: 4.1g, Fiber: 4g, Carbs: 41g, Protein: 4.5g
53.   Spiced Chickpeas Bowls
Preparation Time: 10 minutes
Cooking Time: 30 minutes
Servings: 4
Ingredients:

- 15 oz. canned chickpeas, drained and rinsed
- ¼ tsp cardamom, ground
- ½ tsp cinnamon powder
- 1 and ½ tsps. turmeric powder
- 1 tsp. coriander, ground
- 1 tbsp. olive oil
- A pinch of salt and black pepper
- ¾ cup Greek yogurt
- ½ cup green olives, pitted and halved
- ½ cup cherry tomatoes, halved
- 1 cucumber, sliced

Directions:
Spread the chickpeas on a lined baking sheet, add the cardamom, cinnamon, turmeric, coriander, the oil, salt, and pepper, toss and bake at 375°F for 30 minutes.

In a bowl, combine the roasted chickpeas with the rest of the ingredients, toss and serve for breakfast.

Nutrition: Calories 519, Fat: 34.5g, Fiber: 13.3g, Carbs: 49.8g, Protein: 12g

54.   Avocado Spread
Preparation Time: 5 minutes
Cooking Time: 0 minutes
Servings: 8
Ingredients:

- 2 avocados, peeled, pitted, and roughly chopped
- 1 tbsp. sun-dried tomatoes, chopped
- 2 tbsps. lemon juice
- 3 tbsps. cherry tomatoes, chopped
- ¼ cup red onion, chopped
- 1 tsp. oregano, dried
- 2 tbsps. parsley, chopped
- 4 kalamata olives, pitted and chopped
- A pinch of salt and black pepper

Directions:

Put the avocados in a bowl and mash with a fork.

Add the rest of the ingredients, stir to combine, and serve as a morning spread.

Nutrition: Calories 110, Fat: 10g, Fiber: 3.8g, Carbs: 5.7g, Protein: 1.2g

55.   Greek Beans Tortillas
Preparation Time: 5 minutes
Cooking Time: 20 minutes
Servings: 4
Ingredients:

- 1 red onion, chopped
- 2 garlic cloves, minced
- 1 tbsp. olive oil
- 1 green bell pepper, sliced
- 3 cups canned pinto beans, drained and rinsed
- 2 red chili peppers, chopped
- 4 tbsp parsley, chopped
- 1 tsp. cumin, ground
- A pinch of salt and black pepper
- 4 whole wheat Greek tortillas
- 1 cup cheddar cheese, shredded

Directions:

Heat up a pan with the oil over medium heat, add the onion and sauté for 5 minutes.

Add the rest of the ingredients except the tortillas and the cheese, stir and cook for 15 minutes.

Divide these beans mix on each Greek tortilla, also divide the cheese, roll the tortillas, and serve for breakfast.

Nutrition: Calories 673, Fat: 14.9g, Fiber: 23.7g, Carbs: 75.4g, Protein: 39g

56.   Baked Cauliflower Hash
Preparation Time: 10 minutes
Cooking Time: 25 minutes
Servings: 4
Ingredients:

- 4 cups cauliflower florets
- 1 tbsp. olive oil
- 2 cups white mushrooms, sliced
- 1 cup cherry tomatoes, halved
- 1 yellow onion, chopped
- 2 garlic cloves, minced
- ¼ tsp garlic powder
- 3 tbsps. basil, chopped
- 3 tbsps. mint, chopped
- 1 tbsp. dill, chopped

Directions:
Spread the cauliflower florets on a baking sheet lined with parchment paper, add the rest of the ingredients, introduce in the oven at 350 ° F and bake for 25 minutes.

Divide the hash between plates and serve for breakfast.

Nutrition: Calories 367, Fat: 14.3g, Fiber: 3.5g, Carbs: 16.8g, Protein: 12.2g

57.   Eggs, Mint and Tomatoes
Preparation Time: 10 minutes
Cooking Time: 15 minutes
Servings: 2
Ingredients:

- 2 eggs, whisked
- 2 tomatoes, cubed
- 2 tsps. olive oil
- 1 tbsp. mint, chopped
- 1 tbsp. chives, chopped
- Salt and black pepper to the taste

Directions:
Heat up a pan with the oil over medium heat, add the tomatoes and the rest of the ingredients except the eggs, stir and cook for 5 minutes.

Add the eggs, toss, cook for 10 minutes more, divide between plates, and serve.

Nutrition: Calories 300, Fat: 15.3g, Fiber: 4.5g, Carbs: 17.7g, Protein: 11g

58.   Bacon, Spinach and Tomato Sandwich
Preparation Time: 5 minutes
Cooking Time: 0 minutes
Servings: 1
Ingredients:

- 2 whole-wheat bread slices, toasted
- 1 tbsp. Dijon mustard
- 3 bacon slices
- Salt and black pepper to the taste
- 2 tomato slices
- ¼ cup baby spinach

Directions:
Spread the mustard on each bread slice, divide the bacon and the rest of the ingredients on one slice, top with the other one, cut in half and serve for breakfast.

Nutrition: Calories 246, Fat: 11.2g, Fiber: 4.5g, Carbs: 17.5g, Protein: 8.3g

SIDE DISHES

59.   Bulgur, Kale and Cheese Mix

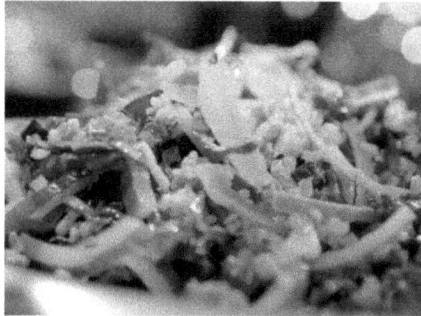

Preparation Time: 10 minutes
Cooking Time: 10 minutes
Servings: 6
Ingredients:

- 4 oz. bulgur
- 4 oz. kale, chopped

- 1 tbsp. mint, chopped
- 3 spring onions, chopped
- 1 cucumber, chopped
- A pinch of allspice, ground
- 2 tbsps. olive oil
- Zest and juice of ½ lemon
- 4 oz. feta cheese, crumbled

Directions:
Put bulgur in a bowl, cover with hot water, aside for 10 minutes and fluff with a fork.

Heat up a pan with the oil over medium heat, add the onions and the allspice and cook for 3 minutes.

Add the bulgur and the rest of the ingredients, cook everything for 5-6 minutes more, divide between plates and serve.

Nutrition: Calories 200, Fat: 6.7g, Fiber: 3.4g, Carbs: 15.4g, Protein: 4.5g

60.   Spicy Green Beans Mix

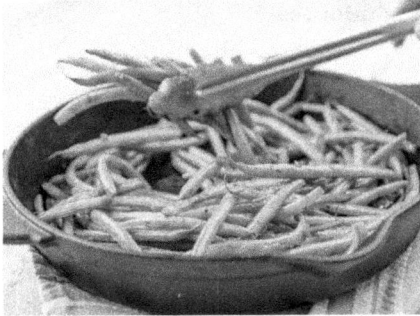

Preparation Time: 5 minutes
Cooking Time: 15 minutes
Servings: 4
Ingredients:

- 4 tsps. olive oil
- 1 garlic clove, minced
- ½ tsp hot paprika
- ¾ cup veggie stock
- 1 yellow onion, sliced
- 1 lb. green beans, trimmed and halved
- ½ cup goat cheese, shredded
- 2 tsp balsamic vinegar

Directions:

Heat up a pan with the oil over medium heat, add the garlic, stir and cook for 1 minute.

Add the green beans and the rest of the ingredients, toss, cook everything for 15 minutes more, divide between plates and serve as a side dish.

Nutrition: Calories 188, Fat: 4g, Fiber: 3g, Carbs: 12.4g, Protein: 4.4g

61.   Beans and Rice

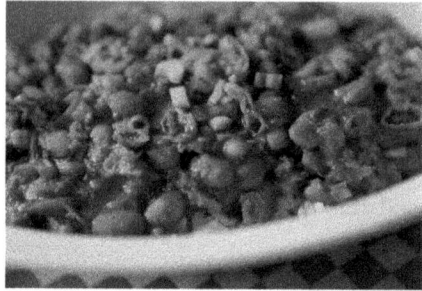

Preparation Time: 10 minutes
Cooking Time: 55 minutes
Servings: 6
Ingredients:

- 1 tbsp. olive oil
- 1 yellow onion, chopped
- 2 celery stalks, chopped
- 2 garlic cloves, minced
- 2 cups brown rice
- 1 and ½ cup canned black beans, rinsed and drained
- 4 cups water
- Salt and black pepper to the taste

Directions:
Heat up a pan with the oil over medium heat, add the celery, garlic, and the onion, stir and cook for 10 minutes.

Add the rest of the ingredients, stir, bring to a simmer, and cook over medium heat for 45 minutes.

Divide between plates and serve.

Nutrition: Calories 224, Fat: 8.4g, Fiber: 3.4g, Carbs: 15.3g, Protein: 6.2g

62.   Tomato and Millet Mix
Preparation Time: 10 minutes
Cooking Time: 20 minutes
Servings: 6
Ingredients:

- 3 tbsps. olive oil
- 1 cup millet
- 2 spring onions, chopped
- 2 tomatoes, chopped
- ½ cup cilantro, chopped
- 1 tsp. chili paste
- 6 cups cold water
- ½ cup lemon juice
- Salt and black pepper to the taste

Directions:
Heat up a pan with the oil over medium heat, add the millet, stir, and cook for 4 minutes.

Add the water, salt, and pepper. Stir then bring to a simmer over medium heat cook for 15 minutes.

Add the rest of the ingredients, toss, divide the mix between plates and serve as a side dish.

Nutrition: Calories 222, Fat: 10.2g, Fiber: 3.4g, Carbs: 14.5g, Protein: 2.4g

63. Quinoa and Greens Salad
Preparation Time: 10 minutes
Cooking Time: 0 minutes
Servings: 4
Ingredients:

- 1 cup quinoa, cooked
- 1 medium bunch collard greens, chopped
- 4 tbsps. walnuts, chopped
- 2 tbsps. balsamic vinegar
- 4 tbsps. tahini paste
- 4 tbsps. cold water
- A pinch of salt and black pepper
- 1 tbsp. olive oil

Directions:
In a bowl, mix the tahini with the water and vinegar and whisk.

In a bowl, mix the quinoa with the rest of the ingredients and the tahini dressing, toss, divide the mix between plates and serve as a side dish.

Nutrition: Calories 175, Fat: 3g, Fiber: 3g, Carbs: 5g, Protein: 3g

64. Veggies and Avocado Dressing
Preparation Time: 10 minutes
Cooking Time: 0 minutes
Servings: 4
Ingredients:

- 3 tbsps. pepitas, roasted
- 3 cups water
- 2 tbsps. cilantro, chopped
- 4 tbsps. parsley, chopped
- 1 and ½ cups corn
- 1 cup radish, sliced
- 2 avocados, peeled, pitted and chopped
- 2 mangos, peeled and chopped
- 3 tbsps. olive oil
- 4 tbsps. Greek yogurt
- 1 tsp. balsamic vinegar
- 2 tbsps. lime juice
- Salt and black pepper to the taste

Directions:

In your blender, mix the olive oil with avocados, salt, pepper, lime juice, the yogurt and the vinegar and pulse.

In a bowl, mix the pepitas with the cilantro, parsley and the rest of the ingredients, and toss.

Add the avocado dressing, toss, divide the mix between plates and serve as a side dish.

Nutrition: Calories 403, Fat: 30.5g, Fiber: 10g, Carbs: 23.5g, Protein: 3.5g

65. Cauliflower Quinoa
Preparation Time: 5 minutes
Cooking Time: 10 minutes
Servings: 4
Ingredients:

- 1 ½ cup quinoa, coked
- 3 tbsps. olive oil
- 3 cups cauliflower florets
- 2 spring onions, chopped
- Salt and pepper to the taste
- 1 tbsp. red wine vinegar
- 1 tbsp. parsley, chopped
- 1 tbsp. chives, chopped

Directions:

Heat up a pan with the oil over medium-high heat, add the spring onions and cook for 2 minutes.

Add the cauliflower, quinoa and the rest of the ingredients, toss, cook over medium heat for 8-9 minutes, divide between plates and serve as a side dish.

Nutrition: Calories 220, Fat: 16.7g, Fiber: 5.6g, Carbs: 6.8g, Protein: 5.4g

66. Mixed Veggies and Chard

Preparation Time: 10 minutes
Cooking Time: 20 minutes
Servings: 4
Ingredients:

- ½ cup celery, chopped
- ½ cup carrot, chopped
- ½ cup red onion, chopped
- ½ cup red bell pepper, chopped
- 1 tbsp. olive oil
- 1 cup veggie stock
- ½ cup black olives, pitted and chopped
- 10 oz. ruby chard, torn
- Salt and black pepper to the taste
- 1 tsp. balsamic vinegar

Directions:
Heat up a pan with the oil over medium-high heat, add the celery, carrot, onion, bell pepper, salt, and pepper, stir and sauté for 5 minutes.

Add the rest of the ingredients, toss, cook over medium heat for 15 minutes more, divide between plates and serve as a side dish.

Nutrition: Calories 150, Fat: 6.7g, Fiber: 2.6g, Carbs: 6.8g, Protein: 5.4g

67. Spicy Broccoli and Almonds
Preparation Time: 10 minutes
Cooking Time: 30 minutes
Servings: 4
Ingredients:

- 1 broccoli head, florets separated
- 2 garlic cloves, minced
- 1 tbsp. olive oil
- 1 tbsp. chili powder
- Salt and black pepper to the taste
- 1 tbsp. mint, chopped
- 2 tbsps. almonds, toasted and chopped

Directions:
In a roasting pan, combine the broccoli with the garlic, oil and the rest of the ingredients, toss, introduce in the oven and cook at 390°F for 30 minutes.

Divide the mix between plates and serve as a side dish.

Nutrition: Calories 156, Fat: 5.4g, Fiber: 1.2g, Carbs: 4.3g, Protein: 2g

68. Balsamic Asparagus

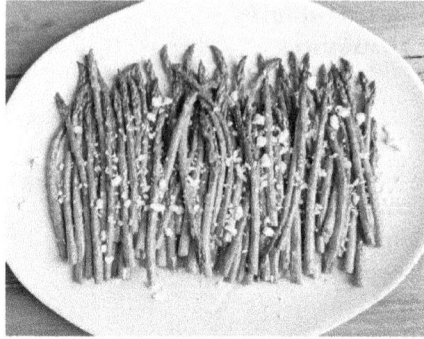

Preparation Time: 10 minutes
Cooking Time: 15 minutes
Servings: 4
Ingredients:

- 3 tbsps. olive oil
- 3 garlic cloves, minced
- 2 tbsps. shallot, chopped
- Salt and black pepper to the taste
- 2 tsps. balsamic vinegar
- 1½ pound asparagus, trimmed

Directions:
Heat up a pan with the oil over medium-high heat, add the garlic and the shallot and sauté for 3 minutes.

Add the rest of the ingredients, cook for 12 minutes more, divide between plates, and serve as a side dish.

Nutrition: Calories 100, Fat: 10.5g, Fiber: 1.2g, Carbs: 2.3g, Protein: 2.1g

69. Lime Cucumber Mix
Preparation Time: 10 minutes
Cooking Time: 0 minutes
Servings: 8
Ingredients:

- 4 cucumbers, chopped
- ½ cup green bell pepper, chopped
- 1 yellow onion, chopped
- 1 chili pepper, chopped
- 1 garlic clove, minced
- 1 tsp. parsley, chopped
- 2 tbsps. lime juice
- 1 tbsp. dill, chopped

- Salt and black pepper to the taste
- 1 tbsp. olive oil

Directions:
In a large bowl, mix the cucumber with the bell peppers and the rest of the ingredients, toss, and serve as a side dish.

Nutrition: Calories 123, Fat: 4.3g, Fiber: 2.3g, Carbs: 5.6g, Protein: 2g

70.   Walnuts Cucumber Mix
Preparation Time: 5 minutes
Cooking Time: 0 minutes
Servings: 2
Ingredients:

- 2 cucumbers, chopped
- 1 tbsp. olive oil
- Salt and black pepper to the taste
- 1 red chili pepper, dried
- 1 tbsp. lemon juice
- 3 tbsps. walnuts, chopped
- 1 tbsp. balsamic vinegar
- 1 tsp. chives, chopped

Directions:
In a bowl, mix the cucumbers with the oil and the rest of the ingredients, toss, and serve as a side dish.

Nutrition: Calories 121, Fat: 2.3g, Fiber: 2.0g, Carbs: 6.7g, Protein: 2.4g

71.   Cheesy Beet Salad
Preparation Time: 10 minutes
Cooking Time: 1 hour
Servings: 4
Ingredients:

- 4 beets, peeled and cut into wedges
- 3 tbsps. olive oil
- Salt and black pepper to the taste
- ¼ cup lime juice
- 8 slices goat cheese, crumbled
- ⅓ cup walnuts, chopped
- 1 tbsp. chives, chopped

Directions:
In a roasting pan, combine the beets with the oil, salt, and pepper, toss and bake at 400 ° F for 1 hour.

Cool the beets down, transfer them to a bowl, add the rest of the ingredients, toss, and serve as a side salad.

Nutrition: Calories 156, Fat: 4.2g, Fiber: 3.4g, Carbs: 6.5g, Protein: 4g

72.   Rosemary Beets
Preparation Time: 10 minutes
Cooking Time: 20 minutes
Servings: 4
Ingredients:

- 4 medium beets, peeled and cubed
- ⅓ cup balsamic vinegar
- 1 tsp. rosemary, chopped
- 1 garlic clove, minced
- ½ tsp Italian seasoning
- 1 tbsp. olive oil

Directions:
Heat up a pan with the oil over medium heat, add the beets and the rest of the ingredients, toss, and cook for 20 minutes.

Divide the mix between plates and serve as a side dish.

Nutrition: Calories 165, Fat: 3.4g, Fiber: 4.5g, Carbs: 11.3g, Protein: 2.3g

73.   Squash and Tomatoes Mix
Preparation Time: 10 minutes
Cooking Time: 20 minutes
Servings: 6
Ingredients:

- 5 medium squash, cubed
- A pinch of salt and black pepper
- 3 tbsps. olive oil
- 1 cup pine nuts, toasted
- ¼ cup goat cheese, crumbled
- 6 tomatoes, cubed
- ½ yellow onion, chopped
- 2 tbsps. cilantro, chopped
- 2 tbsps. lemon juice

Directions:
Heat up a pan with the oil over medium heat, add the onion and pine nuts and cook for 3 minutes.

Add the squash and the rest of the ingredients, cook everything for 15 minutes, divide between plates and serve as a side dish.

Nutrition: Calories 200, Fat: 4.5g, Fiber: 3.4g, Carbs: 6.7g, Protein: 4g

74.   Balsamic Eggplant Mix

Preparation Time: 10 minutes
Cooking Time: 20 minutes
Servings: 6
Ingredients:

- ⅓ cup chicken stock
- 2 tbsps. balsamic vinegar
- A pinch of salt and black pepper
- 1 tbsp. lime juice
- 2 big eggplants, sliced
- 1 tbsp. rosemary, chopped
- ¼ cup cilantro, chopped
- 2 tbsps. olive oil

Directions:

In a roasting pan, combine the eggplants with the stock, vinegar, and the rest of the ingredients, introduce the pan in the oven and bake at 390 ° F for 20 minutes.

Divide the mix between plates and serve as a side dish.

Nutrition: Calories 201, Fat: 4.5g, Fiber: 3g, Carbs: 5.4g, Protein: 3g

75. Sage Barley Mix
Preparation Time: 10 minutes
Cooking Time: 45 minutes
Servings: 4
Ingredients:

- 1 tbsp. olive oil
- 1 red onion, chopped
- 1 tbsp. leaves, chopped
- 1 garlic clove, minced
- 14 oz. barley
- ½ tbsp parmesan, grated
- 6 cups veggie stock
- Salt and black pepper to the taste

Directions:

Heat up a pan with the oil over medium heat, add the onion and garlic, stir and sauté for 5 minutes.

Add the sage, barley, and the rest of the ingredients except the parmesan. Stir, bring to a simmer, and cook for 40 minutes,

Add the parmesan, stir, divide between plates.

Nutrition: Calories 210, Fat: 6.5g, Fiber: 3.4g, Carbs: 8.6g, Protein: 3.4g

76. Chickpeas and Beets Mix
Preparation Time: 10 minutes

Cooking Time: 25 minutes
Servings: 4
Ingredients:

- 3 tbsps. capers, drained and chopped
- Juice of 1 lemon
- Zest of 1 lemon, grated
- 1 red onion, chopped
- 3 tbsps. olive oil
- 14 oz. canned chickpeas, drained
- 8 oz. beets, peeled and cubed
- 1 tbsp. parsley, chopped
- Salt and pepper to the taste

Directions:
Heat up a pan with the oil over medium heat, add the onion, lemon zest, lemon juice and the capers and sauté for 5 minutes.

Add the rest of the ingredients, stir, and cook over medium-low heat for 20 minutes more.

Divide the mix between plates and serve as a side dish.

Nutrition: Calories 199, Fat: 4.5g, Fiber: 2.3g, Carbs: 6.5g, Protein: 3.3g

77.   Creamy Sweet Potatoes Mix

Preparation Time: 10 minutes
Cooking Time: 1 hour
Servings: 4
Ingredients:

- 4 tbsps. olive oil
- 1 garlic clove, minced
- 4 medium sweet potatoes, pricked with a fork
- 1 red onion, sliced
- 3 oz. baby spinach
- Zest and juice of 1 lemon
- A small bunch dill, chopped
- 1 ½ tbsps. Greek yogurt
- 2 tbsps. tahini paste
- Salt and black pepper to the taste

Directions:
Put the potatoes on a baking sheet lined with parchment paper, introduce in the oven at 350°F and cook them for 1 hour.

Peel the potatoes, cut them into wedges and put them in a bowl.

Add the garlic, the oil and the rest of the ingredients, toss, divide the mix between plates and serve.

Nutrition: Calories 214, Fat: 5.6g, Fiber: 3.4g, Carbs: 6.5g, Protein: 3.1g

78. Cabbage and Mushrooms Mix
Preparation Time: 10 minutes
Cooking Time: 15 minutes
Servings: 2
Ingredients:

- 1 yellow onion, sliced
- 2 tbsps. olive oil
- 1 tbsp. balsamic vinegar
- ½ pound white mushrooms, sliced
- 1 green cabbage head, shredded
- 4 spring onions, chopped
- Salt and black pepper to the taste

Directions:
Heat up a pan with the oil over medium heat, add the yellow onion and the spring onions and cook for 5 minutes.
Add the rest of the ingredients, cook everything for 10 minutes, divide between plates and serve.

Nutrition: Calories 199, Fat: 4.5g, Fiber: 2.4g, Carbs: 5.6g, Protein: 2.2g

79. Lemon Mushroom Rice
Preparation Time: 10 minutes
Cooking Time: 30 minutes
Servings: 4
Ingredients:

- 2 cups chicken stock
- 1 yellow onion, chopped
- ½ pound white mushrooms, sliced
- 2 garlic cloves, minced
- 8 oz. wild rice
- Juice and zest of 1 lemon
- 1 tbsp. chives, chopped
- 6 tbsps. goat cheese, crumbled
- Salt and black pepper to the taste

Directions:
Heat up a pot with the stock over medium heat, add the rice, onion, and the rest of the ingredients except the chives and the cheese, bring to a simmer and cook for 25 minutes.
Add the remaining ingredients, cook everything for 5 minutes, divide between plates and serve as a side dish.

Nutrition: Calories 222, Fat: 5.5g, Fiber: 5.4g, Carbs: 12.3g, Protein: 5.6g

80.   Paprika and Chives Potatoes
Preparation Time: 10 minutes
Cooking Time: 1 hour and 8 minutes
Servings: 4
Ingredients:

- 4 potatoes, scrubbed and pricked with a fork
- 1 tbsp. olive oil
- 1 celery stalk, chopped
- 2 tomatoes, chopped
- 1 tsp. sweet paprika
- Salt and black pepper to the taste
- 2 tbsps. chives, chopped

Directions:
Arrange the potatoes on a baking sheet lined with parchment paper, introduce in the oven and bake at 350°F for 1 hour.

Cool the potatoes down, peel and cut them into larger cubes.

Heat up a pan with the oil over medium heat, add the celery and the tomatoes and sauté for 2 minutes.

Add the potatoes and the rest of the ingredients, toss, cook everything for 6 minutes, divide the mix between plates and serve as a side dish.

Nutrition: Calories 233, Fat: 8.7g, Fiber: 4.5g, Carbs: 14.4g, Protein: 6.4g

81.   Lemony Carrots
Preparation Time: 10 minutes
Cooking Time: 40 minutes
Servings: 4
Ingredients:

- 3 tbsps. olive oil
- 2 pounds baby carrots, trimmed
- Salt and black pepper to the taste
- ½ tsp lemon zest, grated
- 1 tbsp. lemon juice
- ⅓ cup Greek yogurt
- 1 garlic clove, minced
- 1 tsp. cumin, ground
- 1 tbsp. dill, chopped

Directions:
In a roasting pan, combine the carrots with the oil, salt, pepper, and the rest of the ingredients except the dill, toss and bake at 400°F for 20 minutes.

Reduce the temperature to 375°F and cook for 20 minutes more.

Divide the mix between plates, sprinkle the dill on top and serve.

Nutrition: Calories 192, Fat: 5.4g, Fiber: 3.4g, Carbs: 7.3g, Protein: 5.6g

82. Oregano Potatoes
Preparation Time: 10 minutes
Cooking Time: 40 minutes
Servings: 4
Ingredients:

- 6 red potatoes, peeled and cut into wedges
- Salt and black pepper to the taste
- 2 tbsps. olive oil
- 1 tsp. lemon zest, grated
- 1 tsp. oregano, dried
- 1 tbsp. chives, chopped
- ½ cup chicken stock

Directions:
In a roasting pan, combine the potatoes with salt, pepper, the oil, and the rest of the ingredients except the chives, toss, introduce in the oven and cook at 425°F for 40 minutes.
Divide the mix between plates, sprinkle the chives on top and serve as a side dish.
Nutrition: Calories 245, Fat: 4.5g, Fiber: 2.8g, Carbs: 7.1g, Protein: 6.4g

83. Baby Squash and Lentils Mix
Preparation Time: 10 minutes
Cooking Time: 10 minutes
Servings: 4
Ingredients:

- 2 tbsps. olive oil
- ½ tsp sweet paprika
- 10 oz. baby squash, sliced
- 1 tbsp. balsamic vinegar
- 15 oz. canned lentils, drained and rinsed
- Salt and black pepper to the taste
- 1 tbsp. dill, chopped

Directions:
Heat up a pan with the oil over medium heat, add the squash, lentils, and the rest of the ingredients, toss and cook over medium heat for 10 minutes.
Divide the mix between plates and serve as a side dish.
Nutrition: Calories 438, Fat: 8.4g, Fiber: 32.4g, Carbs: 65.5g, Protein: 22.4g

84. Parmesan Quinoa and Mushrooms
Preparation Time: 10 minutes
Cooking Time: 20 minutes

Servings: 4
Ingredients:

- 1 cup quinoa, cooked
- ½ cup chicken stock
- 2 tbsps. olive oil
- 6 oz. white mushrooms, sliced
- 1 tsp. garlic, minced
- Salt and black pepper to the taste
- ½ cup parmesan, grated
- 2 tbsps. cilantro, chopped

Directions:
Heat up a pan with the oil over medium heat, add the garlic and mushrooms, stir and sauté for 10 minutes.

Add the quinoa and the rest of the ingredients, toss, cook over medium heat for 10 minutes more, divide between plates and serve as a side dish.

Nutrition: Calories 233, Fat: 9.5g, Fiber: 6.4g, Carbs: 27.4g, Protein: 12.5g

85.   Chives Rice Mix
Preparation Time: 5 minutes
Cooking Time: 5 minutes
Servings: 4
Ingredients:

- 3 tbsps. avocado oil
- 1 cup Arborio rice, cooked
- 2 tbsps. chives, chopped
- Salt and black pepper to the taste
- 2 tsps. lemon juice

Directions:
Heat up a pan with the avocado oil over medium high heat, add the rice and the rest of the ingredients, toss, cook for 5 minutes, divide the mix between plates and serve as a side dish.

Nutrition: Calories 236, Fat: 9g, Fiber: 12.4g, Carbs: 17.5g, Protein: 4.5g

86.   Green Beans and Peppers Mix
Preparation Time: 10 minutes
Cooking Time: 10 minutes
Servings: 4
Ingredients:

- 2 tbsps. olive oil
- 1 ½ pounds green beans, trimmed and halved
- Salt and black pepper to the taste

- 2 red bell peppers, cut into strips
- 1 tbsp. lime juice
- 2 tbsps. rosemary, chopped
- 1 tbsp. dill, chopped

Directions:
Heat up a pan with the oil over medium heat, add the bell peppers and the green beans, toss and cook for 5 minutes.

Add the rest of the ingredients, toss, cook for 5 minutes more, divide between plates and serve as a side dish.

Nutrition: Calories 222, Fat: 8.6g, Fiber: 3.4g, Carbs: 8.6g, Protein: 3.4g

87.   Garlic Snap Peas Mix
Preparation Time: 10 minutes
Cooking Time: 10 minutes
Servings: 4
Ingredients:

- ½ cup walnuts, chopped
- 2 tsps. lime juice
- ¼ cup olive oil
- 1 and ½ tsps. garlic, minced
- ½ cup veggie stock
- 1 lb. sugar snap peas
- Salt and black pepper to the taste
- 1 tbsp. chives, chopped

Directions:
Heat up a pan with the stock over medium heat, add the snap peas and cook for 5 minutes.

Add the rest of the ingredients except the chives, cook for 5 minutes more and divide between plates.

Sprinkle the chives on top and serve as a side dish.

Nutrition: Calories 200, Fat: 7.6g, Fiber: 3.5g, Carbs: 8.5g, Protein: 4.3g

LUNCH RECIPES

88.   Avocado & Tuna Tapas

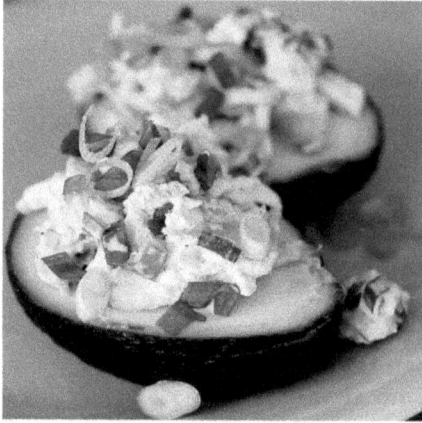

Preparation Time: 10 minutes
Cooking Time: 10 minutes
Servings: 4
Ingredients:

- 12 oz. can Solid white tuna packed in water
- 3 + more for garnish Green onions
- ½ Red bell pepper
- Garlic salt and black pepper as desired
- 1 tbsp. Mayonnaise
- 1 dash Balsamic vinegar
- 2 Ripe avocados

Directions:

Drain the tuna thoroughly. Remove the pit and slice the avocados into halves.

Chop the bell pepper, and thinly slice the onions. Whisk the vinegar, red pepper, onions, salt, pepper, mayonnaise, and tuna.

Load the avocado halves with the tuna.

Top it off with a portion of green onions and black pepper before Servings.

Nutrition: Calories 194, Fat: 18.2g, Protein: 23.9g

89.   Cannellini Bean Lettuce Wraps
Preparation Time: 10 minutes
Cooking Time: 15 minutes
Servings: 4
Ingredients:

- 1 tbsp. Olive oil
- ½ cup Red onion

- 1 medium/ ¾ cup Tomatoes
- ¼ tsp Freshly cracked black pepper
- ¼ cup Fresh curly parsley
- 15 oz. can Great Northern beans or cannellini beans
- ½ cup Prepared hummus
- 8 Romaine lettuce leaves

Directions:

Drain and rinse the vegetables and beans. Chop the tomatoes and onion into fine pieces.

Add the oil into a skillet to heat using the medium heat temperature setting.

Chop and toss in the onions, tomatoes, and pepper to sauté for six. Stir occasionally.

Pour in the drained beans and simmer them for three additional minutes.

Mix in the parsley after removing it from the burner.

Spread the hummus over each of the leaves of lettuce. Spread the bean mixture to the center of each leaf. Fold it over to make a wrap to serve.

Nutrition: Calories 235, Fat: 20g, Protein: 4g

90. Easy Farfalle with Fresh Tomatoes
Preparation Time: 15 minutes
Cooking Time: 25-30 minutes
Servings: 4
Ingredients:

- 4/2 lb. total weight Tomatoes
- ½ cup Fresh basil
- 3 tbsp. Red onion
- 1 clove Garlic ()
- 3 tbsp. Olive oil
- 1 tbsp. Red wine vinegar
- ¼ tsp. Black pepper
- ¾ tsp. Salt
- ½ lb. Farfalle pasta

Directions:

Peel and remove the seeds from the tomatoes and dice them into ½-inch pieces. Cut the basil into slender ribbons, using the whole leaves for garnishing. Chop/mince the garlic and onion.

Prepare the sauce in a large mixing container using the tomatoes, onion, basil oil, garlic, vinegar, pepper, and salt. Toss to mix.

Prepare a large pot of water (about ¾ full) and wait for it to boil. Toss in the farfalle and simmer until it's al dente (10 min.) Pour it into a colander to drain.

Divide the pasta and sauce between the bowls and serve.

Nutrition: Calories 212.5, Fat: 11.2g, Protein: 4.2g

91.   Fried Rice with Spinach - Peppers & Artichokes

Preparation Time: 10 minutes

Cooking Time: 15-20 minutes

Servings: 4

Ingredients:

- 1 ½ cups Cooked rice
- 10 oz. Frozen chopped spinach
- 6 oz. Marinated artichoke hearts
- 4 oz. Roasted red peppers
- ½ tsp. Minced garlic
- ½ cup Crumbled feta cheese with herbs
- 2 tbsp Olive oil

Directions:

Prepare the vegetables. Mince the garlic. Thaw and drain the frozen spinach. Drain and quarter the artichoke hearts. Drain and chop the roasted red peppers.

Heat a skillet on the stovetop to warm the oil using the medium heat setting. Toss in the garlic to sauté for two minutes.

Toss in the rice and continue cooking for about two minutes until well heated.

Fold in the spinach and continue cooking for three more minutes.

Add the red peppers and artichoke hearts. Simmer for two minutes.

Stir in the feta cheese and serve immediately.

Nutrition: Calories 244, Fat: 12.9g, Protein: 9.3g

92.   Gigantes (Greek Lima Beans)

Preparation Time: 1 hour

Cooking Time: 10 hours

Servings: 8

Ingredients:

- 16 oz. pkg. Dried lima beans
- 2 - 16 oz. cans Chopped tomatoes with juice
- 1 cup Olive oil
- 3 cloves Minced garlic
- Sea salt as desired
- 1 tsp. Freshly chopped dill
- Also Needed: 9 x 13 baking dish

Directions:

Pour the beans into a large saucepan with water to fill two inches over the top of the beans. Set them aside to soak overnight.

Set the oven at 375°F.

Place the saucepan over medium heat and wait for it to boil. Once it's boiling, lower the temperature setting to med-low and simmer for 20 minutes. Dump the water and drain the beans in a colander.

Pour and fold the beans into the baking dish with the dill, salt, oil, garlic, and tomatoes.

Bake the beans for 1.5 to 2 hours. Add water as needed, stirring occasionally.

Nutrition: Calories 449, Fat: 27.5g, Protein: 13g

93. Gluten-Free Spanish Rice

Preparation Time: 15 minutes

Cooking Time: 40 minutes

Servings: 6

Ingredients:

- 1 tbsp. Olive oil
- 2 cloves Garlic
- ½ cup Medium onion
- ½ cup Medium green bell pepper
- 1 cup Long-grain rice - regular/uncooked
- ¼ tsp. Sea salt
- ¼ tsp. Crushed red pepper
- 1 ¾ cups Chicken broth
- 1 14.5 oz. can Undrained - Diced fire-roasted tomatoes
- Also Needed: 3-quart saucepan

Directions:

Heat the oil in the saucepan using the medium temperature setting.

Chop/dice the onion, garlic, and bell pepper and toss them into the skillet for about five minutes, stirring constantly.

Add in the red pepper, salt, broth (reduced sodium is best), rice, and tomatoes. Wait for it to boil. Reduce the temperature setting and cook until the rice is tender before Servings (20-25 min.).

Nutrition: Calories 170, Fat: 2.5g, Protein: 4g

94. Greek Baked Zucchini & Potatoes - Briam

Preparation Time: 30 minutes

Cooking Time: 2 hours

Servings: 4

Ingredients:

- 2 lb. Potatoes
- 4 large Zucchini

- 4 small Red onions
- 6 pureed Ripe tomatoes
- ½ cup Olive oil
- Optional: 2 tbsp. Freshly chopped parsley
- Black pepper & Sea salt to taste
- Also Needed: 9 by 13-inch or larger baking dish

Directions:
Thinly slice the zucchini, onions, and potatoes.
Set the oven to reach 400°F.
Chop and spread the red onions, zucchini, and potatoes in the baking pan. Cover with pureed tomatoes, parsley, and olive oil.
Sprinkle using the salt and pepper. Toss until evenly coated. Bake them for approximately one hour or until the veggies are moist and softened.
Cool them slightly and serve at room temperature.
Nutrition: Calories 534, Fat: 28.3g, Protein: 11.3g

95. Chickpeas Soup

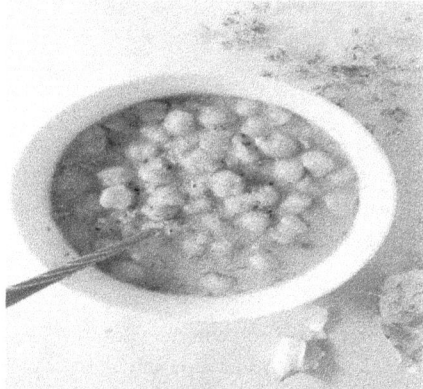

Preparation Time: 10 minutes
Cooking Time: 1 hour
Servings: 4
Ingredients:

- 3 tomatoes, cubed
- 2 yellow onions, chopped
- 2 tbsps. olive oil
- 4 celery stalks, chopped
- ½ cup parsley, chopped
- 2 garlic cloves, minced
- 16 oz. canned chickpeas, drained and rinsed

- 6 cups water
- 1 tsp. cumin, ground
- Juice of ½ lemon
- 1 tsp. turmeric powder
- ½ tsp cinnamon powder
- ½ tsp ginger, grated
- Salt and black pepper to the taste

Directions:

Heat up a pot with the oil over medium heat, add the onion and the garlic and sauté for 5 minutes.

Add the tomatoes, celery, cumin, turmeric, cinnamon, and the ginger, stir and sauté for 5 minutes more.

Add the remaining ingredients, bring the soup to a boil over medium heat and simmer for 50 minutes.

Ladle the soup into bowls and serve.

Nutrition: Calories 300, Fat: 15.4g, Fiber: 4.5g, Carbs: 29.5g, Protein: 15.4g

96. Tomato Soup

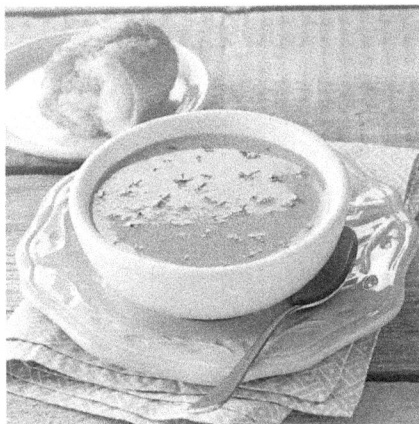

Preparation Time: 10 minutes
Cooking Time: 55 minutes
Servings: 8
Ingredients:

- 4 pounds tomatoes, halved
- 2 tbsps. olive oil
- 6 garlic cloves, minced
- 1 yellow onion, chopped
- Salt and black pepper to the taste

- 4 cups chicken stock
- ½ tsp red pepper flakes
- ½ cup basil, chopped
- ½ cup parmesan, grated

Directions:

Arrange the tomatoes in a roasting pan, add half of the oil, salt and pepper, toss, and bake at 400°F for 20 minutes.

Heat up a pot with the rest of the oil over medium heat, add the onion and sauté for 5 minutes.

Add the tomatoes and the rest of the ingredients except the basil and the parmesan, bring to a simmer and cook for 30 minutes.

Blend the soup using an immersion blender, add the basil and the parmesan, stir, divide into bowls, and serve.

Nutrition: Calories 237, Fat: 10g, Fiber: 3.4g, Carbs: 15.3g, Protein: 7.4g

97. Oyster Stew

Preparation Time: 10 minutes

Cooking Time: 1 hour and 10 minutes

Servings: 6

Ingredients:

- 2 garlic cloves, minced
- ¼ cup jarred roasted red peppers
- 2 tsps. oregano, chopped
- 1 lb. lamb meat, ground
- 1 tbsp. red wine vinegar
- Salt and black pepper to the taste
- 1 tsp. red pepper flakes
- 2 tbsps. olive oil
- 1 ½ cups chicken stock
- 36 oysters, shucked
- 1 ½ cups canned black eyed peas, drained

Directions:

Heat up a pot with the oil over medium heat, add the meat and the garlic and brown for 5 minutes.

Add the peppers and the rest of the ingredients, bring to a simmer, and cook for 15 minutes.

Divide the stew into bowls and serve.

Nutrition: Calories 264, Fat: 9.3g, Fiber: 1.2g, Carbs: 2.3g, Protein: 1.2g

98. Potatoes and Lentils Stew

Preparation Time: 10 minutes

Cooking Time: 35 minutes

Servings: 4

Ingredients:

- 4 cups water
- 1 cup carrots, sliced
- 1 yellow onion, chopped
- 1 tbsp. olive oil
- 1 cup celery, chopped
- 2 garlic cloves, minced
- 2 pounds gold potatoes, cubed
- 1 ½ cup lentils, dried
- ½ tsp smoked paprika
- ½ tsp oregano, dried
- Salt and black pepper to the taste
- 14 oz. canned tomatoes, chopped
- ½ cup cilantro, chopped

Directions:

Heat up a pot with the oil over medium- high heat, add the onion, garlic, celery, and carrots. Stir and cook for 5 minutes.

Add the rest of the ingredients except the cilantro, stir, bring to a simmer, and cook over medium heat for 25 minutes.

Add the cilantro, divide the stew into bowls and serve.

Nutrition: Calories 325, Fat: 17.3g, Fiber: 6.8g, Carbs: 26.4g, Protein: 16.4g

99.   Chicken Salad

Preparation Time: 30 minutes

Cooking Time: 45 minutes

Servings: 4

Ingredients:

- 1 ½ pounds chicken breast, skinless, boneless
- 1 tbsp. dill, chopped
- Zest of 2 lemons, grated
- Juice of 2 lemons
- 3 tbsps. olive oil
- 1 tbsp. oregano, chopped
- 3 tbsps. parsley, chopped
- A pinch of salt and black pepper

For the barley:

- 2 and ½ cups chicken stock
- 1 cup barley
- 1 tsp. oregano, dried
- Zest of 1 lemon, grated

- Juice of 1 lemon
- ¼ cup olive oil
- 2 red leaf lettuce heads, chopped
- 1 red onion, sliced
- 1 pint of cherry tomatoes, sliced
- 2 avocados, peeled, pitted and sliced

Directions:

Put the chicken breasts in a bowl, add the dill, zest of 2 lemons, juice of 2 lemons, 3 tbsps. oil, 1 tbsp. oregano, parsley, salt and pepper, toss, cover the bowl and leave aside for 30 minutes.

Heat up your grill over medium-high heat, add the chicken, cook for 6 minutes on each side, cool down, slice, and put in a bowl.

Put the stock in a pot, add the barley, salt, and pepper. Bring to a simmer over medium heat, cook for 45 minutes, then drain and put in the same bowl with the chicken.

Add the dried oregano, zest of 1 lemon, juice of 1 lemon, ¼ cup oil, the lettuce, onion, tomatoes, and the avocados, toss and serve.

Nutrition: Calories 342, Fat: 17.4g, Fiber: 16.5g, Carbs: 27.7g, Protein: 26.4g

100.   **Chicken Skillet**
Preparation Time: 10 minutes
Cooking Time: 35 minutes
Servings: 6
Ingredients:

- 6 chicken thighs, bone-in and skin-on
- Juice of 2 lemons
- 1 tsp. oregano, dried
- 1 red onion, chopped
- Salt and black pepper to the taste
- 1 tsp. garlic powder
- 2 garlic cloves, minced
- 2 tbsps. olive oil
- 2 ½ cups chicken stock
- 1 cup white rice
- 1 tbsp. oregano, chopped
- 1 cup green olives, pitted and sliced
- ⅓ cup parsley, chopped
- ½ cup feta cheese, crumbled

Directions:

Heat up a pan with the oil over medium heat, add the chicken thighs skin side down, cook for 4 minutes on each side and transfer to a plate.

Add the garlic and the onion to the pan, stir and sauté for 5 minutes.

Add the rice, salt, pepper, the stock, oregano, and lemon juice, stir, cook for 1-2 minutes more, and take off the heat.

Add the chicken to the pan, introduce the pan in the oven and bake at 375°F for 25 minutes.

Add the cheese, olives, and the parsley, divide the whole mix between plates and serve for lunch.

Nutrition: Calories 435, Fat: 18.5g, Fiber: 13.6g, Carbs: 27.8g, Protein: 25.6g

101. **Green Beans & Feta**

Preparation Time: 10 minutes

Cooking Time: 15 minutes

Servings: 8

Ingredients:

- 2 tbsp. Olive oil
- 1 lb. Freshly trimmed green beans
- 2 tbsp. Red onion
- 1 tbsp. Tarragon vinegar
- ½ tsp. Salt
- ¼ tsp. Pepper
- 1 clove Garlic
- ½ cup or 2 oz. Crumbled feta cheese
- Also Needed: 6-quart saucepan

Directions:

Add one inch of water into the pan and add the beans.

Finely chop the onion and garlic and add the rest of the fixings (omit the cheese) to simmer for eight to ten minutes with the lid off. Drain.

Scoop the beans into a Servings dish and add the cheese.

Toss and serve warm.

Nutrition: Calories 80, Fat: 5g, Protein: 2g

102. **Kale - Mediterranean-Style**

Preparation Time: 10 minutes

Cooking Time: 15 minutes

Servings: 6

Ingredients:

- 12 cups Chopped kale
- 1 tbsp./as needed Olive oil
- 1 tbsp. Minced garlic
- Salt and black pepper as preferred
- 1 tsp. Soy sauce
- 2 tbsp. Lemon juice

Directions:

Prepare a saucepan with a steamer insert. Pour in plenty of water to cover the bottom.

Put a lid on the pot and boil using the high-temperature setting.

Toss in the kale. Once it boils, time for 7-10 minutes. Drain.

Whisk the soy sauce, lemon juice, garlic, oil, black pepper, and salt. Toss in the steamed kale. Toss until coated and serve.

Nutrition: Calories 91, Fat: 3.2g, Protein: 4.6g

103.   Mediterranean Endive Boats

Preparation Time: 10 minutes

Cooking Time: 10 minutes

Servings: 8

Ingredients:

- ⅓ cup Chopped sun-dried tomatoes
- 0.66 cup Chickpeas
- 1 tbsp. Olive oil
- ¼ cup Crumbled feta
- 3 Chopped basil leaves
- 2 tbsp. Balsamic reduction

Directions:

Rinse and drain the chickpeas.

Combine the oil, with the drained chickpeas, and tomatoes.

Cut the base of the endive and pull the leaves apart. (It should make eight.)

Arrange the leaves on the Servings platter and add the chickpea mixture.

Garnish it with the crumbled feta and top it off with chopped basil and a spritz of balsamic reduction.

Nutrition: Calories 715, Fat: 30g, Protein: 32g

104.   Mediterranean Nachos

Preparation Time: 10 minutes

Cooking Time: 10 minutes

Servings: 6

Ingredients:

- 2 tbsp. Kalamata olives
- 2 tbsp. + 2 tsp. oil Sun-dried tomatoes in oil
- 1 medium Drained Roma- small plum tomato
- 1 tbsp. Green onion
- 4 oz./30 chips approx. Tortilla chips
- 4 oz. Feta cheese

Directions:

Prep the fixings. Thinly slice/chop the onion olives, and tomatoes. Mix the sun-dried tomatoes, olives, oil, onions, and plum tomato. Set them aside for now.

Place the tortillas (single-layered) on a microwavable platter. Crumble the feta over the chips.

Cook in the microwave for one minute on high.

Rotate the dish and continue cooking for another 30 to 60 seconds or until it's bubbly.

Spoon the tomato mixture over the chips and serve.

Nutrition: Calories 170, Fat: 11g, Protein: 4g

105.   Mediterranean Potatoes
Preparation Time: 15 minutes
Cooking Time: 45-50 minutes
Servings: 4
Ingredients:

- 4-5 Medium potatoes
- 1 tbsp. Olive oil
- 1 tbsp. Butter, melted
- 6 tsp Greek seasoning
- ⅛ tsp Garlic seasoning
- Also Needed: 9 x 13-inch casserole dish

Directions:
Set the oven temperature to 350°F.
Cube the potatoes and toss them into the dish with the rest of the fixings.
Bake them for 30-40 minutes. Turn occasionally.
Serve when the potatoes are browned to your liking.
Nutrition: Calories 207.8, Fat: 6.3g, Protein: 3.8g

106.   Melitzanes Imam/Greek Eggplant Dish
Preparation Time: 30 minutes
Cooking Time: 1 hour 15 minutes
Servings: 2
Ingredients:

- 1 Eggplant
- 14.5 oz. can Diced tomatoes, drained
- 1 tbsp. Tomato paste
- 1 Medium onion
- 1 tbsp./to taste Minced garlic
- 1 tsp. Ground cinnamon
- Pepper & salt as desired
- 3 tbsp. Olive oil

Directions:

Set the oven to reach 350°F.

Slice the eggplant - lengthwise - in half. Cut out the halves leaving about a one-inch shell. Set the flesh aside.

Arrange the shells on a baking pan. Lightly spritz the eggplant using oil and bake until softened (30 min.).

Chop the leftover eggplant into small pieces.

Prepare a skillet using the medium temperature setting with two tbsps. of oil.

Dice and add the onion, garlic, and chopped eggplant to sauté for a few minutes.

Dump the tomato paste and tomatoes and simmer using the low-heat temperature setting.

Transfer the shells to the countertop, and spoon in the tomato/eggplant mixture. Sprinkle using cinnamon and bake for another 30 minutes and serve.

Nutrition: Calories 314, Fat: 20.8g, Protein: 5.3g

107.   Red Mediterranean Potato Salad
Preparation Time: 15 minutes
Cooking Time: 25 minutes
Servings: 12
Ingredients:

- 1 ½ lb. Red potatoes, halved
- 3 slices Bacon
- ¾ cup Grape tomatoes - red/yellow
- ¼ cup Chopped onion
- ¼ cup Sliced olives
- ½ cup Fat-free Italian dressing
- 1 tbsp. Cider vinegar
- 1 tbsp. Italian parsley
- Also Needed: 3-quart saucepan

Directions:
Pour about one inch of water into the pan and let it boil.

Slice and toss in the potatoes. Place a lid on the pot and cook them using the medium temperature setting for 10-15 minutes until tender. Drain and slightly cool.

Slice the halved potatoes into ¾-inch cubes and toss them into a salad dish.

Prepare a microwave-safe platter with a layer of paper towels. Add in the bacon and cook on high for two to three minutes. Crumble them.

Stir the tomatoes, bacon, onion, and olives in with the potatoes.

Whisk the vinegar and dressing. Pour over the potatoes and gently toss.

Chop the parsley to sprinkle the salad and serve or chill.

Nutrition: Calories 60, Fat: 1.5g, Protein: 2g

108.   Savory Mediterranean Orzo

Preparation Time: 15 minutes
Cooking Time: 45 minutes
Servings: 12
Ingredients:

- 4 cups Chicken broth, reduced sodium
- 16 oz. pkg Orzo pasta
- 1 Medium onion
- 2 tbsp. Olive oil
- 4 cloves Garlic
- 8 oz./2 cups Crumbled feta cheese - divided
- 7 ½ oz. jar Roasted sweet red peppers
- 10 oz. pkg Frozen - chopped spinach
- 1 small Yellow summer squash, finely chopped
- ½ tsp. each Salt and black pepper
- Also Needed: 13 by 9-inch baking dish

Directions:
Grease the baking dish and set it to the side for now.

Pour water into a large saucepan and wait for it to boil. Stir in orzo; cook over medium heat until tender (six to eight minutes). Place the pan on the countertop off the burner.

Prepare a pan with oil. Dice and sauté the onion until tender. Mince and add the garlic, sautéing it for one minute longer.

Drain and chop the jarred peppers. Thaw and squeeze the spinach to remove the liquids. Stir one cup of cheese, squash, red peppers, spinach, salt, and pepper into the orzo mixture.

Dump the mixture into the baking dish, sprinkling it with the rest of the cheese. Bake it without the lid, at 350° F for 20 to 25 minutes until it's thoroughly heated.

Nutrition: Calories: 233, Fat: 6g, Protein: 10g

109.   **Spinach Pie**
Preparation Time: 20 minutes
Cooking Time: 60 minutes
Servings: 6
Ingredients:

- ½ cup Melted butter
- 10 oz. pkg. Frozen spinach
- ½ cup Fresh parsley
- ½ cup Green onions
- ½ cup Fresh dill
- ½ cup Crumbled feta cheese
- 4 oz. Cream cheese

- 4 oz. Cottage cheese
- 2 tbsp. grated Parmesan
- 2 Large eggs
- Pepper and salt as desired
- 40 sheets Phyllo dough

Directions:
Heat the oven setting at 350° F.
Mince/chop the onions, dill, and parsley. Thaw the spinach and sheets of dough. Dab the spinach dry by squeezing.
Combine the spinach, scallions, eggs, cheeses, parsley, dill, pepper, and salt in a blender until it's creamy.
Prepare the small phyllo triangles by filling them with one tsp of the spinach mixture.
Lightly brush the outside of the triangles with butter and arrange them with the seam-side facing downwards on an ungreased baking tray.
Place them in the heated oven to bake until golden brown and puffed (20-25 min.). Serve piping hot.
Nutrition: Calories 555, Fat: 21.3g, Protein: 18.7g
110.   Tasty Chicken and Cucumber Salad
Preparation Time: 20 minutes
Cooking Time: 20 minutes
Servings: 4
Ingredients:

- 2 (6-inch) pitas
- 2 cups thinly sliced fennel bulb
- 1 cup shredded skinless, boneless rotisserie chicken breast
- ½ cup chopped fresh flat-leaf parsley
- ¼ cup vertically sliced red onion
- ½ English cucumber, halved lengthwise and thinly sliced
- ½ teaspoon salt, divided
- ¼ teaspoon black pepper, divided
- ¼ cup fresh lemon juice
- 1 tablespoon white wine vinegar
- ½ teaspoon chopped fresh oregano
- 3 tablespoons extra-virgin olive oil

Directions:
Preheat oven to 350°F.
Arrange pitas on a baking sheet. Bake at 350°F for 12 minutes or until toasted and cool for 1 minute. Then, tear into bite-sized pieces.
Combine the pita pieces, fennel, chicken breast, parsley, red onion, and cucumber. Sprinkle with salt and pepper.

Combine juice, vinegar, and oregano. Gradually add oil while stirring with a whisk.

Drizzle dressing over pita mixture; toss to coat. Serve immediately.

Nutrition: Calories 257, Fat: 11.6g, Carbs: 23.3g, Fiber: 2.7g, Protein: 15.6g

III.　　　**Tomato Sauce and Mussels**

Preparation Time: 15 minutes

Cooking Time: 15 minutes

Servings: 4

Ingredients:

- 1 tablespoon extra-virgin olive oil
- 1 tablespoon unsalted butter
- 2 tablespoons shallot, finely chopped
- 1 oz. prosciutto, diced
- 2 teaspoons garlic, finely chopped
- ½ teaspoon red pepper, crushed
- 1 cup chopped boxed or canned San Marzano tomatoes (such as Pomi)
- ½ cup dry white wine
- 1 teaspoon granulated sugar
- ⅜ tsp kosher salt
- 2 pounds mussels, scrubbed and debearded
- 2 tbsps. Chopped fresh flat-leaf parsley
- Whole-wheat baguette slices, toasted

Directions:

Heat olive oil and butter in a large Dutch oven over medium-high until butter melts and starts to foam, about 1 minute.

Add shallot and prosciutto; cook, stirring occasionally, until shallot is translucent and prosciutto is crisp, about 5 minutes.

Add garlic and crushed red pepper; cook, stirring often, until fragrant, about 1 minute.

Add tomatoes, wine, sugar, and salt; bring to a simmer.

Add mussels to sauce. Cover and cook until mussels start to open, 4 to 5 minutes. (Discard any mussels that do not open.)

Stir in 1 tablespoon parsley.

Lightly toss, and spoon into 4 bowls.

Top with remaining parsley and, if desired, lemon wedges.

Serve with bread.

Nutrition: Calories 376, Fat: 10g, Carbs: 26g, Fiber: 2g. Sugars: 4g. Protein: 38g

II2.　　　**Sweet Bean Pasta**

Preparation Time: 20 minutes

Cooking Time: 20 minutes

Servings: 8
Ingredients:

- 1 package (12 ounces) uncooked whole wheat or brown rice penne pasta
- 2 tablespoons olive oil
- 4 cups sliced leeks (white portion only)
- 1 cup sliced sweet onion
- 4 garlic cloves, sliced
- 1 tablespoon minced fresh sage or 1 tsp. rubbed sage
- 1 large sweet potato, peeled and cut into ½-inch cubes
- 1 medium bunch Swiss chard (about 1 pound), cut into 1-inch slices
- 1 can (15 ½ ounces) great northern beans, rinsed and drained
- ¾ teaspoon salt
- ¼ teaspoon chili powder
- ¼ teaspoon crushed red pepper flakes
- ⅛ teaspoon ground nutmeg
- ⅛ teaspoon pepper
- ⅓ cup finely chopped fresh basil
- 2 cups marinara sauce, warmed

Directions:
Cook pasta according to package directions. Drain, ¾ cup pasta water.
In a 6-qt. stockpot, heat oil over medium heat; saute leeks and onion until tender for about 5-7 minutes.
Add garlic and sage; cook and stir 2 minutes.
Add potato and chard; cook, covered, over medium-low heat 5 minutes
Stir in beans, seasonings and reserved pasta water; cook, covered, until potato and chard are tender, about 5 minutes.
Add pasta, basil and vinegar; toss and heat through. Serve with sauce.
Nutrition: Calories 369, Fat: 6g, Carbs: 67g, Protein: 14g

113.   **Chickpeas Spanish Spinach**
Preparation time: 5 minutes
Cook time: 15 minutes
Servings: 4
Ingredients:

- Extra virgin olive oil
- 1 head of garlic (12 cloves)
- 3 tbsp. sweet paprika
- 6 cups spinach (250 g)
- ½ cup water (125 ml)
- 3 ½ cups cooked chickpeas (650 g)
- Sea salt (optional)

Directions:

Cook the garlic (diced) in a saucepan with a little bit of extra virgin olive oil over medium heat until golden brown.

Add the paprika, stir and add the spinach (finely chopped).

Add the water and salt to taste (optional) and cook for about 5 minutes. You can use oil instead of water to cook the spinach.

Add the cooked chickpeas, stir, add more oil if you want (you can add more paprika and salt too) and cook for 5 minutes more.

Nutrition: Calories 555, Fat: 21.3g, Protein: 18.7g

114.   **Sweet Cabbage Rolls**

Preparation Time: 1 hour + chilling

Cooking Time: 50 minutes

Servings: 12 rolls

Ingredients:

- 12 cabbage leaves
- 2 pounds ground beef
- ¾ tsp salt
- ¼ teaspoon pepper
- 2 cups cooked long grain rice
- 2 large eggs, lightly beaten

For the Sauce:

- ¼ cup butter, cubed
- 1 large onion, halved and thinly sliced
- 2 celery ribs, chopped
- 2 ½ cups water
- 2 cans (one 15 ounces, one 8 ounces) tomato sauce
- 2 tablespoons lemon juice
- 2 teaspoons sugar
- 2 teaspoons dried parsley flakes
- 1 teaspoon salt
- ¼ teaspoon pepper

Directions:

In batches, cook cabbage leaves in boiling water 3-5 minutes or until crisp-tender.

Drain; cool slightly. Trim the thick vein from the bottom of each cabbage leaf, making a V-shaped cut.

Meanwhile, in a large skillet, cook beef, salt and pepper over medium heat 8-10 minutes or until no longer pink, breaking into crumbles; drain.

Stir in rice and bananas (substitute for an egg).

In another skillet, heat butter over medium-high heat. Add onion and celery; cook and stir 6-8 minutes or until tender. Stir in water, tomato sauce, lemon juice, sugar, parsley, salt and pepper.

Bring to a boil. Reduce heat; simmer, uncovered, 15-20 minutes or until thickened.

Spoon about ½ cup meat mixture onto each cabbage leaf.

Pull together cut edges of leaf to overlap; fold over filling.

Fold in sides and roll up. Transfer to a greased 13 x 9-inches baking dish.

Pour sauce over rolls. Refrigerate, covered, overnight.

Remove from refrigerator 30 minutes before baking.

Preheat oven to 350°F. Bake, covered, 50-60 minutes or until heated through.

Freeze option: Cover and freeze unbaked cabbage rolls. To use, partially thaw in refrigerator overnight. Remove from refrigerator 30 minutes before baking.

Preheat oven to 350°F.

Bake casserole as directed, increasing time as necessary to heat through and for a thermometer inserted in center to read 165°F.

Nutrition: Calories 492, Fat: 28g, Carbs: 28g, Protein: 33g

115.   **Sweet Potato Ragout and Tenderloin**
Preparation Time: 1 hour
Cooking Time: 20 minutes
Servings: 6
Ingredients:

- 2 tbsps. olive oil
- 1 large onion, chopped
- 2 garlic cloves, minced
- 1 large navel orange
- ¼ cup packed brown sugar
- ⅛ teaspoon plus ½ teaspoon salt, divided
- 1 can (15 ¾ ounces) cut sweet potatoes in syrup, undrained
- 1 can (14 ½ ounces) diced tomatoes, undrained
- 2 medium tart apples, peeled and chopped
- 2 pork tenderloins (¾ pound each)
- ½ teaspoon pepper

Directions:
In a large skillet, heat oil over medium heat.

Add onion; cook and stir 4-5 minutes or until softened.

Reduce heat to medium-low; cook 20-25 minutes or until golden brown, stirring occasionally.

Add garlic; cook 1 minute longer.

Finely grate peel from orange. Cut orange crosswise in half; squeeze juice from orange.

Stir brown sugar, vinegar, salt, orange peel and orange juice into onion mixture.

Bring to a boil; cook 6-8 minutes or until liquid is almost evaporated.

Stir in sweet potatoes, tomatoes and apples.

Return to a boil. Reduce heat; simmer, uncovered, 20-25 minutes or until apples are tender and liquid is almost evaporated, stirring occasionally.

Sprinkle pork with pepper and remaining salt.

Grill, covered, over medium heat 18-22 minutes or until a thermometer reads 145°, turning occasionally.

Let stand 5 minutes before slicing. Serve with ragout.

Nutrition: Calories 344, Fat: 9g, Carbs: 42g, Protein: 25g

116.   Better Brussels Sprouts

Preparation Time: 20 minutes

Cooking Time: 20 minutes

Servings: 6

Ingredients:

- 3 tablespoons coconut oil
- 1 package (16 ounces) fresh halved Brussels sprouts
- ⅓ cup sliced onions
- ½ cup coarsely chopped cashews
- 1 teaspoon granulated garlic
- Salt and pepper to taste

Directions:

In a large heavy skillet or wok, heat coconut oil over medium heat.

Add Brussels sprouts; cook and stir 5 minutes.

Add onion slices; cook 3 minutes longer, stirring every 20-30 seconds.

Add cashews and garlic; cook 1-minute longer. Sprinkle with salt and pepper.

Nutrition: Calories 161, Fat: 13g, Carbs: 11g, Protein: 5g

117.   Carrot Honey Loaf

Preparation Time: 20 minutes

Cooking Time: 1 hour

Servings: 1 loaf (16 slices)

Ingredients:

- 2 large eggs, room temperature
- ¾ cup canola oil
- ¾ cup honey
- 2 teaspoons vanilla extract
- 1 cup all-purpose flour
- 1 cup whole wheat flour
- 2 teaspoons baking powder

- 2 teaspoons ground cinnamon
- 1 teaspoon ground nutmeg
- ½ teaspoon salt
- ¼ teaspoon baking soda
- 2 cups grated carrots (about 3 large carrots)

Directions:

Preheat oven to 350°F.

Combine eggs, oil, honey and vanilla; beat until smooth

oIn another bowl, whisk next 7 ingredients for 30 seconds. Stir flour mixture into egg mixture just until combined. Add carrots; mix well.

Pour batter into a lightly greased 9 x 5-in. loaf pan; bake until a toothpick inserted in center of loaf comes out clean, about 1 hour. Cool 10 minutes before removing to a wire rack.

Nutrition: Calories 212, Carbs: 26g, Protein: 3g

118.   **Mushroom and Sweet Potato Potpie**

Preparation Time: 15 minutes

Cooking Time: 1 hour.

Servings: 8

Ingredients:

- ⅓ cup olive oil, divided
- 1 pound sliced fresh shiitake mushrooms
- 1 pound sliced baby portobello mushrooms
- 2 large onions, chopped
- 2 garlic cloves, minced
- 1 teaspoon minced fresh rosemary, plus more for topping
- 1 bottle (12 ounces) porter or stout beer
- 1 ½ cups mushroom broth or vegetable broth, divided
- 2 bay leaves
- 1 tablespoon balsamic vinegar
- 2 tablespoons reduced-sodium soy sauce
- ¼ cup cornstarch
- 3 to 4 small sweet potatoes, peeled and thinly sliced
- ¾ teaspoon coarsely ground pepper
- ½ teaspoon salt

Directions:

Preheat oven to 400°F.

In a Dutch oven, heat oil over medium heat

Add shiitake mushrooms and cook in batches until dark golden brown, 8-10 minutes; remove with a slotted spoon.

Repeat with 1 tbsp. oil and the portobello mushrooms.

In same pan, heat 1 tablespoon oil over medium heat. Add onions; cook and stir 8-10 minutes or until tender. Add garlic and rosemary; cook 30 seconds longer. Stir in beer, broth, bay leaves, soy sauce, and sauteed mushrooms.

Bring to a boil. Reduce heat; simmer, uncovered, for 10 minutes.

In a small bowl, mix cornstarch and remaining broth until smooth; stir into mushroom mixture.

Return to a boil, stirring constantly; cook and stir until thickened for 1-2 minutes.

Remove and discard bay leaves; transfer mushroom mixture to 8 greased 8-oz. ramekins.

Layer sweet potatoes in a circular pattern on top of each ramekin; brush with remaining oil and sprinkle with pepper, salt and additional rosemary.

Bake, covered, until potatoes are tender, 20-25 minutes.

Remove cover and bake until potatoes are lightly browned, or for 8-10 minutes.

Let stand 5 minutes before serving.

Nutrition: Calories 211, Fat: 10g, Carbs: 26g, Protein: 5g

119. **Badger State Stuffing**

Preparation Time: 35 minutes

Cooking Time: 50 minutes + standing

Servings: 8 cups

Ingredients:

- ½ pound bacon strips, diced
- ½ pound sliced fresh mushrooms
- 1 medium onion, diced
- 1 cup chopped celery (about 3 stalks)
- 1 cup chopped carrot (about 4 medium carrots)
- 2 garlic cloves, minced
- 1 can (8 ounces) sauerkraut, rinsed and well drained
- ½ cup amber beer or chicken broth
- 5 cups cubed sourdough bread (½-inch cubes)
- 1 cup dried cherries or dried cranberries
- 1 large egg
- 1 ¼ cups chicken broth
- 3 tablespoons minced fresh parsley
- 1 teaspoon poultry seasoning
- ½ teaspoon pepper

Directions:

Preheat oven to 350°F.

In a large skillet, cook bacon over medium heat until crisp, stirring occasionally.

Remove with a slotted spoon; drain on paper towels.

Discard drippings, reserving 3 tablespoons in pan.

Add mushrooms, onion, celery and carrot to drippings; cook and stir over medium-high heat until tender, 8-10 minutes.

Add garlic; cook 1 minute longer. Stir in sauerkraut and beer.

Bring to a boil; cook, uncovered, until liquid is reduced by half.

In a large bowl, combine bread cubes, cherries, bacon and sauerkraut mixture.

In a small bowl, whisk egg, broth, parsley, poultry seasoning and pepper. Gradually stir into bread mixture.

Transfer to a greased 2-qt. baking dish.

Bake, covered, 20 minutes.

Uncover; bake until lightly browned, 30-35 minutes longer.

Let stand 10 minutes before serving.

Nutrition: Calories 271, Fat: 11g, Carbs: 35g, Protein: 9g

120.   Tomato and Halloumi Platter

Preparation Time: 5 minutes

Cooking Time: 4 minutes

Servings: 4

Ingredients:

- 1 lb. tomatoes, sliced
- ½ pound halloumi, cut into 4 slices
- 2 tbsps. parsley, chopped
- 1 tbsp. basil, chopped
- 2 tbsps. olive oil
- A pinch of salt and black pepper
- Juice of 1 lemon

Directions:

Brush the halloumi slices with half of the oil, put them on your preheated grill and cook over medium-high heat and cook for 2 minutes on each side.

Arrange the tomato slices on a platter, season with salt and pepper, drizzle the lemon juice and the rest of the oil all over, top with the halloumi slices, sprinkle the herbs on top and serve for lunch.

Nutrition: Calories 181, Fat: 7.3g, Fiber: 1.4g, Carbs: 4.6g, Protein: 1.1g

121.   Chickpeas and Millet Stew

Preparation Time: 10 minutes

Cooking Time: 1 hour and 5 minutes

Servings: 4

Ingredients:

- 1 cup millet
- 2 tbsps. olive oil
- A pinch of salt and black pepper

- 1 eggplant, cubed
- 1 yellow onion, chopped
- 14 oz. canned tomatoes, chopped
- 14 oz. canned chickpeas, drained and rinsed
- 3 garlic cloves, minced
- 2 tbsps. harissa paste
- 1 bunch cilantro, chopped
- 2 cups water

Directions:

Put the water in a pan, bring to a simmer over medium heat, add the millet, simmer for 25 minutes, take off the heat, fluff with a fork and leave aside for now.

Heat up a pan with half of the oil over medium heat, add the eggplant, salt, and pepper. Stir and cook for 10 minutes and transfer to a bowl.

Add the rest of the oil to the pan, heat up over medium heat again, add the onion and sauté for 10 minutes.

Add the garlic, more salt and pepper, the harissa paste, chickpeas, tomatoes and return the eggplant, stir and cook over low heat for 15 minutes more.

Add the millet, toss, divide the mix into bowls, sprinkle the cilantro on top and serve.

Nutrition: Calories 671, Fat: 15.6g, Fiber: 27.5g, Carbs: 87.5g, Protein: 27.1g

122.   **Tuna and Couscous**

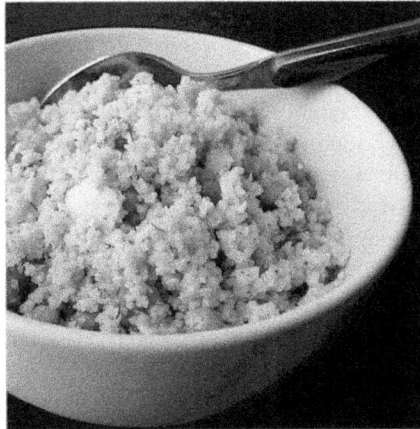

Preparation Time: 10 minutes
Cooking Time: 0 minutes
Servings: 4
Ingredients:

- 1 cup chicken stock
- 1 ¼ cups couscous
- A pinch of salt and black pepper
- 10 oz. canned tuna, drained and flaked
- 1 pint of cherry tomatoes, halved
- ½ cup pepperoncini, sliced
- ⅓ cup parsley, chopped
- 1 tbsp. olive oil
- ¼ cup capers, drained
- Juice of ½ lemon

Directions:
Put the stock in a pan, bring to a boil over medium-high heat, add the couscous, stir, take off the heat, cover, leave aside for 10 minutes, fluff with a fork and transfer to a bowl.

Add the tuna and the rest of the ingredients, toss, and serve for lunch right away.

Nutrition: Calories 253, Fat: 11.5g, Fiber: 3.4g, Carbs: 16.5g, Protein: 23.2g

123. **Chicken Stuffed Peppers**
Preparation Time: 10 minutes
Cooking Time: 0 minutes
Servings: 6
Ingredients:

- 1 cup Greek yogurt
- 2 tbsps. mustard
- Salt and black pepper to the taste
- 1 lb. rotisserie chicken meat, cubed
- 4 celery stalks, chopped
- 2 tbsps. balsamic vinegar
- 1 bunch scallions, sliced
- ¼ cup parsley, chopped
- 1 cucumber, sliced
- 3 red bell peppers, halved and deseeded
- 1 pint of cherry tomatoes, quartered

Directions:
In a bowl, mix the chicken with the celery and the rest of the ingredients except the bell peppers and toss well.

Stuff the peppers halves with the chicken mix and serve for lunch.

Nutrition: Calories 266, Fat: 12.2g, Fiber: 4.5g, Carbs: 15.7g, Protein: 3.7g

124. **Turkey Fritters and Sauce**
Preparation Time: 10 minutes
Cooking Time: 30 minutes

Servings: 4
Ingredients:

- 2 garlic cloves, minced
- 1 egg
- 1 red onion, chopped
- 1 tbsp. olive oil
- ¼ tsp red pepper flakes
- 1 lb. turkey meat, ground
- ½ tsp oregano, dried
- Cooking spray

For the sauce:

- 1 cup Greek yogurt
- 1 cucumber, chopped
- 1 tbsp. olive oil
- ¼ tsp garlic powder
- 2 tbsps. lemon juice
- ¼ cup parsley, chopped

Directions:
Heat up a pan with 1 tbsp. oil over medium heat, add the onion and the garlic, sauté for 5 minutes, cool down and transfer to a bowl.
Add the meat, turkey, oregano and pepper flakes, stir and shape medium fritters out of this mix.
Heat up another pan greased with cooking spray over medium-high heat, add the turkey fritters and brown for 5 minutes on each side.
Introduce the pan in the oven and bake the fritters at 375 ° F for 15 minutes more.
Meanwhile, in a bowl, mix the yogurt with the cucumber, oil, garlic powder, lemon juice and parsley and whisk well.
Divide the fritters between plates, spread the sauce all over and serve for lunch.
Nutrition: Calories 364, Fat: 16.8g, Fiber: 5.5g, Carbs: 26.8g, Protein: 23.4g
125.   Stuffed Eggplants
Preparation Time: 10 minutes
Cooking Time: 35 minutes
Servings: 4
Ingredients:

- 2 eggplants, halved lengthwise and ⅔ of the flesh scooped out
- 3 tbsps. olive oil
- 1 red onion, chopped

- 2 garlic cloves, minced
- 1 pint of white mushrooms, sliced
- 2 cups kale, torn
- 2 cups quinoa, cooked
- 1 tbsp. thyme, chopped
- Zest and juice of 1 lemon
- Salt and black pepper to the taste
- ½ cup Greek yogurt
- 3 tbsps. parsley, chopped

Directions:

Rub the inside of each eggplant half with half of the oil and arrange them on a baking sheet lined with parchment paper.

Heat up a pan with the rest of the oil over medium heat, add the onion and the garlic and sauté for 5 minutes.

Add the mushrooms and cook for 5 minutes more.

Add the kale, salt, pepper, thyme, lemon zest and juice, stir, cook for 5 minutes more and take off the heat.

Stuff the eggplant halves with the mushroom mix, introduce them in the oven and bake 400 ° F for 20 minutes.

Divide the eggplants between plates, sprinkle the parsley and the yogurt on top and serve for lunch.

Nutrition: Calories 512, Fat: 16.4g, Fiber: 17.5g, Carbs: 78g, Protein: 17.2g

126.   Salmon Bowls
Preparation Time: 10 minutes
Cooking Time: 40 minutes
Servings: 4
Ingredients:

- 2 cups farro
- Juice of 2 lemons
- ⅓ cup olive oil + 2 tbsps.
- Salt and black pepper
- 1 cucumber, chopped
- ¼ cup balsamic vinegar
- 1 garlic clove, minced
- ¼ cup parsley, chopped
- ¼ cup mint, chopped
- 2 tbsps. mustard
- 4 salmon fillets, boneless

Directions:

Put water in a large pot, bring to a boil over medium-high heat, add salt and the farro, stir, simmer for 30 minutes, drain, transfer to a bowl, add the lemon juice, mustard, garlic, salt, pepper and ⅓ cup oil, toss and leave aside for now.

In another bowl, mash the cucumber with a fork, add the vinegar, salt, pepper, the parsley, dill and mint, and whisk well.

Heat up a pan with the rest of the oil over medium heat, add the salmon fillets skin side down, cook for 5 minutes on each side, cool them down and break into pieces.

Add over the farro, add the cucumber dressing, toss, and serve for lunch.

Nutrition: Calories 281, Fat: 12.7g, Fiber: 1.7g, Carbs: 5.8g, Protein: 36.5g

127.   Spicy Potato Salad
Preparation Time: 10 minutes
Cooking Time: 15 minutes
Servings: 4
Ingredients:

- 1 and ½ pounds baby potatoes, peeled and halved
- A pinch of salt and black pepper
- 2 tbsps. harissa paste
- 6 oz. Greek yogurt
- Juice of 1 lemon
- ¼ cup red onion, chopped
- ¼ cup parsley, chopped

Directions:
Put the potatoes in a pot, add water to cover, add salt, bring to a boil over medium-high heat, cook for 12 minutes, drain, and transfer them to a bowl.

Add the harissa and the rest of the ingredients, toss, and serve for lunch.

Nutrition: Calories 354, Fat: 19.2g, Fiber: 4.5g, Carbs: 24.7g, Protein: 11.2g

128.   Chicken and Rice Soup
Preparation Time: 10 minutes
Cooking Time: 35 minutes
Servings: 4
Ingredients:

- 6 cups chicken stock
- 1 and ½ cups chicken meat, cooked and shredded
- 1 bay leaf
- 1 yellow onion, chopped
- 2 tbsps. olive oil
- ⅓ cup white rice
- 1 egg, whisked
- Juice of ½ lemon
- 1 cup asparagus, trimmed and halved
- 1 cup carrots, chopped

- ½ cup dill, chopped
- Salt and black pepper to the taste

Directions:
Heat up a pot with the oil over medium heat, add the onions and sauté for 5 minutes.

Add the stock, dill, the rice, and the bay leaf, and stir. Bring to a boil over medium heat and cook for 10 minutes.

Add the rest of the ingredients except the egg and the lemon juice, stir and cook for 15 minutes more.

Add the egg whisked with the lemon juice gradually. Whisk the soup and cook for 2 minutes more. Divide into bowls and serve.

Nutrition: Calories 263, Fat: 18.5g, Fiber: 4.5g, Carbs: 19.8g, Protein: 14.5g

129.   **Fish Soup**
Preparation Time: 10 minutes
Cooking Time: 20 minutes
Servings: 4
Ingredients:

- 2 tbsps. olive oil
- 1 tbsp. garlic, minced
- ½ cup tomatoes, crushed
- 1 yellow onion, chopped
- 1 quart of veggie stock
- 1 lb. cod, skinless, boneless and cubed
- ¼ tsp rosemary, dried
- A pinch of salt and black pepper

Directions:
Heat up a pot with the oil over medium heat, add the onion and the garlic and sauté for 5 minutes.

Add the rest of the ingredients, toss, simmer over medium heat for 15 minutes more, divide into bowls and serve for lunch.

Nutrition: Calories 198, Fat: 8.1g, Fiber: 1g, Carbs: 4.2g, Protein: 26.4g

130.   **Lamb and Potatoes Stew**
Preparation Time: 10 minutes
Cooking Time: 1 hour and 20 minutes
Servings: 4
Ingredients:

- 2 pounds lamb shoulder, boneless and cubed
- Salt and black pepper to the taste
- 1 yellow onion, chopped
- 3 tbsps. olive oil

- 3 tomatoes, grated
- 2 cups chicken stock
- 2 and ½ pounds gold potatoes, cubed
- ¾ cup green olives, pitted and sliced
- 1 tbsp. cilantro, chopped

Directions:

Heat up a pot with the oil over medium-high heat, add the lamb, and brown for 5 minutes on each side.

Add the onion and sauté for 5 minutes more.

Add the rest of the ingredients, bring to a simmer, and cook over medium heat and cook for 1 hour and 10 minutes.

Divide the stew into bowls and serve.

Nutrition: Calories 411, Fat: 17.4g, Fiber: 8.4g, Carbs: 25.5g, Protein: 34.3g

131.   **Ground Pork and Tomatoes Soup**

Preparation Time: 10 minutes

Cooking Time: 40 minutes

Servings: 4

Ingredients:

- 1 lb. pork meat, ground
- Salt and black pepper to the taste
- 2 garlic cloves, minced
- 2 tsps. thyme, dried
- 2 tbsps. olive oil
- 4 cups beef stock
- A pinch of saffron powder
- 15 oz. canned tomatoes, crushed
- 1 tbsp. parsley, chopped

Directions:

Heat up a pot with the oil over medium heat, add the meat and the garlic and brown for 5 minutes.

Add the rest of the ingredients except the parsley, bring to a simmer and cook for 25 minutes.

Divide the soup into bowls, sprinkle the parsley on top and serve.

Nutrition: Calories 372, Fat: 17.3g, Fiber: 5.5g, Carbs: 28.4g, Protein: 17.4g

DINNER RECIPES

132.   **Fig and Prosciutto Pita Bread Pizza**

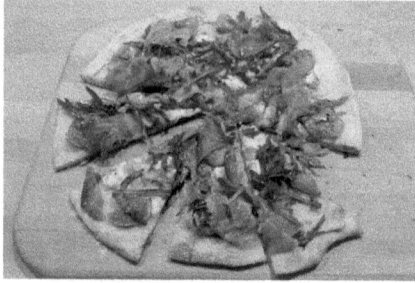

Preparation Time: 5 minutes
Cooking Time: 20 minutes
Servings: 6
Ingredients:

- 4 pita breads
- 8 figs, quartered
- 8 slices prosciutto
- 8 oz. mozzarella, crumbled

Directions:
Place the pita breads on a baking tray.
Top with crumbled cheese then figs and prosciutto.
Bake in the preheated oven at 350F for 8 minutes.
Serve the pizza right away.
Nutrition: Calories 445, Fat: 13.7g, Carbs: 41.5g, Protein: 39.0g
133.   **Spaghetti in Clam Sauce**

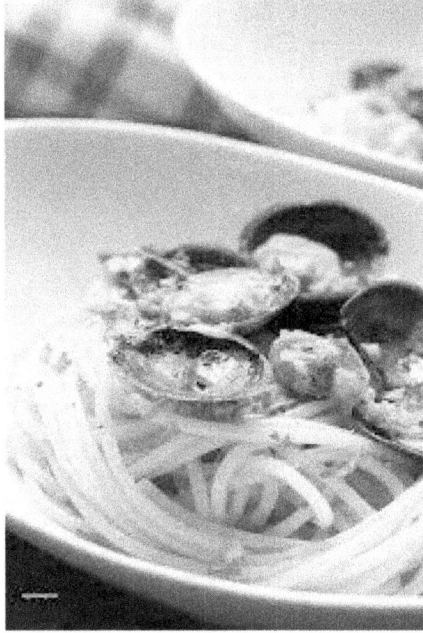

Preparation Time: 5 minutes
Cooking Time: 45 minutes
Servings: 4
Ingredients:

- 8 oz. spaghetti
- 2 tbsps. olive oil
- 2 garlic cloves, minced
- 2 tomatoes, peeled and diced
- 1 cup cherry tomatoes, halved
- 1-pound fresh clams, cleaned and rinsed
- 2 tbsps. white wine
- 1 tsp. sherry vinegar

Directions:

Heat the oil in a heavy saucepan and add the garlic. Cook for 30 seconds until fragrant then add the tomatoes, wine, and vinegar. Bring to a boil and cook for 5 minutes then stir in the clams and continue cooking for 10 more minutes.

In the meantime, bring a large pot of water to a boil with a pinch of salt and add the spaghetti. Cook them for 8 minutes just until al dente. Drain well and mix with the clam sauce.

Serve the dish right away.

Nutrition: Calories 305, Fat: 8.8g, Carbs: 48.3g, Protein: 8.1g

134.   **Creamy Fish Gratin**

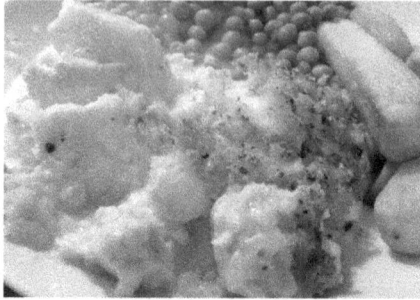

Preparation Time: 5 minutes
Cooking Time: 1 hour
Servings: 6
Ingredients:

- 1 cup heavy cream
- 2 salmon fillets, cubed
- 2 cod fillets, cubed
- 2 sea bass fillets, cubed
- 1 celery stalk, sliced
- Salt and pepper to taste
- ½ cup grated Parmesan
- ½ cup feta cheese, crumbled

Directions:

Combine the cream with the fish fillets and celery in a deep-dish baking pan.

Add salt and pepper to taste then top with the Parmesan and feta cheese.

Cook in the preheated oven at 350F for 20 minutes.

Serve the gratin right away.

Nutrition: Calories:301, Fat:16.1g, Carbs:1.3g, Protein:36.9g

135.   **Broccoli Pesto Spaghetti**

Preparation Time: 5 minutes
Cooking Time: 35 minutes
Servings: 4
Ingredients:

- 8 oz. spaghetti
- 1-pound broccoli, cut into florets
- 2 tbsps. olive oil

- 4 garlic cloves, chopped
- 4 basil leaves
- 2 tbsps. blanched almonds
- 1 lemon, juiced
- Salt and pepper to taste

Directions:

For the pesto, combine the broccoli, oil, garlic, basil, lemon juice and almonds in a blender and pulse until well mixed and smooth.

Cook the spaghetti in a large pot of salty water for 8 minutes or until al dente. Drain well.

Mix the warm spaghetti with the broccoli pesto and serve right away.

Nutrition: Calories 284, Fat: 10.2g, Carbs: 40.2g, Protein: 10.4g

136.   **Spaghetti all'Olio**

Preparation Time: 5 minutes

Cooking Time: 30 minutes

Servings: 4

Ingredients:

- 8 oz. spaghetti
- 3 tbsps. olive oil
- 4 garlic cloves, minced
- 2 red peppers, sliced
- 1 tbsp. lemon juice
- Salt and pepper to taste
- ½ cup grated parmesan cheese

Directions:

Heat the oil in a skillet and add the garlic. Cook for 30 seconds then stir in the red peppers and cook for 1 more minute on low heat, making sure to only infuse them, not to burn or fry them.

Add the lemon juice and remove off heat.

Cook the spaghetti in a large pot of salty water for 8 minutes or as stated on the package, just until they become al dente.

Drain the spaghetti well and mix them with the garlic and pepper oil.

Serve right away.

Nutrition: Calories 268, Fat: 11.9g, Carbs: 34.1g, Protein: 7.1g,

137.   **Quick Tomato Spaghetti**

Preparation Time: 5 minutes

Cooking Time: 15 minutes

Servings: 4

Ingredients:

- 8 oz. spaghetti

- 3 tbsps. olive oil
- 4 garlic cloves, sliced
- 1 jalapeno, sliced
- 2 cups cherry tomatoes
- Salt and pepper to taste
- 1 tsp. balsamic vinegar
- ½ cup grated Parmesan

Directions:
Heat a large pot of water on medium flame. Add a pinch of salt and bring to a boil then add the pasta.

Cook for 8 minutes or until al dente.

While the pasta cooks, heat the oil in a skillet and add the garlic and jalapeno. Cook for 1 minute then stir in the tomatoes, as well as salt and pepper.

Cook for 5-7 minutes until the tomatoes' skins burst.

Add the vinegar and remove off heat.

Drain the pasta well and mix it with the tomato sauce. Sprinkle with cheese and serve right away.

Nutrition: Calories 298, Fat: 13.5g, Carbs: 36.0g, Protein: 9.7g

138.   Creamy Chicken Soup
Preparation Time: 10 minutes
Cooking Time: 1 hour
Servings: 8
Ingredients:

- 2 cups eggplant, cubed
- Salt and black pepper to the taste
- ¼ cup olive oil
- 1 yellow onion, chopped
- 2 tbsps. garlic, minced
- 1 red bell pepper, chopped
- 2 tbsps. hot paprika
- ¼ cup parsley, chopped
- 1 and ½ tbsps. oregano, chopped
- 4 cups chicken stock
- 1 lb. chicken breast, skinless, boneless and cubed
- 1 cup half and half
- 2 egg yolks
- ¼ cup lime juice

Directions:
Heat up a pot with the oil over medium heat, add the chicken, garlic and onion, and brown for 10 minutes.

Add the bell pepper and the rest of the ingredients except the half and half, egg, yolks, and the lime juice, bring to a simmer and cook over medium heat for 40 minutes.

In a bowl, combine the egg yolks with the remaining ingredients with 1 cup of soup, whisk well and pour into the pot.

Whisk the soup, cook for 5 minutes more, divide into bowls and serve.

Nutrition: Calories 312, Fat: 17.4g, Fiber: 5.6g, Carbs: 20.2g, Protein: 15.3g

139.   Chili Oregano Baked Cheese

Preparation Time: 5 minutes

Cooking Time: 35 minutes

Servings: 4

Ingredients:

- 8 oz. feta cheese
- 4 oz. mozzarella, crumbled
- 1 chili pepper, sliced
- 1 tsp. dried oregano
- 2 tbsps. olive oil

Directions:

Place the feta cheese in a small deep-dish baking pan.

Top with the mozzarella then season with pepper slices and oregano.

Cover the pan with aluminum foil and cook in the preheated oven at 350F for 20 minutes.

Serve the cheese right away.

Nutrition: Calories 292, Fat: 24.2g, Carbs:3.7g, Protein: 16.2g

140.   Barley and Chicken Soup

Preparation Time: 10 minutes

Cooking Time: 50 minutes

Servings: 6

Ingredients:

- 1 lb. chicken breasts, skinless, boneless and cubed
- 1 tbsp. olive oil
- Salt and black pepper to the taste
- 2 celery stalks, chopped
- 2 carrots, chopped
- 1 red onion, chopped
- 6 cups chicken stock
- ½ cup parsley, chopped
- ½ cup barley
- 1 tsp. lime juice

Directions:

Heat up a pot with the oil over medium high heat, add the chicken, season with salt and pepper, and brown for cook for 8 minutes.

Add the onion, carrots, and the celery, stir and cook for 3 minutes more. Add the rest of the ingredients except the parsley, bring to a boil and simmer over medium heat for 40 minutes.

Add the parsley, stir, divide the soup into bowls and serve.

Nutrition: Calories 311, Fat: 8.4g, Fiber: 8.3g, Carbs: 17.4g, Protein: 22.3g

141.   **Crispy Italian Chicken**
Preparation Time: 5 minutes
Cooking Time: 40 minutes
Servings: 4
Ingredients:

- 4 chicken legs
- 1 tsp. dried basil
- 1 tsp. dried oregano
- Salt and pepper to taste
- 3 tbsps. olive oil
- 1 tbsp. balsamic vinegar

Directions:

Season the chicken with salt, pepper, basil, and oregano.

Heat the oil in a skillet and add the chicken in the hot oil. Cook on each side for 5 minutes until golden then cover the skillet with a weight – another skillet or a very heavy lid is recommended.

Place over medium heat and cook for 10 minutes on one side then flip the chicken repeatedly, cooking for another 10 minutes until crispy.

Serve the chicken right away.

Nutrition: Calories 262, Fat:13.9g, Carbs:0.3g, Protein:32.6g

142.   **Sea Bass in a Pocket**
Preparation Time: 5 minutes
Cooking Time: 40 minutes
Servings: 4
Ingredients:

- 4 sea bass fillets
- 4 garlic cloves, sliced
- 1 celery stalk, sliced
- 1 zucchini, sliced
- 1 cup cherry tomatoes, halved
- 1 shallot, sliced
- 1 tsp. dried oregano
- Salt and pepper to taste

Directions:

Mix the garlic, celery, zucchini, tomatoes, shallot, and oregano in a bowl. Add salt and pepper to taste.

Take 4 sheets of baking paper and arrange them on your working surface. Spoon the vegetable mixture in the center of each sheet. Top with a fish fillet then wrap the paper well so it resembles a pocket.

Place the wrapped fish in a baking tray and cook in the preheated oven at 350F for 15 minutes. Serve the fish warm and fresh.

Nutrition: Calories 149, Fat: 2.8g, Carbs:5.2g, Protein: 25.2g

143.   Chicken and Chorizo Casserole

Preparation Time: 5 minutes

Cooking Time: 1 hour

Servings: 6

Ingredients:

- 6 chicken thighs
- 4 chorizo links, sliced
- 2 tbsps. olive oil
- 1 cup tomato juice
- 2 tbsps. tomato paste
- 1 bay leaf
- 1 tsp. dried thyme
- Salt and pepper to taste

Directions:

Heat the oil in a skillet and add the chicken. Cook on all sides until golden then transfer the chicken in a deep-dish baking pan. Add the rest of the ingredients and season with salt and pepper.

Cook in the preheated oven at 350°F for 25 minutes. Serve the casserole right away.

Nutrition: Calories 424, Fat: 27.5g, Carbs: 3.6g, Protein: 39.1g

144.   Lamb Stuffed Tomatoes with Herbs

Preparation Time: 5 minutes

Cooking Time: 1 hour

Servings: 6

Ingredients:

- 6 large tomatoes
- 1-pound ground lamb
- ¼ cup white rice
- 2 shallots, chopped
- 2 garlic cloves, minced
- 1 tbsp. chopped dill
- 1 tbsp. chopped parsley

- 1 tbsp. chopped cilantro
- 1 tsp. dried mint
- Salt and pepper to taste
- 1 tbsp. lemon juice
- 2 tbsps. olive oil
- 1 cup vegetable stock

Directions:
Mix the lamb, rice, shallots, garlic, dill, parsley, cilantro, and mint in a bowl. Add salt and pepper to taste.

Remove the top of each tomato then carefully remove the flesh, leaving the skins intact.

Chop the flesh finely and place it in a deep heavy saucepan. Add the lemon juice, as well as salt and pepper to taste.

Stuff the tomatoes with the lamb mixture and place them all in the pan.

Drizzle with oil then pour in the stock.

Cover with a lid and cook on low heat for 35 minutes.

Serve the tomatoes right away.

Nutrition: Calories 248, Fat: 10.7g, Carbs: 14.6g, Protein: 23.7g

145. **Creamy Spinach with Polenta and Poached Egg**
Preparation Time: 5 minutes
Cooking Time: 40 minutes
Servings: 4
Ingredients:

- Creamy spinach:
- 2 tbsps. olive oil
- 2 garlic cloves, minced
- 1 red pepper, chopped
- 4 cups baby spinach
- ½ cup heavy cream
- 1 tbsp. all-purpose flour
- Salt and pepper to taste

For the Polenta:

- ½ cup polenta flour
- 1 ½ cups water
- 1 tbsp. olive oil
- Salt and pepper to taste
- Poached eggs:
- 3 cups water
- 1 tbsp. white wine vinegar
- 4 eggs

Directions:

For the creamy spinach, heat the oil in a skillet and add the garlic and red pepper. Cook on high heat for 1 minute then add the spinach and continue cooking for 5-7 minutes until the spinach is softened and most of the liquid has evaporated.

Mix the cream with the flour and pour it over the spinach.

Cook for 5 more minutes until thickened and creamy.

Adjust the taste with salt and pepper and remove off heat.

For the polenta, heat the water with salt in a saucepan.

When it starts to boil, stir in the oil and polenta flour.

Cook on low heat for 10 minutes.

For the poached eggs, bring the water, vinegar, and a pinch of salt to a boil in a saucepan. Crack open the eggs and drop them in the boiling liquid, one by one, cooking them for 1-2 minutes just until set, but still soft in the center.

To serve, spoon the polenta on Servings plates. Top with creamy spinach and finish with a poached egg.

Nutrition: Calories 231, Fat: 20.7g, Carbs: 5.7g, Protein: 7.3g

146.   Grilled Vegetable Feta Tart

Preparation Time: 5 minutes

Cooking Time: 1 ½ hours

Servings: 8

Ingredients:

For the Crust:

- 2 cups all-purpose flour
- 1 tsp. instant yeast
- ½ tsp salt
- 1 cup water
- 2 tbsps. olive oil

For the Topping:

- 1 zucchini, sliced
- 2 tomatoes, sliced
- 1 shallot, sliced
- 1 tsp. dried basil
- 1 tsp. dried oregano
- 2 garlic cloves, minced
- 2 tbsps. tomato paste
- 4 oz. feta cheese, crumbled

Directions:

For the crust, combine all the ingredients in a bowl and mix well. Knead for a few minutes until elastic.

Allow the dough to rest and rise for 20 minutes then roll it into a thin round of dough.

Place the dough on a baking tray.

Mix the garlic, basil, oregano, and tomato paste in a bowl. Spread the mixture over the dough.

Heat a grill pan over medium flame and place the zucchini and tomatoes on the grill. Cook for a few minutes on all sides until browned.

Top the tart with the vegetables and shallot then sprinkle the cheese on top.

Bake in the preheated oven at 350°F for 25 minutes.

Serve the tart warm and fresh.

Nutrition: Calories 198, Fat: 7.0g, Carbs: 28.0g, Protein: 6.3g

147.   Yogurt Baked Eggplants

Preparation Time: 5 minutes

Cooking Time: 45 minutes

Servings: 4

Ingredients:

- 2 eggplants
- 4 garlic cloves, minced
- 1 tsp. dried basil
- 2 tbsps. lemon juice
- Salt and pepper to taste
- 1 cup Greek yogurt
- 2 tbsps. chopped parsley

Directions:

Cut the eggplants in half and score the halves with a sharp knife.

Season the eggplants with salt and pepper, as well as the basil then drizzle with lemon juice and place the eggplant halves on a baking tray.

Spread the garlic over the eggplants and bake in the preheated oven at 350F for 20 minutes.

When done, place the eggplants on Servings plates and top with yogurt and parsley.

Serve the eggplants right away.

Nutrition: Calories 113, Fat: 1.6g, Carbs: 19.4g, Protein: 8.1g

148.   Asparagus Baked Plaice

Preparation Time: 5 minutes

Cooking Time: 45 minutes

Servings: 4

Ingredients:

- 4 plaice fillets
- 2 cups cherry tomatoes

- 1 bunch asparagus, trimmed and halved
- ½ lemon, juiced
- 2 tbsps. olive oil
- Salt and pepper to taste

Directions:

Combine the tomatoes, asparagus, lemon juice and oil in a deep-dish baking pan. Season with salt and pepper.

Place the fillets on top and cook in the preheated oven at 350F for 15 minutes.

Serve the plaice and the veggies warm and fresh.

Nutrition: Calories 113, Fat: 1.6g, Carbs: 19.4g, Protein: 8.1g

149. **Vegetable Turkey Casserole**

Preparation Time: 5 minutes

Cooking Time: 1 ½ hours

Servings: 8

Ingredients:

- 3 tbsps. olive oil
- 2 pounds turkey breasts, cubed
- 1 sweet onion, chopped
- 3 carrots, sliced
- 2 celery stalks, sliced
- 2 garlic cloves, chopped
- ½ tsp cumin powder
- ½ tsp dried thyme
- 2 cans diced tomatoes
- 1 cup chicken stock
- 1 bay leaf
- Salt and pepper to taste

Directions:

Heat the oil in a deep heavy pot and stir in the turkey.

Cook for 5 minutes until golden on all sides then add the onion, carrot, celery, and garlic. Cook for 5 more minutes then add the rest of the ingredients.

Season with salt and pepper and cook in the preheated oven at 350°F for 40 minutes.

Serve the casserole warm and fresh.

Nutrition: Calories 186, Fat: 7.3g, Protein: 20.1g, Carbs: 9.9g

150. **Mushroom Pilaf**

Preparation Time: 5 minutes

Cooking Time: 50 minutes

Servings: 4

Ingredients:

- 2 tbsps. olive oil
- 1 shallot, chopped
- 2 garlic cloves, minced
- 1 lb. button mushrooms
- 1 cup brown rice
- 2 cups chicken stock
- 1 bay leaf
- 1 thyme sprig
- Salt and pepper to taste

Directions:

Heat the oil in a skillet and stir in the shallot and garlic. Cook for 2 minutes until softened and fragrant.

Add the mushrooms and rice and cook for 5 minutes. Add the stock, bay leaf and thyme, as well as salt and pepper and continue cooking for 20 more minutes on low heat.

Serve the pilaf warm and fresh.

Nutrition: Calories 265, Fat: 8.9g, Carbs: 41.2g, Protein: 7.6g

151.   **Summer Fish Stew**

Preparation Time: 5 minutes

Cooking Time: 1 hour

Servings: 6

Ingredients:

- 3 tbsps. olive oil
- 4 garlic cloves, minced
- 1 red onion, chopped
- 1 celery stalk, sliced
- 2 red bell peppers, cored and diced
- 2 tbsps. tomato paste
- 2 cups cherry tomatoes
- 1 cup vegetable stock
- Salt and pepper to taste
- 4 cod fillets, cubed
- 4 sea bass fillets, cubed
- 2 tbsps. all-purpose flour

Directions:

Season the fish with salt and pepper then sprinkle it with flour.

Heat the oil in a skillet then place the fish and cook it on all sides until golden brown. It just must be golden brown, not cooked through just yet.

Remove the fish on a platter. Add the garlic, onion, and celery in the same skillet as the fish was in and cook for 2 minutes until fragrant.

Stir in the remaining ingredients and season with salt and pepper.

Cook for 10 minutes on low heat then add the fish and cook for another 10 minutes.

Serve the stew warm and fresh.

Nutrition: Calories 318, Fat: 10.1g, Carbs: 10.3g, Protein: 45.1g

152.   **Chorizo White Bean Stew**

Preparation Time: 5 minutes

Cooking Time: 1 hour

Servings: 8

Ingredients:

- 3 tbsps. olive oil
- 4 chorizo links, sliced
- 2 sweet onions, chopped
- 4 garlic cloves, minced
- 2 celery stalks, sliced
- 2 carrots, sliced
- 2 red bell peppers, cored and diced
- 2 tbsps. tomato paste
- 1 can diced tomatoes
- 2 cans white beans, drained
- 1 bay leaf
- 1 tsp. sherry vinegar
- ½ tsp dried oregano
- 1 cup chicken stock
- Salt and pepper to taste

Directions:

Heat the oil in a deep saucepan and stir in the chorizo. Cook for 5 minutes then add the onions and garlic, as well as celery and carrots.

Cook for another 10 minutes to soften.

Add the rest of the ingredients then season with salt and pepper to taste.

Cook on low heat for 35-40 minutes.

Serve the stew right away or freeze it into individual portions for later Servings.

Nutrition: Calories 386, Fat: 17.4g, Carbs: 38.8g, Protein: 20.2g

153.   **Roasted Eggplant Red Pepper Penne**

Preparation Time: 5 minutes

Cooking Time: 40 minutes

Servings: 4

Ingredients:

- 8 oz. penne
- 2 eggplants
- 4 roasted red bell peppers, sliced
- ½ tsp dried oregano
- 2 tbsps. olive oil
- Salt and pepper to taste

Directions:

Heat a large pot of water on medium flame. Add a pinch of salt and bring it to a boil.

Add the penne and cook them until al dente, not more than 8 minutes.

Cut the eggplants in half, season them with salt and pepper and place them in a baking tray.

Cook in the preheated oven at 400°F for 15 minutes.

When done, scoop out the flesh and chop it into fine bits. Mix with the sliced bell peppers, oregano and oil then adjust the taste with salt and pepper.

Stir in the cooked penne and serve the pasta right away.

Nutrition: Calories 292, Fat: 8.8g, Carbs: 47.3g, Protein: 9.1g

154.   Italian Chicken Butternut Pot

Preparation Time: 5 minutes

Cooking Time: 1 hour

Servings: 8

Ingredients:

- 4 chicken breasts, cubed
- 1 tbsp. all-purpose flour
- 3 tbsps. olive oil
- 4 cups butternut squash cubes
- 1 thyme sprig
- 1 rosemary sprig
- 2 garlic cloves, minced
- 1 tsp. dried oregano
- 1 tbsp. balsamic vinegar
- 1 cup vegetable stock
- Salt and pepper to taste

Directions:

Season the chicken with salt and pepper then sprinkle it with flour.

Heat the oil in a pot that can go in the oven then add the chicken.

Cook on all sides for 10 minutes then add the rest of the ingredients.

Season with salt and pepper and cover with a lid.

Cook in the preheated oven at 350F for 35 minutes.

Serve the dish warm and fresh.

Nutrition: Calories 178, Fat: 9.1g, Carbs: 9.4g, Protein: 15.4g

155.   **Sticky Skillet Chicken**
Preparation Time: 5 minutes
Cooking Time: 1 hour
Servings: 4
Ingredients:

- 4 chicken legs
- Salt and pepper to taste
- 3 tbsps. olive oil
- 2 garlic cloves, chopped
- 2 tbsps. honey
- 2 tbsps. lemon juice
- 1 thyme sprig
- 1 rosemary sprig

Directions:
Season the chicken with salt and pepper.
Heat the oil in a skillet and place the chicken in the hot oil.
Fry on each side for 10-15 minutes until golden brown.
Drizzle in the honey and lemon juice then place the herb sprigs on top.
Cover with a lid or aluminum foil and place in the preheated oven at 350F for 20 minutes.
Serve the chicken and the sauce right away.
Nutrition: Calories 316, Fat: 18.0g, Carbs: 9.3g, Protein: 29.1g

156.   **Chicken, Carrots and Lentils Soup**
Preparation Time: 10 minutes
Cooking Time: 1 hour and 10 minutes
Servings: 8
Ingredients:

- 4 tbsps. olive oil
- 2 carrots, chopped
- 1 yellow onion, chopped
- 2 tbsps. tomato paste
- 2 garlic cloves, chopped
- 6 cups chicken stock
- 2 cups brown lentils, dried
- 1 lb. chicken thighs, skinless, boneless and cubed
- Salt and black pepper to the taste

Directions:
Heat up a pot with the oil over medium high heat, add the chicken, onion and the garlic and brown for 10 minutes.

Add the rest of the ingredients, bring the soup to a boil and simmer for 1 hour.

Ladle the soup into bowls and serve for lunch.

Nutrition: Calories 311, Fat: 13.2g, Fiber: 4.3g, Carbs: 17.5g, Protein: 13.4g

157.   **Pork and Rice Soup**
Preparation Time: 5 minutes
Cooking Time: 7 hours
Servings: 4
Ingredients:

- 2 pounds pork stew meat, cubed
- A pinch of salt and black pepper
- 6 cups water
- 1 leek, sliced
- 2 bay leaves
- 1 carrot, sliced
- 3 tbsps. olive oil
- 1 cup white rice
- 2 cups yellow onion, chopped
- ½ cup lemon juice
- 1 tbsp. cilantro, chopped

Directions:

In your slow cooker, combine the pork with the water and the rest of the ingredients except the cilantro, put the lid on and cook on Low for 7 hours.

Stir the soup, ladle into bowls, sprinkle the cilantro on top and serve.

Nutrition: Calories 300, Fat: 15g, Fiber: 7.6g, Carbs: 17.4g, Protein: 22.4g

POULTRY RECIPES

158.   **Italian Chicken & Pasta Skillet**

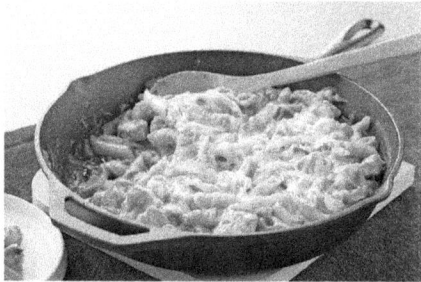

Preparation Time: 10 minutes
Cooking Time: 40-45 minutes

Servings: 4
Ingredients:

- 1 tbsp. Olive oil
- 4 halves Chicken breast
- 2 cloves Garlic
- ½ cup Red cooking wine
- 28 oz. Italian style diced tomatoes
- 8 oz. Seashell pasta
- 5 oz. Freshly chopped spinach
- Shredded mozzarella cheese (1 cup)

Directions:

Pour oil to a large skillet to get warm. Arrange the chicken in the pan to simmer for about five to eight minutes.

Pour in the diced tomatoes and wine. Wait for it to boil using the high heat temperature setting.

Stir in the pasta. Leave the top off and continue cooking. Stir occasionally until the shells are thoroughly cooked (approximately 10 min. after the pasta starts boiling).

Disperse the spinach over the top of the pasta and cover. The spinach should be ready in about five minutes.

Sprinkle using the cheese and simmer for another five minutes or until the cheese is bubbling.

Nutrition: Calories 515, Fat: 13g, Protein: 43g

159. **Lemon Chicken Skewers**

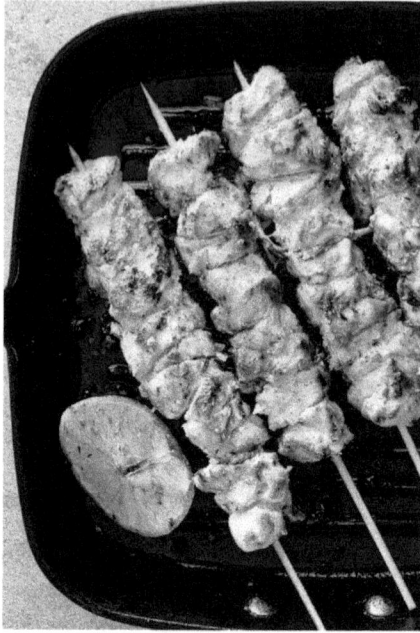

Preparation Time: 10 minutes
Cooking Time: 23-25 minutes
Servings: 6
Ingredients:

- 3 medium - 1.5-inch slices Zucchini
- 2 cloves of garlic, minced
- 3 medium onions, cut into wedges ()
- 12 Cherry tomatoes
- 1 ½ lb. Chicken breasts
- ¼ cup Olive oil
- 1 tbsp. White wine vinegar
- ½ tsp. Sugar
- 3 tbsp. Lemon juice
- 1 tsp. Salt
- 2 tsp Grated lemon zest
- ¼ tsp. Black pepper
- ¼ tsp. Dried oregano

Directions:
Slice the zucchini in half lengthwise and slice into 1.5-inch slices.
Peel the onions and cut them into wedges. Zest the lemon. Cut the chicken into 1.5-inch pieces.

Prepare the marinade. Combine the sugar, pepper, oregano, salt, lemon zest, vinegar, lemon juice, and oil. Reserve ¼ cup for basting. Fold in the chicken and toss to cover.

Add the rest of the marinade in a mixing container with the tomatoes, onions, and zucchini. Put a top or layer of plastic film/foil over the dish and store in the refrigerator overnight (for best results) or a minimum of four hours.

When ready to cook, drain, and trash the marinade. Soak the wooden skewers in water.

Thread the chicken and veggies onto the soaked skewers.

Arrange the skewers on the grill for six minutes using the medium heat setting. It's done when poked with a fork - the juices will run clear.

Nutrition: Calories 219, Fat 6g, Protein: 29g

160. **Slow-Cooked Mediterranean Roasted Turkey Breast**

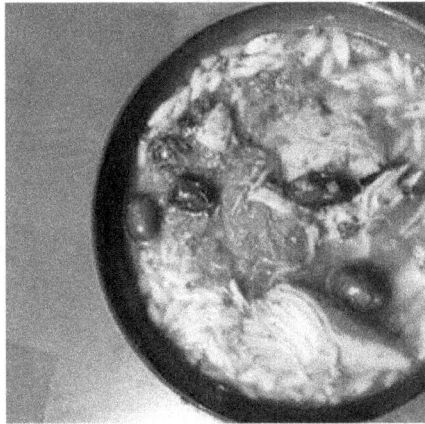

Preparation Time: 45 minutes
Cooking Time: Varied 7.5 + hours
Servings: 8
Ingredients:

- 4 lb. Boneless turkey breast, trimmed
- ½ cup Chicken broth, divided
- 2 tbsp. Fresh lemon juice
- 2 cups onion, chopped
- ½ cup Pitted kalamata olives
- ½ cup Oil-packed sun-dried tomatoes
- 1 tsp. Greek seasoning - such as McCormick's
- ½ tsp. Salt

- ¼ tsp. Black pepper
- 3 tbsp. All-purpose flour

Directions:

Thinly slice the tomatoes. Arrange the turkey breast, salt, Greek season-ing, tomatoes, olives, onion, lemon juice, and ¼ cup of the chicken broth into the slow cooker. Secure the lid and set the timer for 7 hours on the low setting.

Mix the remainder of the broth with the flour in a small mixing container. Beat/whisk until smooth and add it to the slow cooker at the end of the 7-hour cooking time.

Cover and cook in low for another 30 minutes before serving.

Nutrition: Calories 333, Fat: 4.7g, Protein: 60.6g

161.   **Delicious Roasted Duck**

Preparation Time: 10 minutes

Cooking Time: 4 hours and 50 minutes

Servings: 4

Ingredients:

- 1 medium duck
- 1 celery stalk, chopped
- 2 yellow onions, chopped
- 2 tsps. thyme, dried
- 8 garlic cloves, minced
- 2 bay leaves
- ¼ cup parsley, chopped
- A pinch of salt and black pepper
- 1 tsp. herbs de Provence

For the sauce:

- 1 tbsp. tomato paste
- 1 yellow onion, chopped
- ½ tsp sugar
- ½ cup white wine
- 3 cups water
- 1 cup chicken stock
- 1 and ½ cups black olives, pitted and chopped
- ¼ tsp herbs de Provence

Directions:

In a baking dish, arrange thyme, parsley, garlic and 2 onions. Add duck, season with salt, 1 tsp. herbs de Provence and pepper.

Place in the oven at 475°F and roast for 10 minutes. Cover the dish, reduce heat to 275°F and roast duck for 3 hours and 30 minutes.

Meanwhile, heat a pan over medium heat, add 1 yellow onion, stir, and cook for 10 minutes.

Add tomato paste, stock, sugar, ¼ tsp herbs de Provence, olives and water, cover, reduce heat to low and cook for 1 hour.

Transfer duck to a work surface, carve, discard bones, and divide between plates.

Drizzle the sauce all over and serve right away.

Nutrition: Calories 254, Fat: 3g, Fiber: 3g, Carbs: 8g, Protein: 13g

162. **Duck Breast with Apricot Sauce**

Preparation Time: 10 minutes

Cooking Time: 20 minutes

Servings: 4

Ingredients:

- 4 duck breasts, boneless
- Salt and black pepper to taste
- ¼ tsp cinnamon, ground
- ¼ tsp coriander, ground
- 5 tbsps. apricot preserves
- 3 tbsps. chives, chopped
- 2 tbsps. parsley, chopped
- A drizzle of olive oil
- 3 tbsps. apple cider vinegar
- 2 tbsps. red onions, chopped
- 1 cup apricots, chopped
- ¾ cup blackberries

Directions:

Season duck breasts with salt, pepper, coriander, and cinnamon, place them on preheated grill pan over medium high heat, cook for 2 minutes, flip them and cook for 3 minutes more.

Flip duck breasts again, add 3 tbsps. apricot preserves, cook for 1 minute, transfer them to a cutting board, leave aside for 2-3 minutes and slice.

Heat a pan over medium heat, add vinegar, onion, 2 tbsps. apricot preserves, apricots, blackberries, and chives, stir and cook for 3 minutes.

Divide sliced duck breasts between plates and serve with apricot sauce drizzled on top.

Nutrition: Calories 275, Fat: 4g, Fiber: 4g, Carbs: 7g, Protein: 12g

163. **Mediterranean Duck Breast Salad**

Preparation Time: 10 minutes

Cooking Time: 20 minutes

Servings: 4

Ingredients:

- 3 tbsps. white wine vinegar
- 2 tbsps. sugar
- 2 oranges, peeled and cut into segments
- 1 tsp. orange zest, grated
- 1 tbsp. lemon juice
- 1 tsp. lemon zest, grated
- 3 tbsps. shallot, minced
- tbsps. canola oil
- Salt and black pepper to taste
- 2 duck breasts, boneless but skin on, cut into 4 pieces
- 1 head of frisee, torn
- 2 small lettuce heads washed, torn into small pieces
- 2 tbsps. chives, chopped

Directions:

Heat a small saucepan over medium high heat, add vinegar and sugar, stir and boil for 5 minutes and take off heat.

Add orange zest, lemon zest and lemon juice, stir and leave aside for a few minutes. Add shallot, salt and pepper to taste, and the oil, whisk well and leave aside for now.

Pat dry duck pieces, score skin, trim and season with salt and pepper. Heat a pan over medium high heat for 1 minute, arrange duck breast pieces skin side down, brown for 8 minutes, reduce heat to medium and cook for 4 more minutes.

Flip pieces then cook for 3 minutes. Transfer to a cutting board and cover them with foil. Put frisee and lettuce in a bowl, stir and divide between plates.

Slice duck, arrange on top, add orange segments, sprinkle chives, and drizzle the vinaigrette.

Nutrition: Calories 320, Fat: 4g, Fiber: 4g, Carbs: 6g, Protein: 14g

164.   Duck and Orange Sauce

Preparation Time: 10 minutes

Cooking Time: 5 hours

Servings: 6

Ingredients:

- 2 medium ducks, fat trimmed
- 1 tbsp. olive oil
- 1 cup water
- Salt and black pepper to taste
- 2 tomatoes, chopped
- 2 carrots, chopped
- 2 celery stalks, chopped
- 1 leek, chopped
- 2 garlic cloves, minced

- 1 yellow onion, chopped
- 2 bay leaves
- 3 tbsps. white flour
- 1 tsp. thyme, dried
- 2 tbsps. tomato paste
- 1-quart chicken stock
- Juice of 2 oranges
- 3 oranges, peeled and cut into segments
- ⅓ cup sugar
- 2 tbsps. currant jelly
- ⅓ cup cider vinegar
- 2 tbsps. cold butter

Directions:

Pierce the duck skin, season all over with salt and pepper. Arrange them in a roasting pan, add the water, and bake in the oven at 450°F for 20 minutes.

Reduce heat to 350°F, turn the ducks and bake them for 30 minutes more.

Turn ducks again and roast them for 30 minutes more. Meanwhile, heat a pan with the oil over high heat, add carrots, celery, leek, tomatoes, garlic, onion, thyme and bay leaves, stir and cook for 10 minutes.

Add tomato paste, flour, the wine and the stock gradually, bring to a boil, reduce heat to medium low, simmer for 50 minutes, take off heat and strain the sauce into a bowl.

Heat a small pan over medium high heat, add vinegar and sugar, stir and cook for 4 minutes.

Add orange juice and currant jelly, stir and bring to a boil. Add strained sauce, salt and pepper, stir and cook for 8 minutes.

Add butter gradually and stir well again. Take ducks out of the oven, turn them, place in the oven again and cook for 40 more minutes. Take ducks out of the oven again, place them under preheated broiler and broil them for 3 minutes.

Transfer ducks to a platter and keep them warm.

Heat up juices from the pan in a saucepan over medium heat, take off heat and strain them into a bowl.

Add this to orange sauce and stir. Arrange the orange segments next to the ducks and serve with orange sauce on top.

Nutrition: Calories 342, Fat: 13g, Fiber: 4g, Carbs: 17g, Protein: 12g

165. **Duck Breast and Blackberries Mix**

Preparation Time: 10 minutes

Cooking Time: 25 minutes

Servings: 4

Ingredients:

- 4 duck breasts

- 2 tbsps. balsamic vinegar
- 3 tbsps. sugar
- Salt and black pepper to taste
- 1 ½ cups water
- 4 oz. blackberries
- ¼ cup chicken stock
- 1 tbsp. butter
- 2 tsps. corn flour

Directions:
Pat dry duck breasts with paper towels, score the skin, season with salt and pepper to taste, and set aside for 30 minutes.

Put breasts skin side down in a pan, heat over medium heat and cook for 8 minutes.

Flip breasts and cook for 30 more seconds. Transfer duck breasts to a baking dish skin side up, place in the oven at 425°F and bake for 15 minutes.

Take the meat out of the oven and leave aside to cool down for 10 minutes before you cut them.

Meanwhile, put sugar in a pan, heat over medium heat, and melt it, stirring all the time. Take pan off heat, add the water, stock, balsamic vinegar, and the blackberries.

Heat this mix to medium temperature and cook until sauce is reduced to half. Transfer sauce to another pan, add corn flour mixed with water, heat again and cook for 4 minutes until it thickens.

Add salt and pepper, the butter and whisk well.

Slice the duck breasts, divide between plates, and serve with the berries sauce on top.

Nutrition: Calories 320, Fat: 15g, Fiber: 5g, Carbs: 16g, Protein: 11g

166.   Slow Cooked Mediterranean Duck
Preparation Time: 10 minutes
Cooking Time: 5 hours
Servings: 4
Ingredients:

- 1 duck, cut into pieces
- 2 yellow onions, chopped
- 1 celery rib, chopped
- 6 garlic cloves, minced
- 1 and ½ tbsps. thyme, chopped
- ¼ cup parsley, chopped
- A pinch of salt and black pepper
- ½ cup white wine
- ½ tsp sugar
- 1 cup chicken stock

- 1 and ½ cups black olives, pitted and sliced
- ¼ tsp Italian seasoning

Directions:
In your slow cooker, mix the duck with the onions, celery, garlic, thyme, parsley, salt, pepper, wine, sugar, stock, black olives and Italian seasoning.

Toss, cover and cook on high for 5 hours.

Divide the duck pieces and the cooking juices between plates and serve.

Nutrition: Calories 320, Fat: 14g, Fiber: 4g, Carbs: 15g, Protein: 11g

167. **Roasted Turkey**
Preparation Time: 10 minutes
Cooking Time: 2 hours and 20 minutes
Servings: 8
Ingredients:

- 1 cup hot water
- 12 black tea bags
- 2/3 cup brown sugar
- 2 tbsps. butter
- ½ cup cranberry sauce
- 1 large turkey
- 1 onion, cut into 4 wedges
- 1 lemon, cut into 4 wedges
- 2 tbsps. cornstarch
- 1 cup chicken stock
- Salt and black pepper to taste

Directions:
Put the hot water in a bowl, add tea bags, leave aside covered for 5 minutes and discard bags.

Heat a pan with the butter over medium high heat, add sugar and cranberry, stir, and cook until sugar is dissolved.

Add tea, stir, and cook for 15 minutes. Stuff turkey with lemon and onion pieces, place it in a roasting pan and brush it with the tea glaze. Place in the oven at 350 ° F and roast for 2 hours, flipping and basting the turkey with the glaze every 20 minutes.

Put chicken stock in a saucepan and heat up over medium heat. Add cornstarch, salt, and pepper. Stir and cook for 1 minute.

Carve turkey and divide it between plates. Strain gravy and drizzle it over your turkey.

Nutrition: Calories 500, Fat: 13g, Fiber: 1g, Carbs: 20g, Protein: 7g

168. **Herb and Citrus Turkey**
Preparation Time: 30 minutes
Cooking Time: 4 hours

Servings: 10
Ingredients:

- whole turkey, neck and giblets removed
- Zest and juice from 1 lemon
- ½ cup butter
- ½ shallot, chopped
- Sage leaves
- Rosemary, dried
- Thyme, chopped
- 1 garlic clove, minced
- 1 yellow onion, roughly chopped
- Carrots, roughly chopped
- Celery stalks, chopped
- 1 cup dry white wine
- 1 cup chicken stock
- ¼ cup whole wheat flour

Directions:
Place lemon zest and juice in a food processor, add butter, shallot, sage, thyme, rosemary and garlic and pulse.

Lift skin from turkey breast without detaching it, rub it with 3 tbsps. of the herb butter under the skin and secure with toothpicks. Season the cavity and the whole turkey with salt and pepper to taste and place in a baking dish.

Add onion, carrots and celery, tie ends of turkey legs together, rub the turkey with remaining herb butter, add wine and stock to the pan, place in the oven and bake at 425°F for 30 minutes.

Reduce heat to 325°F and bake for 2 hours and 30 minutes. Transfer to a platter, pour veggie drippings through a strainer and reserve 2 ½ cups of drippings.

Heat a pan with the reserved chilled herb butter over medium heat, add flour, stir well, and cook for 2 minutes.

Add reserved pan drippings, bring to a boil, reduce the temperature, and cook for 5 minutes stirring occasionally.

Cut turkey and serve with the gravy you've just prepared.

Nutrition: Calories 287, Fat: 4g, Fiber: 7g, Carbs: 9g, Protein: 12g

169.   Pan Fried Chicken
Preparation Time: 10 minutes
Cooking Time: 40 minutes
Servings: 6
Ingredients:

- 6 chicken breast halves, skinless and boneless
- 2 tsps. olive oil

- ½ cup + 2 tbsps. white wine
- Basil, chopped
- Thyme, chopped
- ½ cup yellow onion, chopped
- Garlic cloves, minced
- ½ cup kalamata olives, pitted and sliced
- ¼ cup parsley, chopped
- Tomatoes, chopped

Directions:

Heat a pan with the oil and 2 tbsps. wine over medium heat, add chicken, cook for 6 minutes on each side and transfer to a plate.

Heat the same pan over medium heat, add garlic, stir, and cook for 1 minute. Add onion, stir, and cook for 3 minutes.

Add tomatoes and remaining wine, stir, bring to a simmer, and cook for 10 minutes.

Add basil and thyme, stir, and cook for 5 minutes more. Add chicken, stir, cover pan, and cook for 10 minutes more.

Add parsley, olives, salt, and pepper. Stir and divide between plates and serve.

Nutrition: Calories 221, Fat: 2g, Fiber: 4g, Carbs: 7g, Protein: 19g

170.   Chicken with Oyster Mushrooms

Preparation Time: 10 minutes

Cooking Time: 25 minutes

Servings: 4

Ingredients:

- 8 chicken breast halves, skinless and boneless
- 6 tbsps. olive oil
- ½ pounds oyster mushrooms
- 1 ½ cups chicken stock
- A pinch of salt and black pepper
- Plum tomatoes, chopped
- ⅔ cup kalamata olives, pitted and sliced
- 1 tbsp. shallot, chopped
- Garlic cloves, minced
- 1 tbsp. capers
- 2 tbsps. butter
- 1 cup cherry tomatoes, red and yellow
- Pine nuts
- 3 tbsps. parsley, chopped

Directions:

Heat a pan with 3 tbsps. oil over medium high heat, add chicken, season with some salt and pepper, cook for 3 minutes on each side and transfer to a plate.

Discard grease from the pan, add remaining oil, heat over medium high heat, add mushrooms, stir, and cook for 3 minutes. Add stock, stir, and cook for 5 minutes more.

Add plum tomatoes, shallot, garlic, olives, and capers, stir, and cook for 7 minutes. Add a pinch of salt and black pepper, also add butter and cherry tomatoes, stir, and cook for a few minutes more.

Divide chicken on plates, add mushroom mix on the side, sprinkle parsley and pine nuts on top and serve.

Nutrition: Calories 241, Fat: 4g, Fiber: 5g, Carbs: 6g, Protein: 16g

171.   Braised Chicken & Artichoke Hearts

Preparation Time: 30 minutes

Cooking Time: 1.5 hours

Servings: 4

Ingredients:

- 1 tbsp. Olive oil
- 4 quarters Chicken legs
- 1 yellow onion
- 4 cloves Garlic
- 1 tbsp. Black pepper
- 1 tsp. Salt
- ½ tsp. Red pepper flakes
- 1 quart of Chicken stock/low-sodium broth
- 10 Canned artichoke hearts
- 2 cups Cherry peppers
- 2 juiced Lemons
- 8 sprigs Fresh thyme
- 16 oz. can Butter beans
- Also Needed: Dutch oven

Directions:

Dice the onion and garlic. Drain the butter beans. Drain the artichokes and cut them in half.

Heat the oven to reach 375°F.

Prepare the pan using the high temperature setting and add the oil.

Sear the chicken until browned or about five minutes per side. Set aside on a warm platter.

Mix in the garlic, onion, pepper flakes, salt, and black pepper. Sauté it for about one minute. Stir in the broth and simmer for about a minute or so. Take the pan off the burner.

Add the chicken back in the Dutch oven, adding the thyme, lemon juice, cherry peppers, and artichoke hearts.

Place the skillet in the oven to bake it for about one hour.

Take the chicken out of the cooker and place it in a warm platter again.

Stir the beans into the pan with the broth and artichoke mixture.

Place each leg quarter in a Servings dish. Add a ladle of the artichoke, bean, and broth mixture over each Servings.

Nutrition: Calories 707, Fat: 34.9g, Protein: 67.9g

172. **Chicken Thighs with Shallots in Red Wine Vinegar**

Preparation Time: 20 minutes

Cooking Time: 35 minutes

Servings: 4

Ingredients:

- 32 oz. / 8 lean Chicken thighs
- Kosher salt and fresh pepper as desired
- 1 cup Chicken broth
- ½ cup Red wine vinegar
- 1 tbsp. Honey
- 1 tsp. Butter
- 1 tbsp. Tomato paste
- 1 large or ¾ cup of Shallot
- 2 cloves Garlic
- 2 tbsp. Light sour cream
- ½ cup Dry white wine
- 2 tbsp. Fresh parsley

Directions:

Trim the thighs and sprinkle them using pepper and salt.

Prepare a medium saucepan with the honey, ¾ cup of the chicken broth, vinegar, and tomato paste. Boil until it's about ¾ cup (about 5 min.). Take the saucepan from the burner.

Prepare a large skillet using the med-low temperature setting. Melt the butter and add the chicken. Cook it for about six to eight minutes. Remove it and set it aside for now.

Thinly slice/toss the garlic and shallots into the pan. Sauté them for five minutes.

Pour the sauce, wine, and broth over the chicken.

Place a lid on the skillet and simmer them until tender (about 20 min.).

Remove the chicken and stir in the sour cream. Stir into the sauce and boil a couple of minutes.

Return the chicken to the skillet and garnish it with parsley.

Nutrition: Calories 353.5, Fat: 11.5g, Protein: 46g

173. **Feta Chicken Burgers**

Preparation Time: 15 minutes

Cooking Time: 30 minutes

Servings: 6
Ingredients:

- ¼ cup Reduced-fat mayonnaise
- ¼ cup Finely chopped cucumber
- ¼ tsp. Black pepper
- 1 tsp. Garlic powder
- ½ cup Chopped roasted sweet red pepper
- ½ tsp. Greek seasoning
- 1 ½ lb. Lean ground chicken
- 1 cup Crumbled feta cheese
- 6 toasted Whole wheat burger buns

Directions:

Heat the broiler to the oven ahead of time. Combine the mayo and cucumber. Set aside.

Whisk each of the seasonings and the red pepper for the burgers. Work in the chicken and the cheese. Shape the mixture into six ½-inch thick patties.

Broil the burgers approximately four inches from the heat source. It should take about three to four minutes per side until the thermometer reaches 165°F.

Serve on the buns with the cucumber sauce. Top it off with tomato and lettuce if desired and serve.

Nutrition: Calories 356, Fat: 14g, Protein: 31g

174.   Grecian Chicken & Pasta Skillet
Preparation Time: 15 minutes
Cooking Time: 40 minutes
Servings: 4
Ingredients:

- 14.5 oz Diced tomatoes, undrained, no-salt-added
- 14.5 oz Chicken broth, reduced sodium
- ¾ lb. Chicken breast, cut into 1-inch pieces
- ½ cup Water or white wine
- 1 clove Garlic
- ½ tsp Dried oregano
- 4 oz Multigrain thin spaghetti
- 7.5 oz. jar Marinated and quartered artichoke hearts
- ¼ cup Roasted sweet bell pepper strips
- ¼ cup Sliced ripe olives
- 2 cups Baby spinach
- 1 Chopped green onion
- 2 tbsp. Fresh parsley
- 1 tbsp. Olive oil

- ½ tsp Grated lemon zest
- 2 tbsp Lemon juice
- ½ tsp Pepper
- Optional: Crumbled reduced-fat feta cheese (as desired)

Directions:
Combine the water/wine, chicken broth, chicken, garlic, oregano, and tomatoes in a large skillet. Drain and coarsely chop the artichoke hearts and add to the skillet.

Toss in the spaghetti and boil for five to seven minutes. Simmer it until the pink is removed from the chicken.

Stir in the spinach, pepper, oil, parsley, green onion, olives, red peppers, and the juice and zest of lemon.

Simmer for another two to three minutes or until the spinach is wilted.

Sprinkle it using the cheese and serve.

Nutrition: Calories 373. Fat: 15g, Protein: 25g

175.   **Greek Penne & Chicken**
Preparation Time: 20 minutes
Cooking Time: 50 minutes
Servings: 4
Ingredients:

- 1 lb. skinless, boneless chicken breast halves
- 16 oz. pkg. Penne pasta
- 1 ½ tbsp Butter
- 16 oz Salted butter
- ½ cup Red onion
- 2 Cloves of garlic
- 14 oz Artichoke hearts in water
- 1 chopped Tomato
- 14.5 oz Hunt's Diced Tomatoes
- ½ cup Crumbled feta cheese
- 3 tbsp Fresh parsley
- Black pepper and salt as desired
- 2 tbsp Lemon juice
- 1 tsp. Dried oregano

Directions:
Slice the chicken into bite-sized pieces.

Prepare the penne until it's al dente and drain it thoroughly.

Melt the butter in a skillet using the med-high temperature setting.

Mince and toss in the garlic and onion. Sauté them for two minutes. Fold in the chicken and continue cooking for another five to six minutes.

Reduce the temperature setting (med-low).

Drain and add the artichoke hearts with the remainder of the fixings.

Simmer for about two to three minutes or until hot.

Chop the parsley and add the salt and pepper to the chicken before Servings.

Nutrition: Calories 685, Fat: 13g. Protein: 47g

176.   Easy and Simple Chicken

Preparation Time: 8 hours and 10 minutes

Cooking Time: 30 minutes

Servings: 8

Ingredients:

- Whole chicken, cut into medium pieces
- A pinch of salt and black pepper
- ½ cup olive oil
- 1 tbsp. rosemary, chopped
- Garlic cloves, minced
- 1 tbsp. thyme, chopped
- 1 tbsp. oregano, chopped
- Juice from 2 lemons

Directions:

In a bowl, mix oil with salt, pepper, garlic, rosemary, thyme, oregano, and lemon juice then whisk well.

Add chicken, toss well, and keep in the fridge for 8 hours.

Place chicken pieces on preheated grill pan over medium heat, cook for 15 minutes on each side, divide between plates, and serve with a side salad.

Nutrition: Calories 287, Fat: 3g, Fiber: 1g, Carbs: 4g, Protein: 20g

177.   Pan Roasted Chicken and Potatoes

Preparation Time: 10 minutes

Cooking Time: 1 hour

Servings: 8

Ingredients:

- 3 pounds potatoes, peeled and roughly chopped
- 2 green bell peppers, chopped
- Yellow onion, chopped
- 4 garlic cloves, minced
- ½ cup black olives, pitted and sliced
- 14 oz. canned tomatoes, chopped
- 16 chicken drumsticks, skinless
- 1 tbsp. mixed herbs, dried
- Feta cheese, crumbled
- ½ cup parsley, chopped

Directions:

Put potatoes in a large saucepan, add water to cover, bring to a boil over medium heat, cook for a couple of minutes, drain and transfer to a large roasting pan.

Add green bell pepper, onion, garlic, tomatoes, olives and herbs and toss.

Add chicken, some salt and pepper, toss again, place in the oven at 400°F and roast for 40 minutes.

Toss everything again and roast for 20 minutes more. Divide on plates, sprinkle parsley and feta on top and serve.

Nutrition: Calories 298, Fat: 3g, Fiber: 3g, Carbs: 7g, Protein: 16g

178.   Chicken with Mustard Sauce

Preparation Time: 10 minutes

Cooking Time: 30 minutes

Servings: 4

Ingredients:

- 8 bacon strips, chopped
- ⅓ cup mustard
- cup yellow onion, chopped
- 1 tbsp. olive oil
- 1 ½ cups chicken stock
- 4 chicken breasts, skinless and boneless
- ¼ tsp sweet paprika

Directions:

In a bowl, mix paprika with mustard, salt and pepper and stir well. Spread this on chicken breasts and massage.

Heat a pan over medium high heat, add bacon, stir, cook until it browns and transfer to a plate.

Heat the same pan with the oil over medium high heat, add chicken breasts, cook for 2 minutes on each side, and transfer to a plate.

Heat the pan once again over medium high heat, add stock, stir, and bring to a simmer.

Add bacon and onions, salt and pepper and stir. Return chicken to pan as well, stir gently and simmer over medium heat for 20 minutes, turning meat halfway.

Divide chicken on plates, drizzle the sauce over it and serve.

Nutrition: Calories 223, Fat: 8g, Fiber: 1g, Carbs: 3g, Protein: 26g

179.   Delicious and Easy Chicken

Preparation Time: 10 minutes

Cooking Time: 1 hour

Servings: 6

Ingredients:

- 8 oz. mushrooms, chopped
- Italian sausage, chopped
- Avocado oil
- 6 cherry peppers, chopped
- 1 red bell pepper, chopped
- 1 red onion, sliced
- Garlic, minced
- 2 cups cherry tomatoes, halved
- Chicken thighs
- Salt and black pepper to taste
- ½ cup chicken stock
- 1 tbsp. balsamic vinegar
- 2 tsps. oregano, dried
- Some chopped parsley for Servings

Directions:

Heat a pan with half of the oil over medium heat, add sausages, stir, brown for a few minutes and transfer to a plate.

Heat the pan again with remaining oil over medium heat, add chicken thighs, season with salt and pepper, cook for 3 minutes on each side and transfer to a plate.

Heat the pan again over medium heat, add cherry peppers, mushrooms, onion, and bell pepper, stir and cook for 4 minutes.

Add garlic, stir, and cook for 2 minutes. Add stock, vinegar, salt, pepper, oregano, and cherry tomatoes and stir.

Add chicken pieces and sausages ones, stir gently, transfer everything to the oven at 400 ° and bake for 30 minutes.

Sprinkle parsley, then divide between plates and serve.

Nutrition: Calories 340 Fat 33 Fiber 3 Carbs 4 Protein 20

180.   Mediterranean Chicken Bites

Preparation Time: 10 minutes

Cooking Time: 10 minutes

Servings: 4

Ingredients:

- 20 oz. canned pineapple slices
- A drizzle of olive oil
- 3 cups chicken thighs, boneless, skinless and cut into medium pieces
- tbsp smoked paprika

Directions:

Heat a pan over medium high heat, add pineapple slices, cook them for a few minutes on each side, transfer to a cutting board, cool them down and cut into medium cubes.

Heat another pan with a drizzle of oil over medium high heat, rub chicken pieces with paprika, add them to the pan and cook for 5 minutes on each side.

Arrange chicken cubes on a platter, add a pineapple piece on top of each and stick a toothpick in each.

Serve right away!

Nutrition: Calories 120, Fat: 3g, Fiber: 1g, Carbs: 5g, Protein: 2g

181. **Orange and Cashew Chicken Salad**

Preparation Time: 10 minutes

Cooking Time: 30 minutes

Servings: 4

Ingredients:

- whole chicken, chopped
- 4 scallions, chopped
- celery stalks, chopped
- 1 cup mandarin orange, chopped
- ¼ cup homemade mayo
- ½ cup yogurts
- 1 cup cashews, toasted and chopped
- A pinch of salt and black pepper

Directions:

Put chicken pieces in a pot, add water to cover, add a pinch of salt, bring to a boil over medium heat and cook for 25 minutes.

Transfer chicken to a cutting board, leave aside to cool down, discard bones, shred meat and put it in a bowl.

Add celery, orange pieces, cashews, scallion, and toss.

Add salt, pepper, mayo, and yogurt, toss to coat well and keep in the fridge until you serve it.

Nutrition: Calories 150, Fat: 3g, Fiber: 3g, Carbs: 7g, Protein: 6g

182. **Grilled Chicken and Peaches**

Preparation Time: 10 minutes

Cooking Time: 1 hour and 10 minutes

Servings: 4

Ingredients:

- whole chicken, cut into medium pieces
- ¾ cup water
- ⅓ cup honey
- Salt and black pepper to taste
- ¼ cup olive oil
- 4 peaches, halved

Directions:

Put the water in a saucepan, bring to a simmer over medium heat, add pepper and honey, whisk well and leave aside.

Rub chicken pieces with the oil, season with salt and pepper, place on preheated grill pan over medium high heat, brush with honey mixture and cook for 15 minutes.

Brush chicken with more honey mix, cook for 15 minutes more and then flip again.

Brush one more time with the honey mix, cover and cook for 20 minutes more.

Divide chicken pieces on plates and keep warm. Brush peaches with remaining honey marinade, place them on your grill pan and cook for 4 minutes.

Flip again and cook for 3 minutes more. Divide between plates next to chicken pieces and serve.

Nutrition: Calories 500, Fat: 14g, Fiber: 3g, Carbs: 15g, Protein: 10g

183.   Mediterranean Chicken and Tomato Dish
Preparation Time: 10 minutes
Cooking Time: 20 minutes
Servings: 4
Ingredients:

- 5 chicken thighs
- Olive oil
- 1 tbsp. thyme, chopped
- Garlic cloves, minced
- 1 tsp. red pepper flakes, crushed
- ½ cup heavy cream
- ¾ cup chicken stock
- ½ cup sun dried tomatoes in olive oil, drained and chopped
- Salt and black pepper to taste
- ¼ cup parmesan cheese, grated
- Basil leaves, chopped for Servings

Directions:

Heat a pan with the oil over medium high heat, add chicken, salt, and pepper to taste, cook for 3 minutes on each side, transfer to a plate and leave aside for now.

Return pan to heat, add thyme, garlic, and pepper flakes. Stir and cook for 1 minute.

Add stock, tomatoes, salt and pepper, heavy cream, and parmesan, stir and bring to a simmer.

Add chicken pieces, stir, place in the oven at 350°F and bake for 15 minutes.

Take pan out of the oven, leave chicken aside for 2-3 minutes, divide between plates and serve with basil sprinkled on top.

Nutrition: Calories 212, Fat: 4g, Fiber: 3g, Carbs: 3g, Protein: 12g

FISH AND SEAFOOD

184.   **Pan-Seared Salmon**

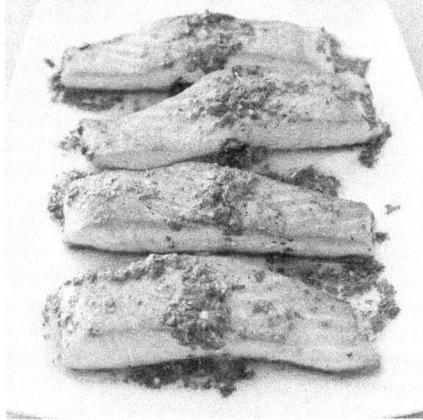

Preparation Time: 10 minutes
Cooking Time: 20 minutes
Servings: 4
Ingredients:

- 4 pieces of 6 oz. each Salmon fillets
- 2 tbsp. Olive oil
- 2 tbsp. Capers
- ⅛ tsp. each Pepper & salt
- 4 slices Lemon

Directions:

Warm a heavy skillet for about three minutes using the medium heat temperature setting.

Lightly spritz the salmon with oil. Arrange them in the pan and increase the temperature setting to high.

Sear for approximately three minutes. Sprinkle with the salt, pepper, and capers.

Flip the salmon over and continue cooking for five minutes or until browned the way you like it.

Garnish with lemon slices and serve.

Nutrition: Calories 371, Fat: 25.1g, Protein: 33.7g

185.   **Pan-Seared Scallops with Pepper & Onions in Anchovy Oil**

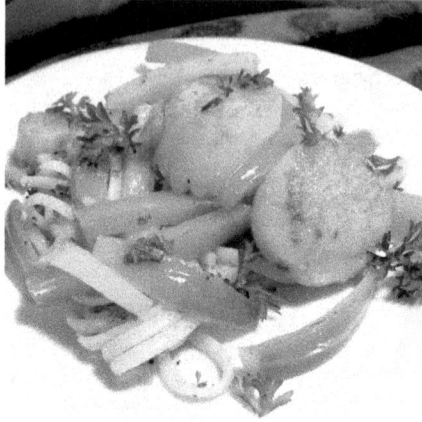

Preparation Time: 30 minutes
Cooking Time: 45 minutes
Servings: 4
Ingredients:

- ⅓ cup Olive oil
- 2 oz. can Anchovy fillets
- 1 lb. Jumbo sea scallops
- 1 large of each Orange & red bell pepper
- 1 Red onion
- 2 cloves Garlic
- 1 tsp. Lime zest
- 1 ½ tsp. Lemon zest
- 1 pinch of Kosher salt & pepper each
- Garnish: 8 sprigs fresh parsley

Directions:
Coarsely chop the peppers and onions. Mince the garlic and anchovy fillet. Zest/mince the lime and lemon.

Heat the oil and anchovies in a large skillet using a med-high temperature setting.

After the anchovies are sizzling, toss in the scallops, and simmer them for about two minutes - without stirring.

Toss the bell peppers, garlic, red onion, lime zest, lemon zest, salt, and pepper into a mixing container. Sprinkle the mixture over the scallops. Cook until they have browned (2 min.).

Flip the scallops, stir, and continue cooking until the scallops have browned thoroughly (4-5 min.).

Top it off using sprigs of parsley before Servings.

Nutrition: Calories 368, Fat: 23.9g, Protein: 24.2g

186.   **Salmon with Warm Tomato-Olive Salad**

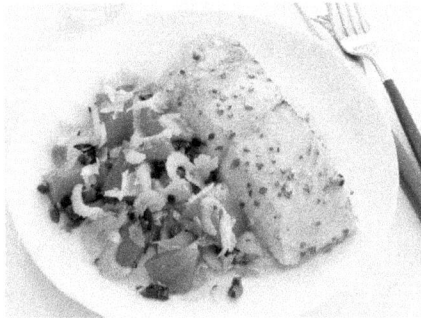

Preparation Time: 15 minutes
Cooking Time: 25 minutes
Servings: 4
Ingredients:

- 4/approx. 4 oz./1¼-inches thick Salmon fillets
- 1 cup Celery
- 2 Medium tomatoes
- ¼ cup Fresh mint
- ½ cup Kalamata olives
- ½ tsp. Garlic
- 1 tsp. + more to taste Salt
- 1 tbsp. Honey
- ¼ tsp. Red pepper flakes
- 2 tbsp. + more for the pan Olive oil
- 1 tsp. Vinegar

Directions:

Slice the tomatoes and celery into 1-inch pieces and mince the garlic. Chop the mint and the olives.

Heat the oven using the broiler setting.

Whisk the oil, vinegar, honey, red pepper flakes, and salt (1 tsp.). Brush the mixture onto the salmon.

Line the broiler pan with a sheet of foil. Spritz the pan lightly with olive oil and add the fillets (skin side downward).

Broil them for four to six minutes until well done.

Meanwhile, make the tomato salad. Mix ½ tsp of the salt with the garlic.

Prepare a small saucepan on the stovetop using the med-high temperature setting. Pour in the rest of the oil and add the garlic mixture with the olives and one tbsp of vinegar. Simmer for about three minutes.

Prepare the Servings dishes. Pour the bubbly mixture into the bowl and add the mint, tomato, and celery. Dust it with the salt as desired and toss.

When the salmon is done, serve with a tomato salad.

Nutrition: Calories 433, Fat: 26g, Protein: 38g

187.   **Shrimp & Penne**

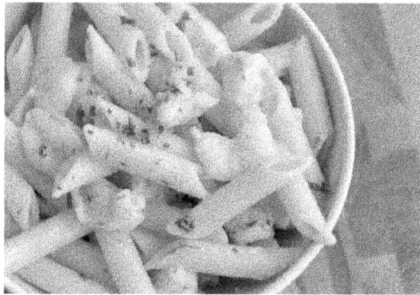

Preparation Time: 20 minutes
Cooking Time: 35 minutes
Servings: 8
Ingredients:

- 16 oz. pkg. Penne pasta
- ¼ tsp. Salt
- 2 tbsp. Olive oil
- 2 - 14.5 oz. cans Diced tomatoes
- 1 tbsp Garlic
- ¼ cup Red onion
- ¼ cup White wine
- 1 lb. Shrimp
- 1 cup Grated parmesan cheese

Directions:

Dice the red onion and garlic. Peel and devein the shrimp.

Add salt to a large soup pot of water and set it on the stovetop to boil. Add the pasta and cook for nine to ten minutes. Drain it thoroughly in a colander.

Empty oil into a skillet. Warm it using the medium temperature setting.

Toss in the garlic and onion to sauté until tender. Pour in the tomatoes and wine. Continue cooking for about ten minutes, stirring occasionally.

Fold in the shrimp and continue cooking for about five minutes or until it's opaque.

Combine the pasta and shrimp and top it off with the cheese to serve.

Nutrition: Fat: 8.5 g Protein: 24.5 g Calories: 385

188. **Tilapia with Avocado & Red Onion**
Preparation Time: 5 minutes
Cooking Time: 15 minutes
Servings: 4
Ingredients:

- 1 tbsp Olive oil
- ¼ tsp Sea salt
- 1 tbsp Fresh orange juice
- Four 4 oz. - more rectangular than square Tilapia fillets
- ¼ cup Red onion
- 1 Sliced avocado
- Also Needed: 9-inch pie plate

Directions:
Combine the salt, juice, and oil to add into the pie dish. Work with one fillet at a time. Place it in the dish and turn to coat all sides.

Arrange the fillets in a wagon wheel-shaped formation. (Each of the fillets should be in the center of the dish with the other end draped over the edge.)

Place a tbsp of the onion on top of each of the fillets and fold the end into the center. Cover the dish with plastic wrap, leaving one corner open to vent the steam.

Place in the microwave using the high heat setting for three minutes. It's done when the center can be easily flaked.

Top the fillets off with avocado and serve.

Nutrition: Calories 200, Fat: 11g, Protein: 22g

189. **Berries and Grilled Calamari**
Preparation Time: 5 minutes
Cooking Time: 5 minutes
Servings: 4
Ingredients:

- ¼ cup dried cranberries
- ¼ cup extra virgin olive oil
- ¼ cup olive oil
- ¼ cup sliced almonds
- ½ lemon, juiced
- ¾ cup blueberries
- 1 ½ pounds calamari tube, cleaned
- 1 granny smith apple, sliced thinly

- 1 tbsp. fresh lemon juice
- 2 tbsps. apple cider vinegar
- 6 cups fresh spinach
- Freshly grated pepper to taste
- Sea salt to taste

Directions:

In a small bowl, make the vinaigrette by mixing well the tbsp of lemon juice, apple cider vinegar, and extra virgin olive oil. Season with pepper and salt to taste. Set aside.

Turn on the grill to medium fire and let the grates heat up for a minute or two.

In a large bowl, add olive oil and the calamari tube. Season calamari generously with pepper and salt.

Place seasoned and oiled calamari onto heated grate and grill until cooked or opaque. This is around two minutes per side.

As you wait for the calamari to cook, you can combine almonds, cranberries, blueberries, spinach, and the thinly sliced apple in a large salad bowl. Toss to mix.

Remove cooked calamari from grill and transfer on a chopping board. Cut into ¼-inch thick rings and throw into the salad bowl.

Drizzle with vinaigrette and toss well to coat salad.

Serve and enjoy!

Nutrition: Calories 567, Fat: 24.5g, Carbs: 30.6g, Protein: 54.8g

190.   Cajun Garlic Shrimp Noodle Bowl
Preparation Time: 7 minutes
Cooking Time: 15 minutes
Servings: 2
Ingredients:

- ½ tsp salt
- 1 onion, sliced
- 1 red pepper, sliced
- 1 tbsp. butter
- 1 tsp. garlic granules
- 1 tsp. onion powder
- 1 tsp. paprika
- 2 large zucchinis, cut into noodle strips
- 20 jumbo shrimps, shells removed and deveined
- 3 cloves garlic, minced
- 3 tbsp ghee
- A dash of cayenne pepper
- A dash of red pepper flakes

Directions:
Prepare the Cajun seasoning by mixing the onion powder, garlic granules, pepper flakes, cayenne pepper, paprika and salt. Toss in the shrimp to coat in the seasoning.

In a skillet, heat the ghee and sauté the garlic. Add in the red pepper and onions and continue sautéing for 4 minutes.

Add the Cajun shrimp and cook until opaque. Set aside.

In another pan, heat the butter and sauté the zucchini noodles for three minutes.

Assemble by the placing the Cajun shrimps on top of the zucchini noodles.

Nutrition: Calories 712, Fat: 30.0g, Carbs: 20.2g, Protein: 97.8g

191.   **Tarragon Cod Fillets**
Preparation Time: 10 minutes
Cooking Time: 12 minutes
Servings: 4
Ingredients:

- 4 cod fillets, boneless
- ¼ cup capers, drained
- 1 tbsp. tarragon, chopped
- Sea salt and black pepper to the taste
- 2 tbsps. olive oil
- 2 tbsps. parsley, chopped
- 1 tbsp. olive oil
- 1 tbsp. lemon juice

Directions:
Heat up a pan with the oil over medium-high heat, add the fish and cook for 3 minutes on each side.

Add the rest of the ingredients, cook everything for 7 minutes more, divide between plates and serve.

Nutrition: Calories 162, Fat: 9.6g, Fiber: 4.3g, Carbs: 12.4g, Protein: 16.5g

192.   **Salmon and Radish Mix**
Preparation Time: 10 minutes
Cooking Time: 15 minutes
Servings: 4
Ingredients:

- 2 tbsps. olive oil
- 1 tbsp. balsamic vinegar
- 1 ½ cup chicken stock
- 4 salmon fillets, boneless
- 2 garlic cloves, minced
- 1 tbsp. ginger, grated

- 1 cup radishes, grated
- ¼ cup scallions, chopped

Directions:
Heat up a pan with the oil over medium-high heat, add the salmon, cook for 4 minutes on each side, and divide between plates

Add the vinegar and the rest of the ingredients to the pan, toss gently, cook for 10 minutes, add over the salmon, and serve.

Nutrition: Calories 274, Fat: 14.5g, Fiber: 3.5g, Carbs: 8.5g, Protein: 22.3g

193.   Smoked Salmon and Watercress Salad
Preparation Time: 5 minutes
Cooking Time: 0 minutes
Servings: 4
Ingredients:

- 2 bunches watercress
- 1 lb. smoked salmon, skinless, boneless and flaked
- 2 tsps. mustard
- ¼ cup lemon juice
- ½ cup Greek yogurt
- Salt and black pepper to the taste
- 1 big cucumber, sliced
- 2 tbsps. chives, chopped

Directions:
In a salad bowl, combine the salmon with the watercress and the rest of the ingredients toss and serve right away.

Nutrition: Calories 244, Fat: 16.7g, Fiber: 4.5g, Carbs: 22.5g, Protein: 15.6g

194.   Salmon and Corn Salad
Preparation Time: 5 minutes
Cooking Time: 0 minutes
Servings: 4
Ingredients:

- ½ cup pecans, chopped
- 2 cups baby arugula
- 1 cup corn
- ¼ pound smoked salmon, skinless, boneless and cut into small chunks
- 2 tbsps. olive oil
- 2 tbsp lemon juice
- Sea salt and black pepper to the taste

Directions:

In a salad bowl, combine the salmon with the corn and the rest of the ingredients, toss and serve right away.

Nutrition: Calories 284, Fat: 18.4g, Fiber: 5.4g, Carbs: 22.6g, Protein: 17.4g

195.   Cod and Mushrooms Mix

Preparation Time: 10 minutes

Cooking Time: 25 minutes

Servings: 4

Ingredients:

- 2 cod fillets, boneless
- 4 tbsps. olive oil
- 4 oz. mushrooms, sliced
- Sea salt and black pepper to the taste
- 12 cherry tomatoes, halved
- 8 oz. lettuce leaves, torn
- 1 avocado, pitted, peeled and cubed
- 1 red chili pepper, chopped
- 1 tbsp. cilantro, chopped
- 2 tbsps. balsamic vinegar
- 1 oz. feta cheese, crumbled

Directions:

Put the fish in a roasting pan, brush it with 2 tbsps. oil, sprinkle salt and pepper all over and broil under medium-high heat for 15 minutes. Meanwhile, heat up a pan with the rest of the oil over medium heat, add the mushrooms, stir, and sauté for 5 minutes.

Add the rest of the ingredients, toss, cook for 5 minutes more and divide between plates.

Top with the fish and serve right away.

Nutrition: Calories 257, Fat: 10g, Fiber: 3.1g, Carbs: 24.3g, Protein: 19.4g

196.   Sesame Shrimp Mix

Preparation Time: 10 minutes

Cooking Time: 0 minutes

Servings: 4

Ingredients:

- 2 tbsp lime juice
- 3 tbsps. teriyaki sauce
- 2 tbsps. olive oil
- 8 cups baby spinach
- 14 oz. shrimp, cooked, peeled and deveined
- 1 cup cucumber, sliced
- 1 cup radish, sliced
- ¼ cup cilantro, chopped

- 2 tsps. sesame seeds, toasted

Directions:
In a bowl, mix the shrimp with the lime juice, spinach, and the rest of the ingredients, toss, and serve cold.

Nutrition: Calories 177, Fat: 9g, Fiber: 7.1g, Carbs: 14.3g, Protein: 9.4g

197.   Creamy Curry Salmon
Preparation Time: 10 minutes
Cooking Time: 20 minutes
Servings: 2
Ingredients:

- 2 salmon fillets, boneless and cubed
- 1 tbsp. olive oil
- 1 tbsp. basil, chopped
- Sea salt and black pepper to the taste
- 1 cup Greek yogurt
- 2 tsps. curry powder
- 1 garlic clove, minced
- ½ tsp mint, chopped

Directions:
Heat up a pan with the oil over medium-high heat, add the salmon and cook for 3 minutes.

Add the rest of the ingredients, toss, cook for 15 minutes more, divide between plates, and serve.

Nutrition: Calories 284, Fat: 14.1g, Fiber: 8.5g, Carbs: 26.7g, Protein: 31.4g

198.   Creamy Bacon-fish Chowder
Preparation Time: 15 minutes
Cooking Time: 30 minutes
Servings: 8
Ingredients:

- 1 ½ lbs. cod
- 1 ½ tsp dried thyme
- 1 large onion, chopped
- 1 medium carrot, coarsely chopped
- 1 tbsp. butter, cut into small pieces
- 1 tsp. salt, divided
- 3 ½ cups baking potato, peeled and cubed
- 3 slices uncooked bacon
- ¾ tsp freshly ground black pepper, divided
- 4 ½ cups water
- 4 bay leaves

- 4 cups 2% reduced-fat milk

Directions:
In a large skillet, add the water and bay leaves and let it simmer. Add the fish. Cover and let it simmer some more until the flesh flakes easily with fork. Remove the fish from the skillet and cut into large pieces. Set aside the cooking liquid.

Place Dutch oven in medium heat and cook the bacon until crisp. Remove the bacon and reserve the bacon drippings. Crush the bacon and set aside.

Stir potato, onion, and carrot in the pan with the bacon drippings, cook over medium heat for 10 minutes. Add the cooking liquid, bay leaves, ½ tsp salt, ¼ tsp pepper and thyme, let it boil. Lower the heat and let simmer for 10 minutes. Add the milk and butter, simmer until the potatoes becomes tender, but do not boil. Add the fish, ½ tsp salt, ½ tsp pepper. Remove the bay leaves.

Serve sprinkled with the crushed bacon.

Nutrition: Calories per Servings: 400 Carbs: 34.5g Protein: 20.8g Fat: 19.7g

199. **Cucumber-basil Salsa on Halibut Pouches**
Preparation Time: 8 minutes
Cooking Time: 17 minutes
Servings: 4
Ingredients:

- 1 lime, thinly sliced into 8 pieces
- 2 cups mustard greens, stems removed
- 2 tsp olive oil
- 4 − 5 radishes trimmed and quartered
- 4 4-oz skinless halibut filets
- 4 large fresh basil leaves
- Cayenne pepper to taste − optional
- Pepper and salt to taste

Salsa Ingredients:

- 1 ½ cups diced cucumber
- 1 ½ finely chopped fresh basil leaves
- 2 tsp fresh lime juice
- Pepper and salt to taste

Directions:
Preheat oven to 400°F.

Prepare parchment papers by making 4 pieces of 15 x 12-inch rectangles. Lengthwise, fold in half and unfold pieces on the table.

Season halibut fillets with pepper, salt, and cayenne—if using cayenne.

Just to the right of the fold going lengthwise, place ½ cup of mustard greens. Add a basil leaf on center of mustard greens and topped with 1 lime slice. Around the greens, layer ¼ of the radishes. Drizzle with ½ tsp of oil, season with pepper and salt. Top it with a slice of halibut fillet.

Just as you would make a calzone, fold parchment paper over your filling and crimp the edges of the parchment paper beginning from one end to the other end. To seal the end of the crimped parchment paper, pinch it.

Repeat process to remaining ingredients until you have 4 pieces of parchment papers filled with halibut and greens.

Place pouches in a baking pan and bake in the oven until halibut is flaky, around 15 to 17 minutes.

While waiting for halibut pouches to cook, make your salsa by mixing all salsa ingredients in a medium bowl.

Once halibut is cooked, remove from oven, and make a tear on top. Be careful of the steam as it is very hot. Equally divide salsa and spoon ¼ of salsa on top of halibut through the slit you have created.

Serve and enjoy.

Nutrition: Calories 335.4, Fat: 16.3g, Carbs: 22.1g, Protein: 20.2g

200.   **Dill Relish on White Sea Bass**

Preparation Time: 5 minutes

Cooking Time: 12 minutes

Servings: 4

Ingredients:

- 1 ½ tbsp chopped white onion
- 1 ½ tsp chopped fresh dill
- 1 lemon, quartered
- 1 tsp. Dijon mustard
- 1 tsp. lemon juice
- 1 tsp. pickled baby capers, drained
- 4 pieces of 4-oz white sea bass fillets

Directions:

Preheat oven to 375°F.

Mix lemon juice, mustard, dill, capers, and onions in a small bowl.

Prepare four aluminum foil squares and place 1 fillet per foil. Squeeze a lemon wedge per fish.

Evenly divide into 4 the dill spread and drizzle over fillet.

Close the foil over the fish securely and pop in the oven. Bake for 10 to 12 minutes or until fish is cooked through.

Remove from foil and transfer to a platter.

Serve and enjoy.

Nutrition: Calories 115, Fat: 1g, Carbs: 12g, Protein: 7g

201.   **Fish and Orzo**

Preparation Time: 10 minutes
Cooking Time: 35 minutes
Servings: 4
Ingredients:

- 1 tsp. garlic, minced
- 1 tsp. red pepper, crushed
- 2 shallots, chopped
- 1 tbsp. olive oil
- 1 tsp. anchovy paste
- 1 tbsp. oregano, chopped
- 2 tbsps. black olives, pitted and chopped
- 2 tbsps. capers, drained
- 15 oz. canned tomatoes, crushed
- A pinch of salt and black pepper
- 4 cod fillets, boneless
- 1 oz. feta cheese, crumbled
- 1 tbsp. parsley, chopped
- 3 cups chicken stock
- 1 cup orzo pasta
- Zest of 1 lemon, grated

Directions:
Heat up a pan with the oil over medium heat, add the garlic, red pepper and the shallots and sauté for 5 minutes.

Add the anchovy paste, oregano, black olives, capers, tomatoes, salt, and pepper, stir, and cook for 5 minutes more.

Add the cod fillets, sprinkle the cheese and the parsley on top, introduce in the oven and bake at 375°F for 15 minutes more.

Meanwhile, put the stock in a pot, bring to a boil over medium heat, add the orzo and the lemon zest, bring to a simmer, cook for 10 minutes, fluff with a fork, and divide between plates.

Top each Servings with the fish mix and serve.

Nutrition: Calories 402, Fat: 21g, Fiber: 8g, Carbs: 21g, Protein: 31g

202.   Baked Sea Bass
Preparation Time: 10 minutes
Cooking Time: 12 minutes
Servings: 4
Ingredients:

- 4 sea bass fillets, boneless
- Sal and black pepper to the taste
- 2 cups potato chips, crushed
- 1 tbsp. mayonnaise

Directions:

Season the fish fillets with salt and pepper, brush with the mayonnaise and dredge each in the potato chips.

Arrange the fillets on a baking sheet lined with parchment paper and bake at 400°F for 12 minutes.

Divide the fish between plates and serve with a side salad.

Nutrition: Calories 228, Fat: 8.6g, Fiber: 0.6g, Carbs: 9.3g, Protein: 25g

203.   **Fish and Tomato Sauce**

Preparation Time: 10 minutes

Cooking Time: 30 minutes

Servings: 4

Ingredients:

- 4 cod fillets, boneless
- 2 garlic cloves, minced
- 2 cups cherry tomatoes, halved
- 1 cup chicken stock
- A pinch of salt and black pepper
- ¼ cup basil, chopped

Directions:

Put the tomatoes, garlic, salt, and pepper in a pan, heat up over medium heat and cook for 5 minutes.

Add the fish and the rest of the ingredients, bring to a simmer, cover the pan, and cook for 25 minutes.

Divide the mix between plates and serve.

Nutrition: Calories 180, Fat: 1.9g, Fiber: 1.4g, Carbs: 5.3g, Protein: 33.8g

204.   **Halibut and Quinoa Mix**

Preparation Time: 10 minutes

Cooking Time: 12 minutes

Servings: 4

Ingredients:

- 4 halibut fillets, boneless
- 2 tbsps. olive oil
- 1 tsp. rosemary, dried
- 2 tsps. cumin, ground
- 1 tbsp. coriander, ground
- 2 tsps. cinnamon powder
- 2 tsps. oregano, dried
- A pinch of salt and black pepper
- 2 cups quinoa, cooked
- 1 cup cherry tomatoes, halved
- 1 avocado, peeled, pitted and sliced

- 1 cucumber, cubed
- ½ cup black olives, pitted and sliced
- Juice of 1 lemon

Directions:

In a bowl, combine the fish with the rosemary, cumin, coriander, cinnamon, oregano, salt and pepper and toss.

Heat up a pan with the oil over medium heat, add the fish, and sear for 2 minutes on each side.

Introduce the pan in the oven and bake the fish at 425°F for 7 minutes.

Meanwhile, in a bowl, mix the quinoa with the remaining ingredients, toss, and divide between plates.

Add the fish next to the quinoa mix and serve right away.

Nutrition: Calories 364, Fat: 15.4g, Fiber: 11.2g, Carbs: 56.4g, Protein: 24.5g

205. **Lemon and Dates Barramundi**

Preparation Time: 10 minutes

Cooking Time: 12 minutes

Servings: 2

Ingredients:

- 2 barramundi fillets, boneless
- 1 shallot, sliced
- 4 lemon slices
- Juice of ½ lemon
- Zest of 1 lemon, grated
- 2 tbsps. olive oil
- 6 oz. baby spinach
- ¼ cup almonds, chopped
- 4 dates, pitted and chopped
- ¼ cup parsley, chopped
- Salt and black pepper to the taste

Directions:

Season the fish with salt and pepper and arrange on 2 parchment paper pieces.

Top the fish with the lemon slices, drizzle the lemon juice, and then top with the other ingredients except the oil.

Drizzle 1 tbsp. oil over each fish mix, wrap the parchment paper around the fish shaping to packets and arrange them on a baking sheet.

Bake at 400°F for 12 minutes, cool the mix a bit, unfold, divide everything between plates and serve.

Nutrition: Calories 232, Fat: 16.5g, Fiber: 11.1g, Carbs: 24.8g, Protein: 6.5g

206. **Fish Cakes**

Preparation Time: 10 minutes
Cooking Time: 10 minutes
Servings: 6
Ingredients:

- 20 oz. canned sardines, drained and mashed well
- 2 garlic cloves, minced
- 2 tbsps. dill, chopped
- 1 yellow onion, chopped
- 1 cup panko breadcrumbs
- 1 egg, whisked
- A pinch of salt and black pepper
- 2 tbsps. lemon juice
- 5 tbsps. olive oil

Directions:

In a bowl, combine the sardines with the garlic, dill, and the rest of the ingredients except the oil, stir well and shape medium cakes out of this mix.

Heat up a pan with the oil over medium-high heat, add the fish cakes, cook for 5 minutes on each side.

Serve the cakes with a side salad.

Nutrition: Calories 288, Fat: 12.8g, Fiber: 10.2g, Carbs: 22.2g, Protein: 6.8g

207.   **Baked Salmon with Dill**
Preparation Time: 10 minutes
Cooking Time: 15 minutes
Servings: 4
Ingredients:

- 4- 6 oz. portions - 1-inch thickness Salmon fillets
- ½ tsp. Kosher salt
- 1½ tbsp. Finely chopped fresh dill
- ⅛ tsp. Black pepper
- 4 Lemon wedges

Directions:

Warm the oven in advance to reach 350°F.

Lightly grease a baking sheet with a misting of cooking oil spray and add the fish. Lightly spritz the fish with the spray along with a shake of salt, pepper, and dill.

Bake it until the fish is easily flaked (10 min.).

Serve with lemon wedges.

Nutrition: Calories 251, Fat: 16g, Protein: 28g

208.   **Couscous with Pepperoncini & Tuna**

Preparation Time: 10 minutes
Cooking Time: 20 minutes
Servings: 4
Ingredients:
For the Couscous:

- 1 cup Chicken broth or water
- 1¼ cups Couscous
- ¾ tsp. Kosher salt

For the Accompaniments:

- 2- 5-oz. cans Oil-packed tuna
- 1 pint - halved Cherry tomatoes
- ½ cup Sliced pepperoncini
- ⅓ cup Chopped fresh parsley
- ¼ cup Capers
- Olive oil for serving
- Black pepper & kosher salt as desired
- 1 quartered Lemon

Directions:
Make the couscous in a small saucepan using water or broth. Prepare it on medium heat temperature setting. Let it sit for about ten minutes.

Toss the tomatoes, tuna, capers, parsley, and pepperoncini into a mixing bowl.

Fluff the couscous when done and dust using the pepper and salt. Spritz it using the oil and serve with the tuna mix and a lemon wedge.

Nutrition: Calories 226, Fat: 1g, Protein: 8g

209.   Herb-Crusted Halibut
Preparation Time: 10 minutes
Cooking Time: 25 minutes
Servings: 4
Ingredients:

- ⅓ cup Fresh parsley
- ¼ cup Fresh dill
- ¼ cup Fresh chives
- 1 tsp. Lemon zest
- ¾ cup Panko breadcrumbs
- 1 tbsp. Olive oil
- ¼ tsp. Freshly cracked black pepper
- 1 tsp. Sea salt
- 4 - 6 oz. Halibut fillets

Directions:
Chop the fresh dill, chives, and parsley. Prepare a baking tray using a sheet of foil. Set the oven to reach 400°F.

Combine the salt, pepper, lemon zest, olive oil, chives, dill, parsley, and the breadcrumbs in a mixing bowl.

Rinse the halibut thoroughly. Use paper towels to dry it before baking.

Arrange the fish on the baking sheet. Spoon the crumbs over the fish and press it into each of the fillets.

Bake it until the top is browned and easily flaked or about 10 to 15 minutes.

Nutrition: Calories 273, Fat: 7g, Protein: 38g

210.   **Marinated Tuna Steak**
Preparation Time: 5 minutes
Cooking Time: 15-20 minutes
Servings: 4
Ingredients:

- 2 tbsp. Olive oil
- ¼ cup Orange juice
- ¼ cup Soy sauce
- 1 tbsp. Lemon juice
- 2 tbsp. Fresh parsley
- 1 Garlic clove
- ½ tsp. Ground black pepper
- ½ tsp. Fresh oregano
- 4 - 4 oz. steaks Tuna steaks

Directions:
Mince the garlic and chop the oregano and parsley.

In a glass container, mix the pepper, oregano, garlic, parsley, lemon juice, soy sauce, olive oil, and orange juice.

Warm the grill using the high heat setting. Grease the grate with oil.

Add to tuna steaks and cook for five to six minutes. Turn and baste with the marinated sauce.

Cook another five minutes or until it's the way you like it. Discard the remaining marinade.

Nutrition: Calories 200, Fat: 7.9g, Protein: 27.4g

211.   **Mediterranean Flounder**
Preparation Time: 25 minutes
Cooking Time: 45 minutes
Servings: 4
Ingredients:

- 5 Roma or plum tomatoes

- 2 tbsp. Extra-virgin olive oil
- Half of 1 Spanish onion
- 2 cloves Garlic
- 1 pinch Italian seasoning
- 24 Kalamata olives
- ¼ cup White wine
- ¼ cup Capers
- 1 tsp. Lemon juice
- 6 leaves Chopped basil
- 3 tbsp. Freshly grated parmesan cheese
- 1 lb. Flounder fillets
- 6 leaves Freshly torn basil

Directions:

Set the oven to reach 425° F. Remove the pit and chop the olives (set aside).

Pour water into a saucepan and bring to boiling. Plunge the tomatoes into the water and remove immediately. Add to a dish of ice water and drain. Remove the skins, chop, and set to the side for now.

Heat a skillet with the oil using the medium temperature heat setting. Chop and toss in the onions. Sauté them for around four minutes.

Dice and add the garlic, tomatoes, and seasoning. Simmer for five to seven minutes.

Stir in the capers, wine, olives, half of the basil, and freshly squeezed lemon juice.

Lower the heat setting and blend in the cheese. Simmer it until the sauce is thickened (15 min.).

Arrange the flounder into a shallow baking tin. Add the sauce and garnish with the remainder of the basil leaves.

Set the timer to bake it for 12 minutes until the fish is easily flaked.

Nutrition: Calories 282, Fat: 15.4g, Protein: 24.4g

212.   Moroccan Fish

Preparation Time: 30 minutes

Cooking Time: 1 hour 25 minutes

Servings: 12

Ingredients:

- 15 oz. can Garbanzo beans
- 2 Red bell peppers
- 1 Large carrot
- 1 tbsp. Vegetable oil
- 1 Onion
- 1 clove Garlic
- 3 chopped/14.5 oz can Tomatoes

- 4 chopped Olives
- ¼ cup Chopped fresh parsley
- ¼ cup Ground cumin
- 3 tbsp. Paprika
- 2 tbsp. Chicken bouillon granules
- 1 tsp. Cayenne pepper
- Salt to your liking
- 5 lbs. Tilapia fillets

Directions:

Drain and rinse the beans. Thinly slice the carrot and onion. Mince the garlic and chop the olives. Discard the seeds from the peppers and slice them into strips.

Warm the oil in a frying pan using the medium temperature setting. Toss in the onion and garlic. Simmer them for approximately five minutes.

Fold in the bell peppers, beans, tomatoes, carrots, and olives.

Continue sautéing them for about five additional minutes.

Sprinkle the veggies with the cumin, parsley, salt, chicken bouillon, paprika, and cayenne.

Stir thoroughly and place the fish on top of the veggies.

Pour in water to cover the veggies.

Lower the heat setting and cover the pan to slowly cook until the fish is flaky (about 40 min.).

Nutrition: Calories 268, Fat: 5g, Protein: 42g

213.   **Niçoise-Style Tuna Salad with Olives & White Beans**

Preparation Time: 10 minutes
Cooking Time: 20-30 minutes
Servings: 4
Ingredients:

- ¾ lb. Green beans
- 12 oz. can Solid white albacore tuna
- 16 oz. can Great Northern beans
- 2¼ oz. Sliced black olives
- ¼ of 1 Thinly sliced medium red onion
- 4 large Hard-cooked eggs
- 1 tsp. Dried oregano
- 6 tbsp. Olive oil
- Black pepper and salt as desired
- ½ tsp. Finely grated lemon zest
- ⅓ cup Water
- 3 tbsp. Lemon juice

Directions:

Drain the can of tuna, Great Northern beans, and black olives. Trim and snap the green beans into halves. Thinly slice the red onion. Cook and peel the eggs until hard-boiled.

Pour the water and salt into a skillet and add the beans. Place a top on the pot and switch the temperature setting to high. Wait for it to boil.

Once the beans are cooking, set a timer for five minutes. Immediately, drain and add the beans to a cookie sheet with a raised edge on paper towels to cool.

Combine the onion, olives, white beans, and drained tuna. Mix them with the zest, lemon juice, oil, and oregano.

Dump the mixture over the salad and gently toss.

Adjust the seasonings to your liking. Portion the tuna-bean salad with the green beans and eggs to serve.

Nutrition: Calories 548, Fat: 30.3g, Protein: 36.3g

214. **Catfish Fillets and Rice**

Preparation Time: 10 minutes

Cooking Time: 55 minutes

Servings: 2

Ingredients:

- 2 catfish fillets, boneless
- 2 tbsps. Italian seasoning
- 2 tbsps. olive oil

For the rice:

- 1 cup brown rice
- 2 tbsps. olive oil
- 1 and ½ cups water
- ½ cup green bell pepper, chopped
- 2 garlic cloves, minced
- ½ cup white onion, chopped
- 2 tsps. Cajun seasoning
- ½ tsp garlic powder
- Salt and black pepper to the taste

Directions:

Heat up a pot with 2 tbsps. oil over medium heat, add the onion, garlic, garlic powder, salt and pepper and sauté for 5 minutes.

Add the rice, water, bell pepper and the seasoning, bring to a simmer and cook over medium heat for 40 minutes.

Heat up a pan with 2 tbsps. oil over medium heat, add the fish and the Italian seasoning, and cook for 5 minutes on each side.

Divide the rice between plates, add the fish on top and serve.
Nutrition: Calories 261, Fat: 17.6g, Fiber: 12.2g, Carbs: 24.8g, Protein: 12.5g
215.   **Halibut Pan**
Preparation Time: 10 minutes
Cooking Time: 20 minutes
Servings: 4
Ingredients:

- 4 halibut fillets, boneless
- 1 red bell pepper, chopped
- 2 tbsps. olive oil
- 1 yellow onion, chopped
- 4 garlic cloves, minced
- ½ cup chicken stock
- 1 tsp. basil, dried
- ½ cup cherry tomatoes, halved
- ⅓ cup kalamata olives, pitted and halved
- Salt and black pepper to the taste

Directions:
Heat up a pan with the oil over medium heat, add the fish, cook for 5 minutes on each side, and divide between plates.

Add the onion, bell pepper, garlic, and tomatoes to the pan, stir and sauté for 3 minutes.

Add salt, pepper and the rest of the ingredients, toss, cook for 3 minutes more, divide next to the fish, and serve.
Nutrition: Calories 253, Fat: 8g, Fiber: 1g, Carbs: 5g, Protein: 28g
216.   **Baked Shrimp Mix**
Preparation Time: 10 minutes
Cooking Time: 32 minutes
Servings: 4
Ingredients:

- 4 gold potatoes, peeled and sliced
- 2 fennel bulbs, trimmed and cut into wedges
- 2 shallots, chopped
- 2 garlic cloves, minced
- 3 tbsps. olive oil
- ½ cup kalamata olives, pitted and halved
- 2 pounds shrimp, peeled and deveined
- 1 tsp. lemon zest, grated
- 2 tsps. oregano, dried
- 4 oz. feta cheese, crumbled
- 2 tbsps. parsley, chopped

Directions:

In a roasting pan, combine the potatoes with 2 tbsps. oil, garlic, and the rest of the ingredients except the shrimp, toss, introduce in the oven and bake at 450°F for 25 minutes.

Add the shrimp, toss, bake for 7 minutes more, divide between plates, and serve.

Nutrition: Calories 341, Fat: 19g, Fiber: 9g, Carbs: 34g, Protein: 10g

217. **Shrimp and Lemon Sauce**

Preparation Time: 10 minutes

Cooking Time: 15 minutes

Servings: 4

Ingredients:

- 1 lb. shrimp, peeled and deveined
- ⅓ cup lemon juice
- 4 egg yolks
- 2 tbsps. olive oil
- 1 cup chicken stock
- Salt and black pepper to the taste
- 1 cup black olives, pitted and halved
- 1 tbsp. thyme, chopped

Directions:

In a bowl, mix the lemon juice with the egg yolks and whisk well.

Heat up a pan with the oil over medium heat, add the shrimp and cook for 2 minutes on each side and transfer to a plate.

Heat up a pan with the stock over medium heat, add some of this over the egg yolks and lemon juice mix and whisk well.

Add this over the rest of the stock, also add salt and pepper, whisk well and simmer for 2 minutes. Add the shrimp and the rest of the ingredients, toss, and serve right away.

Nutrition: Calories 237, Fat: 15.3g, Fiber: 4.6g, Carbs: 15.4g, Protein: 7.6g

218. **Shrimp and Beans Salad**

Preparation Time: 10 minutes

Cooking Time: 4 minutes

Servings: 4

Ingredients:

- 1 lb. shrimp, peeled and deveined
- 30 oz. canned cannellini beans, drained and rinsed
- 2 tbsps. olive oil
- 1 cup cherry tomatoes, halved
- 1 tsp. lemon zest, grated
- ½ cup red onion, chopped

- 4 handfuls baby arugula
- A pinch of salt and black pepper
- For the dressing:
- 3 tbsps. red wine vinegar
- 2 garlic cloves, minced
- ½ cup olive oil

Directions:

Heat up a pan with 2 tbsps. oil over medium-high heat, add the shrimp and cook for 2 minutes on each side.

In a salad bowl, combine the shrimp with the beans and the rest of the ingredients except the ones for the dressing and toss.

In a separate bowl, combine the vinegar with ½ cup oil and the garlic and whisk well.

Pour over the salad, toss, and serve right away.

Nutrition: Calories 207, Fat: 12.3g, Fiber: 6.6g, Carbs: 15.4g, Protein: 8.7g

219.   Pecan Salmon Fillets

Preparation Time: 10 minutes

Cooking Time: 15 minutes

Servings: 6

Ingredients:

- 3 tbsps. olive oil
- 3 tbsps. mustard
- 5 tsps. honey
- 1 cup pecans, chopped
- 6 salmon fillets, boneless
- 1 tbsp. lemon juice
- 3 tsps. parsley, chopped
- Salt and pepper to the taste

Directions:

In a bowl, mix the oil with the mustard and honey and whisk well.

Put the pecans and the parsley in another bowl.

Season the salmon fillets with salt and pepper, arrange them on a baking sheet lined with parchment paper, brush with the honey and mustard mix and top with the pecans mix.

Introduce in the oven at 400°F, bake for 15 minutes, divide between plates, drizzle the lemon juice on top and serve.

Nutrition: Calories 282, Fat: 15.5g, Fiber: 8.5g, Carbs: 20.9g, Protein: 16.8g

220.   Salmon and Broccoli

Preparation Time: 10 minutes

Cooking Time: 20 minutes

Servings: 4

Ingredients:

- 2 tbsps. balsamic vinegar
- 1 broccoli head, florets separated
- 4 pieces salmon fillets, skinless
- 1 big red onion, roughly chopped
- 1 tbsp. olive oil
- Sea salt and black pepper to the taste

Directions:

In a baking dish, combine the salmon with the broccoli and the rest of the ingredients, introduce in the oven and bake at 390°F for 20 minutes.

Divide the mix between plates and serve.

Nutrition: Calories 302, Fat: 15.5g, Fiber: 8.5g, Carbs: 18.9g, Protein: 19.8g

221.   **Salmon and Peach Pan**

Preparation Time: 10 minutes
Cooking Time: 11 minutes
Servings: 4
Ingredients:

- 1 tbsp. balsamic vinegar
- 1 tsp. thyme, chopped
- 1 tbsp. ginger, grated
- 2 tbsps. olive oil
- Sea salt and black pepper to the taste
- 3 peaches, cut into medium wedges
- 4 salmon fillets, boneless

Directions:

Heat up a pan with the oil over medium-high heat, add the salmon and cook for 3 minutes on each side.

Add the vinegar, the peaches, and the rest of the ingredients, cook for 5 minutes more, divide everything between plates and serve.

Nutrition: Calories 293, Fat: 17.1g, Fiber: 4.1g, Carbs: 26.4g, Protein: 24.5g

MEAT RECIPES

222.   **Greek Honey & Lemon Pork Chops**

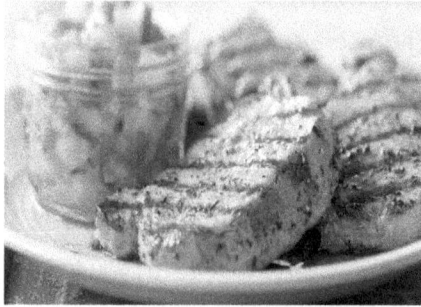

Preparation Time: 60 minutes
Cooking Time: 4 hours 20 minutes
Servings: 4
Ingredients:

- 4 Pork rib chops
- ½ tsp. Salt
- 2 tbsp. Lemon juice
- 1 tbsp. Freshly trimmed mint
- 2 tbsp. Honey
- ¼ tsp. Cayenne pepper
- 1 tbsp. Olive oil
- 2 tbsp. Shredded lemon peel

Directions:
Remove all fat from the pork chops. Snip the fresh mint and shred the lemon peel.

Slice the chops into one-inch-thick chunks and toss them into a large plastic zipper-type resealable bag.

Whisk the rest of the fixings and pour over the pork. Seal the bag.

Rotate the bag a few times and let it marinate for about four hours.

When ready to cook, prepare the grill. Grease the grilling rack with oil, and preheat the grill using the medium heat setting.

Arrange the chops on the grilling rack to grill for five to six minutes per side. The meat thermometer should reach 160°F.

Serve immediately.

Nutrition: Calories: 257, Protein: 29g, Fat: 3g

223.   Pork Stew
Preparation Time: 10 minutes
Cooking Time: 40 minutes
Servings: 6
Ingredients:

- 2 pounds pork meat, boneless and cubed
- 2 yellow onions, chopped
- 1 tbsp. olive oil
- 1 garlic clove, minced
- 3 cups chicken stock
- 2 tbsps. paprika
- 1 tsp. caraway seeds
- Salt and black pepper to taste
- ¼ cup water
- 2 tbsps. white flour
- 1 ½ cups sour cream
- 2 tbsps. dill, chopped

Directions:
Heat a pot with the oil over medium heat, add the pork and brown it for a few minutes.

Add onions, stir, and cook for 3 minutes. Add garlic, stir, and cook 1 minute.

Add stock, caraway seeds, paprika, salt and pepper, bring to a boil, reduce temperature, cover, and cook for 30 minutes.

Add flour mixed with water, stir and boil 2 minutes more.

Take off heat, add dill weed and cream, return to heat, cook the stew for 2 minutes, divide into bowls and serve.

Nutrition: Calories 300, Fat: 12g, Fiber: 4g, Carbs: 9g, Protein: 12g

224.   **Mediterranean Grilled Pork Chops**

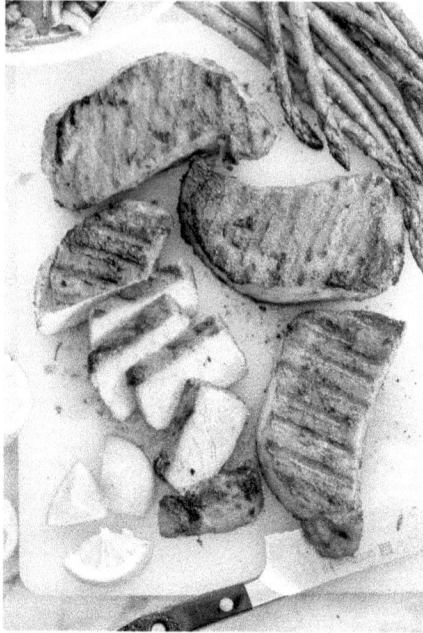

Preparation Time: 1 day
Cooking Time: 20 minutes
Servings: 6
Ingredients:

- 2 pork chops
- ¼ cup olive oil
- 2 yellow onions, sliced
- 2 garlic cloves, minced
- 2 tsps. mustard
- 1 tsp. sweet paprika
- Salt and black pepper to taste
- ½ tsp oregano, dried
- ½ tsp thyme, dried
- A pinch of cayenne pepper

Directions:

In a small bowl, mix oil with garlic, mustard, paprika, black pepper, oregano, thyme, and cayenne and whisk well.

In a bowl, combine onions with meat and mustard mix, toss to coat, cover, and keep in the fridge for 1 day. Place meat on preheated grill pan over medium high heat, season with salt and cook for 10 minutes on each side.

Meanwhile, heat a pan over medium heat, add marinated onions, stir and sauté for 4 minutes.

Divide pork chops on plates, add sautéed onions on top and serve.

Nutrition: Calories 284, Fat: 4g, Fiber: 4g, Carbs: 7g, Protein: 12g

225.   **Simple Pork Stir Fry**

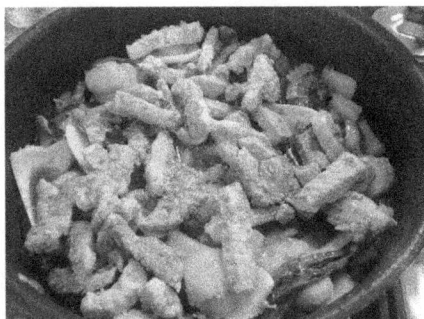

Preparation Time: 10 minutes
Cooking Time: 15 minutes
Servings: 4
Ingredients:

- 4 oz. bacon, chopped
- 4 oz. snow peas
- 2 tbsps. butter
- 1 lb. pork loin, cut into thin strips
- 2 cups mushrooms, sliced
- ¾ cup white wine
- ½ cup yellow onion, chopped
- 3 tbsps. sour cream
- Salt and white pepper to taste

Directions:

Put snow peas in a saucepan, add water to cover, add a pinch of salt, bring to a boil over medium heat, cook until they are soft, drain and leave aside.

Heat a pan over medium high heat, add bacon, cook for a few minutes, drain grease, transfer to a bowl, and also leave aside.

Heat a pan with 1 tbsp. butter over medium heat, add pork strips, salt and pepper to taste, brown for a few minutes and transfer to a plate as well.

Return pan to medium heat, add remaining butter and melt it. Add onions and mushrooms, stir, and cook for 4 minutes.

Add wine, and simmer until it's reduced. Add cream, peas, pork, salt and pepper to taste, stir, heat up, divide between plates, top with bacon and serve.

Nutrition: Calories 310, Fat: 4g, Fiber: 6g, Carbs: 9g, Protein: 10g

226.   Delicious Sausage Kebabs
Preparation Time: 1 hour
Cooking Time: 13 minutes
Servings: 6
Ingredients:

- 1 yellow onion, chopped
- 1 lb. ground pork
- 3 tbsps. parsley, chopped
- 1 tbsp. lemon juice
- 1 garlic clove, minced
- 1 tsp. oregano, dried
- 1 tsp. mint, dried
- Salt and black pepper to taste
- Vegetable oil

For the sauce:

- 2 tbsps. olive oil
- ¼ cup tahini sauce
- ¼ cup water
- 1 tbsp. lemon juice
- 1 garlic clove, minced
- Salt and cayenne pepper to taste

Directions:
In a bowl, mix ground pork with onion, parsley, 1 garlic clove, 1 tbsp. lemon juice, mint, oregano, salt and pepper to taste, stir well and divide into 6 portions.

Shape your kebabs by squeezing each portion on a skewer, cover and keep them in the fridge for 1 hour.

Heat your kitchen grill pan over medium high heat, place kebabs on it, brush them with vegetable oil, cook them for 13 minutes, turning from time to time and transfer to plates.

In a food processor, mix tahini with olive oil, 1 tbsp. lemon juice, 1 garlic clove, water, salt and cayenne pepper and blend well.

Serve your kebabs with this sauce all over.

Nutrition: Calories 250, Fat: 23g, Fiber: 1g, Carbs: 4g, Protein: 14g

227.   Mediterranean Meatloaf
Preparation Time: 10 minutes
Cooking Time: 1 hour and 20 minutes
Servings: 8
Ingredients:

- 1 yellow onion, chopped
- 2 tbsps. olive oil
- 2 garlic cloves, minced
- ¾ cup red wine
- 4 oz. white bread, chopped
- 2 pounds lamb, ground
- 1 cup milk
- ¼ cup feta cheese, crumbled
- 2 eggs
- ⅓ cup kalamata olives, pitted and chopped
- 4 tbsps. oregano, chopped
- Salt and black pepper to taste
- 2 tbsps. honey
- 1 tbsp. Worcestershire sauce
- 2 tsps. lemon zest, grated

Directions:

Heat a pan with 2 tbsps. oil over medium heat, add garlic and onion, stir and cook for 8 minutes.

Add wine, stir, simmer for 5 minutes and transfer everything to a bowl.

Put bread pieces in a bowl, add milk, leave aside for 10 minutes, squeeze bread a bit, chop and add it to onions mix.

Add lamb, eggs, cheese, olives, lemon, zest, oregano, Worcestershire sauce, salt and pepper to onions mix and stir well.

Transfer meatloaf mix to a baking dish, spread honey all over, place in the oven at 375°F and bake for 50 minutes.

Take meatloaf out of the oven, leave aside for 5 minutes, slice and arrange on a platter.

Nutrition: Calories 350, Fat: 23g, Fiber: 1g, Carbs: 17g, Protein: 24g

228. **Pork and Lentil Soup**

Preparation Time: 10 minutes

Cooking Time: 1 hour

Servings: 6

Ingredients:

- 1 small yellow onion, chopped
- 1 tbsp. olive oil
- 1 and ½ tsps. basil, chopped
- 1 and ½ tsps. ginger, grated
- 3 garlic cloves, chopped
- Salt and black pepper to taste
- ½ tsp cumin, ground
- 1 carrot, chopped
- 1 lb. pork chops, bone-in

- 3 oz. brown lentils, rinsed
- 3 cups chicken stock
- 2 tbsps. tomato paste
- 2 tbsps. lime juice
- 1 tsp. red chili flakes, crushed

Directions:
Heat a saucepan with the oil over medium heat, add garlic, onion, basil, ginger, salt, pepper and cumin, stir well and cook for 6 minutes.

Add carrots, stir, and cook 5 more minutes. Add pork and brown for a few minutes.

Add lentils, tomato paste and stock, stir, bring to a boil, cover pan and simmer for 50 minutes.

Transfer pork to a plate, discard bones, shred it and return to pan.

Add chili flakes and lime juice, stir, ladle into bowls, and serve.

Nutrition: Calories 263, Fat: 4g, Fiber: 6g, Carbs: 8g, Protein: 10g

229.   Simple Braised Pork
Preparation Time: 40 minutes
Cooking Time: 1 hour
Servings: 4
Ingredients:

- 2 pounds pork loin roast, boneless and cubed
- 5 tbsps. butter
- Salt and black pepper to taste
- 2 cups chicken stock
- ½ cup dry white wine
- 2 garlic cloves, minced
- 1 tsp. thyme, chopped
- 1 thyme spring
- 1 bay leaf
- ½ yellow onion, chopped
- 2 tbsps. white flour
- ¾ pound pearl onions
- ½ pound red grapes

Directions:
Heat a pan with 2 tbsps. butter over high heat, add pork loin, some salt and pepper, stir, brown for 10 minutes and transfer to a plate.

Add wine to the pan, bring to a boil over high heat and cook for 3 minutes.

Add stock, garlic, thyme spring, bay leaf, yellow onion and return meat to the pan, bring to a boil, cover, reduce heat to low, cook for 1 hour, strain liquid into another saucepan and transfer pork to a plate.

Put pearl onions in a small saucepan, add water to cover, bring to a boil over medium high heat, boil them for 5 minutes, drain, peel them, and leave aside for now.

In a bowl, mix 2 tbsps. butter with flour and stir well. Add ½ cup of strained cooking liquid and whisk well.

Pour this into cooking liquid, bring to a simmer over medium heat and cook for 5 minutes.

Add salt and pepper, chopped thyme, pork and pearl onions, cover, and simmer for a few minutes.

Meanwhile, heat a pan with 1 tbsp. butter, add grapes, stir, and cook them for 1-2 minutes.

Divide pork meat on plates, drizzle the sauce all over and serve with onions and grapes on the side.

Nutrition: Calories 320, Fat: 4g, Fiber: 5g, Carbs: 9g, Protein: 18g

230.   Pork and Chickpea Stew
Preparation Time: 20 minutes
Cooking Time: 8 hours
Servings: 4
Ingredients:

- 2 tbsps. white flour
- ½ cup chicken stock
- 1 tbsp. ginger, grated
- 1 tsp. coriander, ground
- 2 tsps. cumin, ground
- Salt and black pepper to taste
- 2 and ½ pounds pork butt, cubed
- 28 oz. canned tomatoes, drained and chopped
- 4 oz. carrots, chopped
- 1 red onion cut in wedges
- 4 garlic cloves, minced
- ½ cup apricots, cut in quarters
- 1 cup couscous, cooked
- 15 oz. canned chickpeas, drained
- Cilantro, chopped for Servings

Directions:

Put stock in your slow cooker. Add flour, cumin, ginger, coriander, salt, and pepper and stir.

Add tomatoes, pork, carrots, garlic, onion, and apricots, cover cooker and cook on Low for 7 hours and 50 minutes.

Add chickpeas and couscous, cover and cook for 10 more minutes. Divide on plates, sprinkle cilantro, and serve right away.

Nutrition: Calories 216, Fat: 6g, Fiber: 8g, Carbs: 10g, Protein: 20g

231.   Pork and Greens Salad
Preparation Time: 10 minutes
Cooking Time: 15 minutes
Servings: 4
Ingredients:

- 1 lb. pork chops, boneless and cut into strips
- 8 oz. white mushrooms, sliced
- ½ cup Italian dressing
- 6 cups mixed salad greens
- 6 oz. jarred artichoke hearts, drained
- Salt and black pepper to the taste
- ½ cup basil, chopped
- 1 tbsp. olive oil

Directions:
Heat a pan with the oil over medium-high heat, add the pork and brown for 5 minutes.
Add the mushrooms, stir, and sauté for 5 minutes more.
Add the dressing, artichokes, salad greens, salt, pepper, and the basil, cook for 4-5 minutes, divide everything into bowls and serve.
Nutrition: Calories 235, Fat: 6g, Fiber: 4g, Carbs: 14g, Protein: 11g

232.   Pork Strips and Rice
Preparation Time: 10 minutes
Cooking Time: 25 minutes
Servings: 4
Ingredients:

- ½ pound pork loin, cut into strips
- Salt and black pepper to taste
- 2 tbsps. olive oil
- 2 carrots, chopped
- 1 red bell pepper, chopped
- 3 garlic cloves, minced
- 2 cups veggie stock
- 1 cup basmati rice
- ½ cup garbanzo beans
- 10 black olives, pitted and sliced
- 1 tbsp. parsley, chopped

Directions:
Heat a pan with the oil over medium high heat.
Add the pork fillets, stir, cook for 5 minutes, and transfer them to a plate.

Add the carrots, bell pepper and the garlic, stir and cook for 5 more minutes.

Add the rice, the stock, beans, and the olives, stir, cook for 14 minutes, divide between plates, sprinkle the parsley on top and serve.

Nutrition: Calories 220, Fat: 12g, Fiber: 4g, Carbs: 7g, Protein: 11g

233. **Pork and Bean Stew**
Preparation Time: 20 minutes
Cooking Time: 4 hours
Servings: 4
Ingredients:

- 2 pounds pork neck
- 1 tbsp. white flour
- 1 ½ tbsps. olive oil
- 2 eggplants, chopped
- 1 brown onion, chopped
- 1 red bell pepper, chopped
- 3 garlic cloves, minced
- 1 tbsp. thyme, dried
- 2 tsps. sage, dried
- 4 oz. canned white beans, drained
- 1 cup chicken stock
- 12 oz. zucchinis, chopped
- Salt and pepper to taste
- 2 tbsps. tomato paste

Directions:
In a bowl, mix flour with salt, pepper, pork neck and toss.

Heat a pan with 2 tsps. oil over medium high heat, add pork and cook for 3 minutes on each side.

Transfer pork to a slow cooker and leave aside. Heat the remaining oil in the same pan over medium heat, add eggplant, onion, bell pepper, thyme, sage and garlic, stir and cook for 5 minutes.

Add reserved flour, stir, and cook for 1 more minute. Add to pork, then add beans, stock, tomato paste and zucchinis.

Cover and cook on High for 4 hours. Uncover, transfer to plates, and serve.

Nutrition: Calories 310, Fat: 3g, Fiber: 5g, Carbs: 8g, Protein: 12g

234. **Pork with Couscous**
Preparation Time: 10 minutes
Cooking Time: 7 hours
Servings: 6
Ingredients:

- 2 ½ pounds pork loin, boneless and trimmed
- ¾ cup chicken stock
- 2 tbsps. olive oil
- ½ tbsp sweet paprika
- 2 ¼ tsp sage, dried
- ½ tbsp garlic powder
- ¼ tsp rosemary, dried
- ¼ tsp marjoram, dried
- 1 tsp. basil, dried
- 1 tsp. oregano, dried
- Salt and black pepper to taste
- 2 cups couscous, cooked

Directions:

In a bowl, mix oil with stock, paprika, garlic powder, sage, rosemary, thyme, marjoram, oregano, salt and pepper to taste and whisk well. Put pork loin in your crock pot.

Add stock and spice mix, stir, cover, and cook on Low for 7 hours. Slice pork then return to the pot. After, toss with cooking juices.

Divide between plates and serve with couscous on the side.

Nutrition: Calories 310, Fat: 4g, Fiber: 6g, Carbs: 7g, Protein: 14g

235.   **Easy Roasted Pork Shoulder**
Preparation Time: 30 minutes
Cooking Time: 4 hours
Servings: 6
Ingredients:

- 3 tbsps. garlic, minced
- 3 tbsps. olive oil
- 4 pounds pork shoulder
- Salt and black pepper to taste

Directions:

In a bowl, mix olive oil with salt, pepper and oil and whisk well.

Brush pork shoulder with this mix, arrange in a baking dish and place in the oven at 425°F for 20 minutes.

Reduce heat to 325°F and bake for 4 hours.

Take pork shoulder out of the oven, slice and arrange on a platter. Serve with your favorite Mediterranean side salad.

Nutrition: Calories 221, Fat: 4g, Fiber: 4g, Carbs: 7g, Protein: 10g

236.   **Herb Roasted Pork**
Preparation Time: 20 minutes
Cooking Time: 2 hours
Servings: 10

Ingredients:

- 5 ½ pounds pork loin roast, trimmed, chine bone removed
- Salt and black pepper to taste
- 3 garlic cloves, minced
- 2 tbsps. rosemary, chopped
- 1 tsp. fennel, ground
- 1 tbsp. fennel seeds
- 2 tsps. red pepper, crushed
- ¼ cup olive oil

Directions:

In a food processor mix garlic with fennel seeds, fennel, rosemary, red pepper, some black pepper and the olive oil and blend until you obtain a paste.

Place pork roast in a roasting pan, spread 2 tbsps. garlic paste all over and rub well.

Season with salt and pepper, place in the oven at 400°F and bake for 1 hour.

Reduce heat to 325 ° F and bake for another 35 minutes. Carve roast into chops, divide between plates, and serve right away.

Nutrition: Calories 300, Fat: 4g, Fiber: 2g, Carbs: 6g, Protein: 15g

237.   Slow Cooked Beef Brisket

Preparation Time: 10 minutes

Cooking Time: 9 hours

Servings: 8

Ingredients:

- 6 pounds beef brisket
- 2 tbsps. cumin, ground
- 3 tbsps. rosemary, chopped
- 2 tbsps. coriander, dried
- 1 tbsp. oregano, dried
- 2 tsps. cinnamon powder
- 1 cup beef stock
- A pinch of salt and black pepper

Directions:

In a slow cooker, combine the beef with the cumin, rosemary, coriander, oregano, cinnamon, salt, pepper, and stock.

Cover and cook on low for 9 hours. Slice and serve.

Nutrition: Calories 400, Fat: 12g, Fiber: 4g, Carbs: 15g, Protein: 17g

238.   Mediterranean Beef Dish

Preparation Time: 10 minutes

Cooking Time: 15 minutes
Servings: 6
Ingredients:

- 1 lb. beef, ground
- 2 cups zucchinis, chopped
- ½ cup yellow onion, chopped
- Salt and black pepper to taste
- 15 oz. canned roasted tomatoes and garlic
- 1 cup water
- ¾ cup cheddar cheese, shredded
- 1 ½ cups white rice

Directions:

Heat a pan over medium high heat, add beef, onion, salt, pepper, and zucchini, stir, and cook for 7 minutes.

Add water, tomatoes, and garlic, stir and bring to a boil. Add rice, more salt and pepper, stir, cover, take off heat and leave aside for 7 minutes.

Divide between plates and serve with cheddar cheese on top.

Nutrition: Calories 400, Fat: 12g, Fiber: 4g, Carbs: 15g, Protein: 17g

239.   **Mixed Spice Burgers**
Preparation Time: 25 minutes
Cooking Time: 25-30 minutes
Servings: 6/2 chops each
Ingredients:

- 1 Medium onion
- 3 tbsp. Fresh parsley
- 1 Clove of garlic
- ¾ tsp. Ground allspice
- ¾ tsp. Pepper
- ¼ tsp. Ground nutmeg
- ½ tsp. Cinnamon
- ½ tsp. Salt
- 2 tbsp. Fresh mint
- 1.5 lbs. 90% lean ground beef
- Optional: Cold Tzatziki sauce

Directions:

Finely chop/mince the parsley, mint, garlic, and onions.

Whisk the nutmeg, salt, cinnamon, pepper, allspice, garlic, mint, parsley, and onion.

Add the beef and prepare six (6) 2 x 4-inch oblong patties.

Use the medium temperature setting to grill the patties or broil them four inches from the heat source for four to six minutes per side.

When they're done, the meat thermometer will register 160°F. Serve with the sauce if desired.

Nutrition: Calories: 231, Fat: 9g, Protein: 32g

240.   **Crispy Pork Carnitas**

Preparation Time: 45 minutes

Cooking Time: 3 hours 55 minutes

Servings: 6

Ingredients:

- ¼ cup Olive oil
- 3 lbs. Boneless pork butt shoulder
- 8 cloves Garlic
- 1 Orange
- 1 tbsp Kosher salt
- 2 Bay leaves
- 1 tsp Black pepper
- ½ tsp Chinese 5-spice powder
- ¾ tsp Cinnamon
- 1 tsp Ground cumin
- Also Needed: 9 x 13-inch baking dish

Directions:

Set the oven to reach 275°F.

Remove all fat from the pork, slice it into two-inch cubes, and roughly chop the fat. Tear the bay leaves into halves. Mince the garlic. Juice and slice the orange peel into thin strips.

Mix the olive oil, pork, cinnamon, orange peel, garlic, orange juice, bay leaves, black pepper, salt, cumin, and 5-spice powder in a bowl until the pork is thoroughly covered. Dump the mixture into the baking dish.

Arrange the baking dish on a baking tray and cover it tightly using a layer of foil.

Bake until the pork is fork-tender (3.5 hrs.).

Arrange the oven rack about six inches. Heat the oven using the broiler.

Place the meat in a colander placed over a bowl. Remove bay leaves, garlic, and orange peels from the baking dish.

Empty the accumulated juices from the baking dish over the meat in the colander. Return the pork to the baking dish and drizzle the accumulated juices over each piece of meat.

Broil the pork for three minutes. Drizzle more juices over the meat and continue broiling until it's crispy (3-5 min.).

Transfer the pork to a Servings plate with juices over the top and serve.

Nutrition: Calories: 317, Fat: 22.6g, Protein: 25.5g

241.   CJ's Porchetta
Preparation Time: 45 minutes
Cooking Time: 9 hours 45 minutes
Servings: 6
Ingredients:

- 2.5 lbs. Boneless pork shoulder blade roast
- Olive oil
- 1 tbsp. each Black pepper and Kosher salt - divided
- 2 tbsp. Sage leaves
- 2 tbsp. Fresh rosemary
- 6 Garlic cloves
- 2 tsp Fennel seeds
- 1 zested Orange
- 2 tsp Olive oil

For the Vinegar sauce:

- Half of 1 Anchovy fillet
- ¼ cup White wine vinegar
- 1 tsp. Red pepper flakes
- ¼ cup Italian parsley

Directions:
Lightly crush the fennel, mince the garlic, and chop the rosemary and sage.

Place the roast on a cutting block to make a lengthwise (about 1 inch from the edge of the meat - but not cutting it all the way through).

Open the meat (using a sharp knife) flat along with the cut of the roast, so that you can unroll it into a large - flat piece.

Drizzle and rub the cut surface with two tsps. of oil. Dust it with two tsps. of black pepper, salt, sage, rosemary, orange zest, crushed fennel seeds, and garlic.

Push the seasonings in firmly, roll up the roast, and tie it in several places using kitchen twine.

Place the pork roast on a baking tray and sprinkle it using the rest of the salt (1 tsp.). Place the roast in the fridge without a covering/top overnight to dry-age.

Time to Bake: Set the oven temperature at 450°F.

Lightly spritz a baking dish and add the roast. Rub the meat using two tsps. of oil.

Bake it in the hot oven until the outside is seared (15 min.).

Lower the oven temperature setting to 250°F. Roast until an instant-read meat thermometer inserted into the center of the roast reads 145°F (approx. 1 hr.).

Loosely cover the roast with foil and wait for it to rest about ten minutes. Thinly slice it before serving.

Mash the anchovy fillet and mix with the white wine vinegar, red pepper flakes, and parsley.

Stir and scoop the mixture to drizzle it over the pork.

Nutrition: Calories: 266, Fat: 19.1g, Protein: 19.8g

242.   **Delicious Pork & Orzo**
Preparation Time: 15 minutes
Cooking Time: 30 minutes
Servings: 6
Ingredients:

- 1.5 lbs. Pork tenderloin
- 2 tbsp. Olive oil
- 3 quarts Water
- 1¼ cups Uncooked orzo pasta
- ¼ tsp. Salt
- 1 tsp. Coarsely ground pepper
- 6 oz. pkg. Fresh baby spinach
- 1 cup Grape tomatoes
- ¾ cup Feta cheese

Directions:
Rub the pork in pepper and slice the pepper into one-inch cubes.

Prepare a large skillet with oil and warm using the medium temperature setting.

Toss in the pork and cook for eight to ten minutes.

Pour water and salt in a Dutch oven and wait for it to boil. Add the orzo to simmer (lid off) for eight minutes. Stir in the spinach and cook until it's wilted and tender (45-60 sec.). Drain it in a colander.

Cut the tomatoes into halves and add in with the pork and heat, adding in the orzo mixture and crumbled feta cheese.

Nutrition: Calories 372, Fat: 11g, Protein: 31g

243.   **Beef Tartar**
Preparation Time: 10 minutes
Servings: 1
Ingredients:

- 1 shallot, chopped
- 4 oz. beef fillet, minced
- 5 small cucumbers, chopped
- 1 egg yolk

- A pinch of salt and black pepper
- 2 tsps. mustard
- 1 tbsp. parsley, chopped
- 1 parsley spring, roughly chopped for Servings

Directions:
In a bowl, mix meat with shallot, egg yolk, salt, pepper, mustard, cucumbers, and parsley.

Stir well and arrange on a platter.

Garnish with the chopped parsley spring and serve.

Nutrition: Calories 210, Fat: 3g, Fiber: 1g, Carbs: 5g, Protein: 8g

244. **Delicious Lamb Chops**
Preparation Time: 10 minutes
Cooking Time: 6 minutes
Servings: 2
Ingredients:

- 1 red onion, thinly sliced
- Salt and black pepper to taste
- 2 tsps. brown sugar
- 6 lamb chops
- 1 tsp. smoked paprika
- 6 mint leaves, chopped
- 1 tbsp. olive oil

Directions:
Put the onion in a bowl, add some cold water, leave aside for 5 minutes, drain and transfer to another bowl.

Add lamb chops to the bowl, season with salt, pepper, mint, paprika and oil. Toss to coat and leave aside for 10 minutes.

Heat your kitchen grill pan over medium high heat, place lamb chops, grill them for 3 minutes on each side and transfer to a platter.

Serve with watermelon salad on the side.

Nutrition: Calories 460, Fat: 31g, Fiber: 1g, Carbs: 18g, Protein: 34g

245. **Simple and Tasty Braised Beef**
Preparation Time: 30 minutes
Cooking Time: 3 hours and 30 minutes
Servings: 6
Ingredients:
For the ribs:

- 6 beef short ribs
- 1 tbsp. thyme, chopped
- Salt and black pepper to taste

- 3 tbsps. olive oil
- 1 carrot, chopped
- 1 yellow onion, chopped
- 1 celery stalk, chopped
- 1 ½ cups ruby port
- 2 bay leaves
- 2 ½ cups red wine
- 2 tbsps. balsamic vinegar
- 6 cups beef stock
- 4 parsley sprigs
- For the salsa:
- 1 cup parsley, chopped
- 1 tsp. marjoram, chopped
- ¼ cup mint, chopped
- 1 garlic clove, minced
- 1 tbsp. capers, drained
- 1 anchovy
- ¾ cup olive oil
- Salt and black pepper to taste
- ½ cup feta cheese, crumbled

Directions:
In a bowl, mix thyme with salt and pepper, add short ribs, toss to coat, and leave aside for 30 minutes.

Heat a large saucepan with the oil over high heat, add short ribs, sear for 3 minutes on each side and transfer to a bowl.

Heat the pan again over medium heat, add celery, onion, carrot, and bay leaves, stir and cook for 8 minutes.

Add port, vinegar, and wine, stir, bring to a boil and simmer for about 10 minutes.

Add stock, return short ribs, parsley, salt and pepper, cover and bake in the oven at 325 ° F for 3 hours. Take ribs out of the oven and leave aside for 30 minutes.

In a food processor, mix 1 cup parsley with marjoram, mint, 1 garlic clove, capers, anchovy, ¾ cup olive oil, feta cheese, salt and pepper and pulse well.

Divide short ribs into bowls, add some of the cooking liquid and toss with the salsa.

Nutrition: Calories 450, Fat: 45g, Fiber: 2g, Carbs: 18g, Protein: 43g

246.   Spanish Style Spareribs
Preparation Time: 3 hours and 10 minutes
Cooking Time: 1 hour
Servings: 4
Ingredients:

- 1 rack of baby back pork ribs, trimmed
- 2 garlic cloves, minced
- 1 tsp. Spanish paprika
- 3 tbsps. red wine vinegar
- ¼ cup olive oil
- 1 tbsp. oregano, dried
- Salt and black pepper to the taste

Directions:
In a bowl, mix the pork ribs with the garlic, paprika, vinegar, oil, oregano, salt and pepper.

Mix well and refrigerate for 3 hours.

Place the ribs on your preheated BBQ and cook over medium heat for 30 minutes on each side. Serve the ribs with a side salad.

Nutrition: Calories 450, Fat: 34g, Fiber: 1g, Carbs: 2g, Protein: 35g

247.   Tunisian-Style Short Ribs
Preparation Time: 10 minutes
Cooking Time: 3 hours
Servings: 6
Ingredients:

- 3 tbsps. vegetable oil
- 12 beef short ribs
- Salt and black pepper to taste
- 1 cup onions, chopped
- 1 cup carrots, chopped
- 1 cup figs, dried and chopped
- 1 tbsp. ginger, grated
- 3-star anise
- 1 tbsp. garlic, minced
- 2 cinnamon sticks
- 1 cup canned tomatoes, crushed
- 1 cup red wine
- 1 cup chicken stock
- ¼ cup soy sauce
- 2 tbsps. mint, chopped
- 2 tbsps. parsley, chopped

Directions:
Heat a saucepan with 2 tbsps. oil over medium high heat, add short ribs, season with salt and pepper to taste, cook for 4 minutes on each side and transfer to a plate.

Add remaining oil to your saucepan and heat over medium high heat.

Add onions and carrots, salt and pepper, stir and cook for 8 minutes. Add figs, ginger, garlic, cinnamon sticks, star anise, stir and cook for 1 minute.

Add ½ cup wine, stir and cook for 1 minute. Return ribs to the pan, add tomatoes, soy sauce, the remaining wine and stock, stir, bring to a simmer, cover, and place in the oven at 325°F.

Bake for 2 hours and 50 minutes, stirring gently every 40 minutes.

Add salt, pepper, parsley, and mint.

Stir, divide into plates and serve.

Nutrition: Calories 300, Fat: 23g, Fiber: 4g, Carbs: 23g, Protein: 35g

248. **Sautéed Chorizo**

Preparation Time: 10 minutes

Cooking Time: 13 minutes

Servings: 4

Ingredients:

- 1 and 1.2 cups soft chorizo, sliced
- 3 tbsps. olive oil
- ⅓ cup dry red wine
- White bread, cubed

Directions:

Heat a pan with the olive oil over medium high heat, add chorizo, stir, and cook for 4 minutes.

Stir again and cook for 5 minutes more. Add wine, stir, and simmer for 3 minutes.

Pour this into bowls and serve with cubed bread on top.

Nutrition: Calories 340, Fat: 23g, Carbs: 2g, Protein: 21g

249. **Simple Pot Roast**

Preparation Time: 10 minutes

Cooking Time: 3 hours

Servings: 6

Ingredients:

- 2 ½ pounds pork shoulder roast, boneless
- 1 tbsp. olive oil
- Salt and black pepper to taste
- 4 shallots, chopped
- 2 cups beef stock
- 1 ½ cups red wine
- 2 tsps. herbs de provender
- 1 red onion, cut into wedges
- ⅔ cup black olives, pitted
- 12 baby carrots
- 1 cup cherry tomatoes

- 1 zucchini, chopped

Directions:
Heat a large saucepan with the oil over medium high heat; add the pork shoulder, season with salt and pepper, brown for 10 minutes and transfer to a plate.

Add shallots to the pan, stir and sauté for 4 minutes. Add the wine, stir, and simmer for 3-4 minutes.

Add the herbs, stock, and return the pork roast, cover, reduce heat to medium-low and cook for 2 hours and 30 minutes, turning the pork from time to time.

Take roast out of the pan, transfer to a platter, cover and keep warm.

Add carrots, onion and olives to the saucepan, cover and cook for 10 minutes. Add tomatoes and zucchini, cook for 10 minutes, and transfer all veggies next to the roast.

Bring cooking liquid to a boil, cook for 5 minutes, add more salt and pepper and take off heat.

Slice roast and divide between plates and drizzle the sauce on top.

Nutrition: Calories 432, Fat: 12g, Fiber: 2g, Carbs: 13g, Protein: 42g

250.   Simple Grilled Pork Chops
Preparation Time: 30 minutes
Cooking Time: 7 minutes
Servings: 4
Ingredients:

- 8 pork loin chops
- Salt and black pepper to taste
- 1 tbsp. olive oil
- ¼ cup red wine vinegar
- 1 tsp. oregano, dried
- 1 tbsp. garlic, minced
- ¼ cup sweet paprika

Directions:
In a bowl mix paprika with oregano, garlic, salt, pepper, olive oil and vinegar and whisk well.

Spread over pork chops, rub well, and leave aside for 30 minutes.

Heat your kitchen grill pan over medium high heat, place pork chops on it, cook for 3 minutes on each side, transfer to a platter and leave aside for 5 minutes.

Serve right away with your favorite side salad.

Nutrition: Calories 430, Fat: 23g, Fiber: 2g, Carbs: 4g, Protein: 45g

VEGETABLE RECIPES

251.   **Peppers and Lentils Salad**

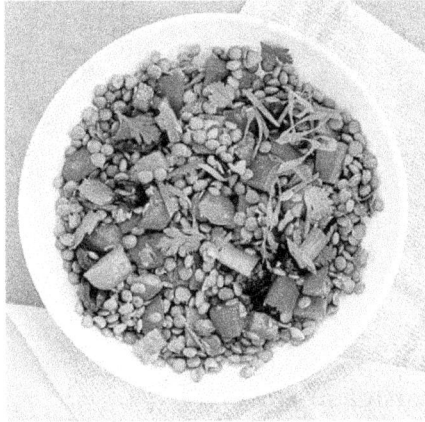

Preparation Time: 10 minutes
Cooking Time: 0 minutes
Servings: 4
Ingredients:

- 14 oz. canned lentils, drained and rinsed
- 2 spring onions, chopped
- 1 red bell pepper, chopped
- 1 green bell pepper, chopped
- 1 tbsp. fresh lime juice
- ⅓ cup coriander, chopped
- 2 tsp balsamic vinegar

Directions:
In a salad bowl, combine the lentils with the onions, bell peppers and the rest of the ingredients, toss and serve.

Nutrition: Calories 200, Fat: 2.45g, Fiber: 6.7g, Carbs: 10.5g, Protein: 5.6g

252.   **Olives and Lentils Salad**

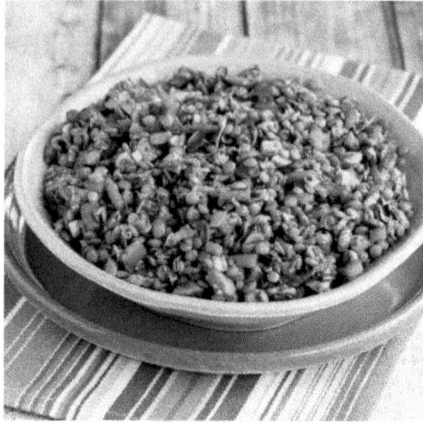

Preparation Time: 10 minutes
Cooking Time: 0 minutes
Servings: 2
Ingredients:

- ⅓ cup canned green lentils, drained and rinsed
- 1 tbsp. olive oil
- 2 cups baby spinach
- 1 cup black olives, pitted and halved
- 2 tbsps. sunflower seeds
- 1 tbsp. Dijon mustard
- 2 tbsps. balsamic vinegar
- 2 tbsps. olive oil

Directions:

In a bowl, mix the lentils with the spinach, olives, and the rest of the ingredients, toss and serve cold.

Nutrition: Calories 279, Fat: 6.5g, Fiber: 4.5g, Carbs: 9.6g, Protein: 12g

253.   Lime Spinach and Chickpeas Salad
Preparation Time: 10 minutes
Cooking Time: 0 minutes
Servings: 4
Ingredients:

- 16 oz. canned chickpeas, drained and rinsed
- 2 cups baby spinach leaves
- ½ tbsp lime juice
- 2 tbsps. olive oil
- 1 tsp. cumin, ground

- A pinch of sea salt and black pepper
- ½ tsp chili flakes

Directions:
In a bowl, mix the chickpeas with the spinach and the rest of the ingredients, toss, and serve cold.

Nutrition: Calories 240, Fat: 8.2g, Fiber: 5.3g. Carbs: 11.6g, Protein: 12g

254.   **Beans and Cucumber Salad**

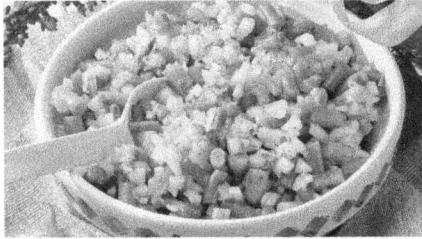

Preparation Time: 10 minutes
Cooking Time: 0 minutes
Servings: 4
Ingredients:

- 15 oz. canned great northern beans, drained and rinsed
- 2 tbsps. olive oil
- ½ cup baby arugula
- 1 cup cucumber, sliced
- 1 tbsp. parsley, chopped
- 2 tomatoes, cubed
- A pinch of sea salt and black pepper
- 2 tbsp balsamic vinegar

Directions:
In a bowl, mix the beans with the cucumber and the rest of the ingredients, toss, and serve cold.

Nutrition: Calories 233, Fat: 9g, Fiber: 6.5g, Carbs: 13g, Protein: 8g

255.   **Tomato and Avocado Salad**

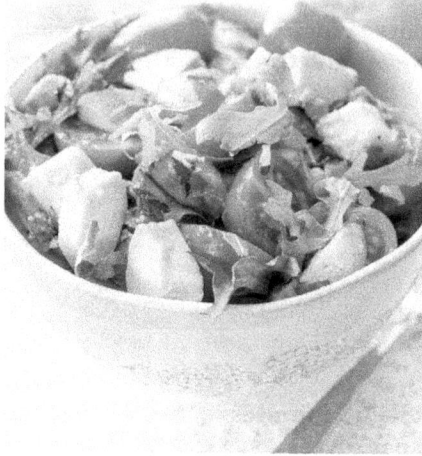

Preparation Time: 10 minutes
Cooking Time: 0 minutes
Servings: 4
Ingredients:

- 1 lb. cherry tomatoes, cubed
- 2 avocados, pitted, peeled and cubed
- 1 sweet onion, chopped
- A pinch of sea salt and black pepper
- 2 tbsps. lemon juice
- 1 and ½ tbsps. olive oil
- A handful basil, chopped

Directions:
In a salad bowl, mix the tomatoes with the avocados and the rest of the ingredients, toss, and serve right away.

Nutrition: Calories 148, Fat: 7.8g, Fiber: 2.9g, Carbs: 5.4g, Protein: 5.5g

256.   Corn and Tomato Salad
Preparation Time: 10 minutes
Cooking Time: 0 minutes
Servings: 4
Ingredients:

- 2 avocados, pitted, peeled and cubed
- 1 pint of mixed cherry tomatoes, halved:
- 2 tbsps. avocado oil
- 1 tbsp. lime juice
- ½ tsp lime zest, grated
- A pinch of salt and black pepper
- ¼ cup dill, chopped

Directions:

In a salad bowl, mix the avocados with the tomatoes and the rest of the ingredients, toss, and serve cold.

Nutrition: Calories 188, Fat: 7.3g, Fiber: 4.9g, Carbs: 6.4g, Protein: 6.5g

257.   **Orange and Cucumber Salad**

Preparation Time: 10 minutes

Cooking Time: 0 minutes

Servings: 4

Ingredients:

- 2 cucumbers, sliced
- 1 orange, peeled and cut into segments
- 1 cup cherry tomatoes, halved
- 1 small red onion, chopped
- 3 tbsps. olive oil
- 4 ½ tsps. balsamic vinegar
- Salt and black pepper to the taste
- 1 tbsp. lemon juice

Directions:

In a bowl, mix the cucumbers with the orange and the rest of the ingredients, toss, and serve

Nutrition: Calories 102, Fat: 7.5g, Fiber: 3g, Carbs: 6.1g, Protein: 3.4g

258.   **Parsley and Corn Salad**

Preparation Time: 10 minutes

Cooking Time: 0 minutes

Servings: 4

Ingredients:

- 1 ½ tsps. balsamic vinegar
- 2 tbsps. lime juice
- 2 tbsps. olive oil
- A pinch of sea salt and black pepper
- Black pepper to the taste
- 4 cups corn
- ½ cup parsley, chopped

- 2 spring onions, chopped

Directions:
In a salad bowl, combine the corn with the onions and the rest of the ingredients, toss and serve cold.
   Nutrition: Calories 121, Fat: 9.5g, Fiber: 1.8g, Carbs: 4.1g, Protein: 1.9g
259.   **Lettuce and Onions Salad**
Preparation Time: 10 minutes
Cooking Time: 0 minutes
Servings: 4
Ingredients:

- ¼ cup lime juice
- 1 garlic clove, minced
- Salt and black pepper to the taste
- 2 tbsps. olive oil
- 1 green head lettuce, chopped
- 2 red onions, chopped
- 4 tomatoes, chopped
- ½ cup cilantro, chopped

Directions:
In a bowl, mix the lettuce with the onions and the rest of the ingredients, toss, and serve right away.
   Nutrition: Calories 103, Fat: 3g, Fiber: 2g, Carbs: 3g, Protein: 2g
260.   **Sweet Potato and Eggplant Mix**
Preparation Time: 10 minutes
Cooking Time: 15 minutes
Servings: 4
Ingredients:

- 2 baby eggplants, cubed
- 2 sweet potatoes, cubed
- 1 tbsp. olive oil
- 1 red onion, cut into wedges
- 1 tsp. hot paprika
- 2 tsps. cumin, ground
- Salt and black pepper to the taste
- 4 cups baby spinach
- ¼ cup lime juice

Directions:
Heat up a pan with the oil over medium-high heat, add the eggplants and the potatoes and sauté for 5 minutes.

Add the rest of the ingredients except the spinach, toss and cook for 10 minutes more.

Add the spinach, toss, divide into bowls and serve.

Nutrition: Calories 200, Fat: 8.3g, Fiber: 3.4g, Carbs: 12.4g, Protein: 4.5g

261.   Tomato and Beans Salad

Preparation Time: 10 minutes

Cooking Time: 0 minutes

Servings: 4

Ingredients:

- 2 tomatoes, cubed
- 2 cups canned black beans, drained and rinsed
- 1 garlic clove, minced
- 1 yellow onion, chopped
- 1 tbsp. olive oil
- Salt and black pepper to the taste
- ¼ tsp cumin, ground

Directions:

In a bowl, combine the tomatoes with the beans and the other ingredients, toss and serve.

Nutrition: Calories 200, Fat: 8.7g, Fiber: 3.4g, Carbs: 6.5g, Protein: 5.4g

262.   Cheese Avocado Salad

Preparation Time: 10 minutes

Cooking Time: 0 minutes

Servings: 4

Ingredients:

- Salt and black pepper to the taste
- 1 tbsp. olive oil
- 2 avocadoes, pitted, peeled and cubed
- ½ tsp lime juice
- 2 oz. feta cheese, crumbled
- 2 scallions, chopped
- 1 tbsp. mint, chopped

Directions:

In a salad bowl, combine the avocados with the scallions and the rest of the ingredients, toss and serve right away.

Nutrition: Calories 222, Fat: 2.4g, Fiber: 3.4g, Carbs: 12.4g, Protein: 4.5g

263.   Mozzarella and Pears Salad

Preparation Time: 10 minutes

Cooking Time: 0 minutes

Servings: 4

Ingredients:

- 1 ½ tsps. orange zest, grated
- ¼ cup orange juice
- 3 tbsps. balsamic vinegar
- 2 tbsps. olive oil
- Salt and black pepper to the taste
- 1 romaine lettuce head, torn
- 2 pears, cored and cut into medium wedges
- 4 oz. mozzarella, shredded

Directions:
In a salad bowl, combine the lettuce with the pears and the other ingredients, toss and serve cold.

Nutrition: Calories 200, Fat: 4.5g, Fiber: 4.2g, Carbs: 10.4g, Protein: 3.4g

264.   Radish and Corn Salad
Preparation Time: 10 minutes
Cooking Time: 0 minutes
Servings: 2
Ingredients:

- 1 tbsp. lemon juice
- 1 jalapeno, chopped
- 2 tbsps. olive oil
- ¼ tsp oregano, dried
- A pinch of sea salt and black pepper
- 2 cups fresh corn
- 6 radishes, sliced

Directions:
In a salad bowl, combine the corn with the radishes and the rest of the ingredients, toss and serve cold.

Nutrition: Calories 134, Fat: 4.5g, Fiber: 1.8g, Carbs: 4.1g, Protein: 1.9g

265.   Arugula and Corn Salad
Preparation Time: 10 minutes
Cooking Time: 0 minutes
Servings: 4
Ingredients:

- 1 red bell pepper, thinly sliced
- 2 cups corn
- Juice of 1 lime
- Zest of 1 lime, grated
- 8 cups baby arugula

- A pinch of sea salt and black pepper

Directions:
In a salad bowl, mix the corn with the arugula and the rest of the ingredients, toss, and serve cold.
Nutrition: Calories 172, Fat: 8.5g, Fiber: 1.8g, Carbs: 5.1g, Protein: 1.4g
266. **Balsamic Bulgur Salad**
Preparation Time: 30 minutes
Cooking Time: 0 minutes
Servings: 4
Ingredients:

- 1 cup bulgur
- 2 cups hot water
- 1 cucumber, sliced
- A pinch of sea salt and black pepper
- 2 tbsps. lemon juice
- 2 tbsps. balsamic vinegar
- ¼ cup olive oil

Directions:
In a bowl, mix bulgur with the water, cover, leave aside for 30 minutes, fluff with a fork and transfer to a salad bowl.
Add the rest of the ingredients, toss, and serve.
Nutrition: Calories 171, Fat: 5.1g, Fiber: 6.1g, Carbs: 11.3g, Protein: 4.4g
267. **Lettuce and Cucumber Salad**
Preparation Time: 10 minutes
Cooking Time: 0 minutes
Servings: 4
Ingredients:

- 2 tbsps. olive oil
- 2 cucumbers, sliced
- 1 romaine lettuce head, torn
- 1 medium tomato, chopped
- ½ tsp sumac
- 1 cup parsley, chopped
- Juice of 1 lime

Directions:
In a bowl, mix the cucumbers with the lettuce and the rest of the ingredients, toss, and serve.
Nutrition: Calories 133, Fat: 5.1g, Fiber: 1.1g, Carbs: 1.3g, Protein: 4.4g
268. **Dill Cucumber and Tomato Salad**

Preparation Time: 20 minutes
Cooking Time: 0 minutes
Servings: 6
Ingredients:

- 1 lb. tomatoes, cubed
- 1 lb. cucumbers, chopped
- 1 red onion, sliced
- 2 tbsps. dill, chopped
- Salt and black pepper to the taste
- 3 tbsps. olive oil
- 3 tbsps. lemon juice

Directions:
In a large salad bowl mix the tomatoes with the cucumbers and the rest of the ingredients, toss, and serve after keeping in the fridge for 20 minutes.
Nutrition: Calories 70, Fat: 1.8g, Fiber: 1.1g, Carbs: 4.4g, Protein: 6.6g

269.   Corn, Carrot and Rice Salad
Preparation Time: 10 minutes
Cooking Time: 0 minutes
Servings: 4
Ingredients:

- ½ cup brown rice, cooked
- 2 tbsps. olive oil
- 1 red onion, sliced
- 2 carrots, grated
- ½ cup mint, chopped
- Juice of 1 lime
- ½ cup corn
- Salt and black pepper to the taste

Directions:
In a salad bowl, combine the rice with the onion and the rest of the ingredients, toss and serve cold.
Nutrition: Calories 145, Fat: 5.8g, Fiber: 6.1g, Carbs: 9.4g, Protein: 6.6g

270.   Cashews and Red Cabbage Salad
Preparation Time: 10 minutes
Cooking Time: 0 minutes
Servings: 4
Ingredients:

- 1 lb. red cabbage, shredded
- 2 tbsps. coriander, chopped

- ½ cup cashews, halved
- 2 tbsps. olive oil
- 1 tomato, cubed
- A pinch of salt and black pepper
- 1 tbsp. white vinegar

Directions:
In a salad bowl, combine the cabbage with the coriander and the rest of the ingredients, toss and serve cold.
Nutrition: Calories 210, Fat: 6.3g, Fiber: 5.2g, Carbs: 5.5g, Protein: 8g
271. **Apples and Pomegranate Salad**
Preparation Time: 10 minutes
Cooking Time: 0 minutes
Servings: 4
Ingredients:

- 3 big apples, cored and cubed
- 1 cup pomegranate seeds
- 3 cups baby arugula
- 1 cup walnuts, chopped
- 1 tbsp. olive oil
- 1 tsp. white sesame seeds
- 2 tbsps. apple cider vinegar
- Salt and black pepper to the taste

Directions:
In a bowl, mix the apples with the arugula and the rest of the ingredients, toss, and serve cold.
Nutrition: Calories 160, Fat: 4.3g, Fiber: 5.3g, Carbs: 8.7g, Protein: 10g
272. **Cranberry Bulgur Mix**
Preparation Time: 10 minutes
Cooking Time: 0 minutes
Servings: 4
Ingredients:

- 1 ½ cups hot water
- 1 cup bulgur
- Juice of ½ lemon
- 4 tbsps. cilantro, chopped
- ½ cup cranberries, chopped
- 1 ½ tsps. curry powder
- ¼ cup green onions, chopped
- ½ cup red bell peppers, chopped
- ½ cup carrots, grated

- 1 tbsp. olive oil
- A pinch of salt and black pepper

Directions:
Put bulgur into a bowl, add the water, stir, cover, leave aside for 10 minutes, fluff with a fork and transfer to a bowl.

Add the rest of the ingredients, toss, and serve cold.

Nutrition: Calories 300, Fat: 6.4g, Fiber: 6.1g, Carbs: 7.6g, Protein: 13g

273.   Peas and Couscous Salad
Preparation Time: 10 minutes
Cooking Time: 0 minutes
Servings: 6
Ingredients:

- 2 cups couscous, cooked
- 3 tbsps. olive oil
- 1 cup sweet peas
- ¼ cup parsley, chopped
- 1 tbsp. mint, chopped
- Salt and black pepper to the taste

Directions:
In a salad bowl, combine the couscous with the peas, and the other ingredients, toss and serve.

Nutrition: Calories 210, Fat: 2g, Fiber: 2g, Carbs: 4g, Protein: 7g

274.   Yogurt Cucumber Salad
Preparation Time: 1 hour
Cooking Time: 0 minutes
Servings: 4
Ingredients:

- 2 garlic cloves, minced
- Salt and white pepper to the taste
- 1 tbsp. wine vinegar
- 1 cup Greek yogurt
- 1 tbsp. dill, chopped
- 3 medium cucumbers, sliced
- 1 tbsp. avocado oil
- 1 tbsp. chives, chopped

Directions:
In a bowl, mix the cucumbers with the garlic, salt, pepper, and the rest of the ingredients, toss and keep in the fridge for 1 hour before serving.

Nutrition: Calories 210, Fat: 11.3g, Fiber: 6.4g, Carbs: 7.5g, Protein: 3.4g

275.   **Greek Potato and Corn Salad**
Preparation Time: 10 minutes
Cooking Time: 20 minutes
Servings: 2
Ingredients:

- 2 medium potatoes, peeled and cubed
- 2 shallots, chopped
- 1 tbsp. olive oil
- 2 cups corn
- 1 tbsp. dill, chopped
- 1 tbsp. balsamic vinegar
- Salt and black pepper to the taste

Directions:
Put the potatoes in a pot, add water to cover, bring to a simmer over medium heat, cook for 20 minutes, drain and transfer to a bowl.

Add the shallots and the other ingredients, toss, and serve cold.

Nutrition: Calories 198, Fat: 5.3g, Fiber: 6.5g, Carbs: 11.6g, Protein: 4.5g

276.   **Parsley Tomato Mix**
Preparation Time: 10 minutes
Cooking Time: 10 minutes
Servings: 4
Ingredients:

- 4 medium tomatoes, roughly cubed
- 1 garlic clove, minced
- 1 tbsp. olive oil
- ½ tsp sweet paprika
- Salt and black pepper to the taste
- ½ bunch parsley, chopped

Directions:
Heat up a pot with the olive oil over medium heat, add the tomatoes and the garlic and sauté for 5 minutes.

Add the rest of the ingredients, toss, cook for 3-4 minutes more, divide into bowls, and serve.

Nutrition: Calories 220, Fat: 9.4g, Fiber: 5.3g, Carbs: 6.5g, Protein: 4.6g

277.   **Garlic Cucumber Mix**
Preparation Time: 15 minutes
Cooking Time: 0 minutes
Servings: 4
Ingredients:

- 2 cucumbers, sliced
- 2 spring onions, chopped
- 2 tbsps. olive oil
- 3 garlic cloves, grated
- 1 tbsp. thyme, chopped
- Salt and black pepper to the taste
- 3 ½ oz. goat cheese, crumbled

Directions:
In a salad bowl, mix the cucumbers with the onions and the rest of the ingredients, toss, and serve after keeping it in the fridge for 15 minutes.
Nutrition: Calories 140, Fat: 5.4g, Fiber: 4.3g, Carbs: 6.5g, Protein: 4.8g
278. **Jalapeno Tomato salad**
Preparation Time: 10 minutes
Cooking Time: 0 minutes
Servings: 4
Ingredients:

- 6 big tomatoes, peeled and cut into wedges
- 2 tbsps. olive oil
- 1 yellow onion, chopped
- 2 jalapenos, chopped
- 1 green bell pepper, chopped
- 2 garlic cloves, minced
- Salt and black pepper to the taste
- A splash of balsamic vinegar
- 1 tbsp. basil, chopped

Directions:
In a salad bowl, combine the tomatoes with the jalapeno, onion, and the rest of the ingredients, toss and serve right away.
Nutrition: Calories 200 Fat 5.6 Fiber 3.4 Carbs 11.5 Protein 6.5
279. **Broccoli and Mushroom Salad**
Preparation Time: 10 minutes
Cooking Time: 0 minutes
Servings: 4
Ingredients:

- ½ pound white mushrooms, sliced
- 1 broccoli head, florets separated and steamed
- 1 garlic clove, minced
- 1 tbsp. balsamic vinegar
- 1 yellow onion, chopped
- 1 tbsp. olive oil

- A pinch of sea salt and black pepper
- A pinch of red pepper flakes

Directions:
In a bowl, mix the broccoli with the mushrooms and the other ingredients, toss, and serve cold.

Nutrition: Calories 183, Fat: 6.5g, Fiber: 4.2g, Carbs: 8.5g, Protein: 4g

280.   Avocado and Mushroom Mix
Preparation Time: 10 minutes
Cooking Time: 10 minutes
Servings: 4
Ingredients:

- 1 yellow onion, chopped
- 1 tbsp. balsamic vinegar
- 2 tbsps. olive oil
- 12 oz. mushrooms, sliced
- 2 avocados, pitted, peeled and cubed
- 1 garlic clove, minced
- A pinch of salt and black pepper

Directions:
Heat up a pan with half of the oil over medium-high heat, add the mushrooms, sauté for 10 minutes and transfer to a bowl.

Add the rest of the ingredients, toss, and serve.

Nutrition: Calories 187, Fat: 4.3g, Fiber: 4.2g, Carbs: 11.6g, Protein: 4g

281.   Saffron Zucchini Mix
Preparation Time: 10 minutes
Cooking Time: 10 minutes
Servings: 4
Ingredients:

- 2 zucchinis, sliced
- A pinch of sea salt and black pepper
- 1 tbsp. white vinegar
- 1 tbsp. olive oil
- 1 tsp. saffron powder

Directions:
Heat up a pan with the oil over medium heat, add the zucchinis and sauté for 8 minutes.

Add the rest of the ingredients, toss, cook for 2 minutes more, divide between plates, and serve.

Nutrition: Calories 150, Fat: 5.2g, Fiber: 4.3g, Carbs: 5g, Protein: 4g

282.   **Hemp and Cucumber Salad**
Preparation Time: 10 minutes
Cooking Time: 0 minutes
Servings: 2
Ingredients:

- 2 cucumbers, roughly cubed
- 2 green onions, chopped
- 1 tbsp. dill, chopped
- 1 tbsp. lemon juice
- A pinch of sea salt and black pepper
- ½ cup hemp seeds
- A drizzle of olive oil

Directions:
In a salad bowl, combine the cucumbers with the onions and the rest of the ingredients, toss and serve cold.
Nutrition: Calories 153, Fat: 4g, Fiber: 5g, Carbs: 6g, Protein: 3.4g

283.   **Minty Cauliflower Mix**
Preparation Time: 10 minutes
Cooking Time: 0 minutes
Servings: 2
Ingredients:

- ½ cups walnuts, chopped
- 2 cups cauliflower florets, steamed
- 1 tsp. ginger, grated
- 1 garlic clove, minced
- 1 tbsp. mint, chopped
- Juice of ½ lemon
- A pinch of sea salt and black pepper

Directions:
In a salad bowl, combine the cauliflower with the walnuts and the rest of the ingredients, toss and serve.
Nutrition: Calories 199, Fat: 5.6g, Fiber: 4.5g, Carbs: 8.4g, Protein: 3.5g

284.   **Leeks Salad**
Preparation Time: 10 minutes
Cooking Time: 0 minutes
Servings: 4
Ingredients:

- 1 tbsp. olive oil
- 4 leeks, sliced

- 3 garlic cloves, grated
- A pinch of sea salt and white pepper
- ½ tsp apple cider vinegar
- A drizzle of olive oil
- 1 tbsp. dill, chopped

Directions:

In a salad bowl, combine the leeks with the garlic and the rest of the ingredients, toss and serve cold.

Nutrition: calories 71, fat 2.1, fiber 1.1, carbs 1.3, protein 2.4

285.   **Snow Peas Salad**

Preparation Time: 6 hours

Cooking Time: 10 minutes

Servings: 4

Ingredients:

- 3 cups snow peas, trimmed
- 1 and ¼ cup bean sprouts
- 1 tbsp. basil, chopped
- 1 tbsp. lime juice
- 1 tsp. ginger, grated
- 2 spring onions, chopped
- 2 garlic cloves, minced

Directions:

Put the snow peas in a pot, add water to cover, bring to a simmer and cook over medium heat for 10 minutes.

Drain the peas, transfer them to a bowl, add the sprouts and the rest of the ingredients, toss, and keep in the fridge for 6 hours before Servings.

Nutrition: Calories 200, Fat: 8.6g, Fiber: 3g, Carbs: 5.4g, Protein: 3.4g

286.   **Parsley Couscous and Cherries Salad**

Preparation Time: 10 minutes

Cooking Time: 0 minutes

Servings: 6

Ingredients:

- 2 cups hot water
- 1 cup couscous
- ½ cup walnuts, roasted and chopped
- ½ cup cherries, pitted
- ½ cup parsley, chopped
- A pinch of sea salt and black pepper
- 1 tbsp. lime juice
- 2 tbsps. olive oil

Directions:

Put the couscous in a bowl, add the hot water, cover, leave aside for 10 minutes, fluff with a fork and transfer to a bowl.

Add the rest of the ingredients, toss, and serve.

Nutrition: Calories 200, Fat: 6.71g, Fiber: 7.3g, Carbs: 8.5g, Protein: 5g

287.   **Mango and Cucumber Salad**

Preparation Time: 10 minutes

Cooking Time: 0 minutes

Servings: 4

Ingredients:

- 1 avocado, pitted, peeled and chopped
- ½ pound cucumbers, sliced
- 2 mangos, peeled and cubed
- 1 tbsp. olive oil
- 1 garlic clove, minced
- 2 tbsps. lime juice
- 1 tsp. mustard
- A pinch of salt and black pepper

Directions:

In a salad bowl, combine the cucumbers with the mangos and the rest of the ingredients, toss and serve.

Nutrition: Calories 190, Fat: 6g, Fiber: 2g, Carbs: 6.6g, Protein: 8g

288.   **Fennel and Zucchini Mix**

Preparation Time: 10 minutes

Cooking Time: 15 minutes

Servings: 4

Ingredients:

- 1 cup fennel bulb, chopped
- 1 sweet onion, chopped
- 1 tbsp. olive oil
- 3 garlic cloves, minced
- 5 cups zucchini, roughly cubed
- 1 cup veggie stock
- Salt and black pepper the taste
- 2 tsps. white wine vinegar
- 1 tsp. lemon juice

Directions:

Heat up a pan with the oil over medium heat, add the onion and the garlic, toss and sauté for 5 minutes.

Add the rest of the ingredients, toss, cook for 10 minutes more, divide into bowls, and serve.

Nutrition: Calories 193, Fat: 3g, Fiber: 2.4g, Carbs: 3g, Protein: 2.3g

289.   Bell Peppers Salad

Preparation Time: 10 minutes

Cooking Time: 0 minutes

Servings: 6

Ingredients:

- 2 green bell peppers, cut into thick strips
- 2 red bell peppers, cut into thick strips
- 2 tbsps. olive oil
- 1 garlic clove, minced
- ½ cup goat cheese, crumbled
- A pinch of salt and black pepper

Directions:

In a bowl, mix the bell peppers with the garlic and the other ingredients, toss, and serve.

Nutrition: Calories 193, Fat: 4.5g, Fiber: 2g, Carbs: 4.3g, Protein: 3g

290.   Zucchini and Corn

Preparation Time: 10 minutes

Cooking Time: 15 minutes

Servings: 4

Ingredients:

- Salt and black pepper to the taste
- 2 tbsps. olive oil
- 2 zucchinis, quartered and cubed
- 1 yellow onion, chopped
- 1 cup corn kernels
- 3 tbsps. mint, chopped
- 2 tsps. balsamic vinegar

Directions:

Heat up a pan with the oil over medium-high heat, add the zucchinis and sauté for 5 minutes.

Add the rest of the ingredients, toss, cook for 10 minutes more, divide into bowls, and serve.

Nutrition: Calories 120, Fat: 1.8g, Fiber: 1.1g, Carbs: 1.4g, Protein: 2.6g

291.   Lime Beans Salad

Preparation Time: 1 hour

Cooking Time: 0 minutes

Servings: 4

Ingredients:

- 10 oz. canned cannellini beans, drained and rinsed
- 15 oz. canned kidney beans, drained
- Salt and black pepper to the taste
- 1 garlic clove, minced
- 10 oz. corn
- ½ cup olive oil
- 1 red onion, chopped
- 2 tbsps. lime juice
- ½ tbsp cumin, ground
- ¼ cup cilantro, chopped

Directions:
In a bowl, mix the beans with salt, pepper, the garlic, and the rest of the ingredients, toss and serve.

Nutrition: Calories 190, Fat: 11.8g, Fiber: 4.1g, Carbs: 5.4g, Protein: 6.6g

292.   **Lemony Arugula Salad**
Preparation Time: 10 minutes
Cooking Time: 0 minutes
Servings: 4
Ingredients:

- 1 tbsp. capers, drained and chopped
- 1 ½ tbsps. balsamic vinegar
- 1 tsp. lemon zest, grated
- 1 tbsp. lemon juice
- 1 tbsp. olive oil
- 1 tsp. parsley, chopped
- Salt and black pepper to the taste
- 4 cups baby arugula

Directions:
In a salad bowl, combine the arugula with the capers and the rest of the ingredients, toss and serve.

Nutrition: Calories 143, Fat: 3g, Fiber: 1.2g, Carbs: 3.4g, Protein: 4.5g

293.   **Raisins, Endives and Herbs Salad**
Preparation Time: 10 minutes
Cooking Time: 0 minutes
Servings: 4
Ingredients:

- 2 tbsps. olive oil
- 1 cup raisins

- 2 tbsps. lemon juice
- ¼ cup chives, chopped
- ¾ cup parsley, chopped
- ¼ cup cilantro, chopped
- Salt and black pepper to the taste
- 1 cup endives, shredded
- ¼ cup dill, chopped
- ¼ cup mint leaves, torn
- 1 tbsp. sesame seeds, toasted

Directions:
1. In a salad bowl, combine the raisins with the lemon juice, oil, chives, and the rest of the ingredients, toss and serve cold.
Nutrition: Calories 63, Fat: 2.7g, Fiber: 0.4g, Carbs: 2.8g, Protein: 0.7g

294.   Radish Salad
Preparation Time: 10 minutes
Cooking Time: 0 minutes
Servings: 4
Ingredients:

- 1 tbsp. lemon zest, grated
- Salt and black pepper to the taste
- 2 tbsps. parsley, chopped
- A drizzle of olive oil
- 1 lb. red radishes, roughly cubed
- 1 small red onion, thinly sliced
- ⅓ cup black olives, pitted and halved
- Salt and black pepper to the taste
- 1 tsp. oregano, chopped

Directions:
In a salad bowl, combine the radishes with the onion, olives, and the rest of the ingredients, toss and serve cold.
Nutrition: Calories 68, Fat: 4.2g, Fiber: 2.3g, Carbs: 3.4g, Protein: 2.4g

295.   Capers and Spinach Salad
Preparation Time: 10 minutes
Cooking Time: 0 minutes
Servings: 4
Ingredients:

- 3 garlic cloves, minced
- 2 ½ tbsps. olive oil
- 2 tsps. balsamic vinegar
- 1 tbsp. oregano, chopped

- Salt and black pepper to the taste
- 2 tbsps. parsley, chopped
- 1 tbsp. capers, chopped
- 1 tsp. thyme, chopped
- ¼ tsp red chili flakes
- 4 cups baby spinach

Directions:
In a bowl, mix the spinach with the capers, garlic, and the other ingredients, toss and serve cold.
Nutrition: Calories 92, Fat: 3.4g, Fiber: 2.3g, Carbs: 2.9g, Protein: 2.3g
296.   **Orange Potato Salad**
Preparation Time: 10 minutes
Cooking Time: 40 minutes
Servings: 4
Ingredients:

- 4 sweet potatoes
- 3 tbsps. olive oil
- ⅓ cup orange juice
- ½ tsp sumac, ground
- 1 tbsp. red wine vinegar
- Salt and black pepper to the taste
- 1 tbsp. orange zest, grated
- 2 tbsps. mint, chopped
- ⅓ cup walnuts, chopped
- ⅓ cup pomegranate seeds

Directions:
Put the potatoes on a lined baking sheet, introduce them in the oven at 350°F, bake for 40 minutes, cool them down, peel, cut into wedges and transfer to a bowl.
Add the rest of the ingredients, toss, and serve cold.
Nutrition: Calories 138, Fat: 3.5g, Fiber: 6.2g, Carbs: 10.4g, Protein: 6.5g
297.   **Spinach and Avocado Salad**
Preparation Time: 5 minutes
Cooking Time: 0 minutes
Servings: 4
Ingredients:

- 2 tbsps. olive oil
- 3 tbsps. balsamic vinegar
- 1 tsp. basil, dried
- 3 avocados, peeled, pitted and cubed

- 2 cups baby spinach
- Salt and black pepper to the taste
- 1 small red onion, chopped
- 1 tbsp. dill, chopped

Directions:
In a bowl, mix the avocados with the spinach, basil, and the rest of the ingredients, toss, and serve right away.
Nutrition: Calories 53, Fat: 0.3g, Fiber: 0.5g, Carbs: 11g, Protein: 1g
298.   **Mint Cabbage Salad**
Preparation Time: 10 minutes
Cooking Time: 0 minutes
Servings: 4
Ingredients:

- 1 small red onion, chopped
- 1 tbsp. olive oil
- 2 tbsps. lemon juice
- 1 tbsp. lemon zest, grated
- Salt and black pepper to the taste
- 1 green cabbage head, shredded
- ½ cup mint, chopped
- ¼ cup pistachios, chopped

Directions:
In a salad bowl, combine the cabbage with the mint, pistachios, and the rest of the ingredients, toss and serve cold.
Nutrition: Calories 101, Fat: 4.1g, Fiber: 3.1g, Carbs: 4.5g, Protein: 4.6g
299.   **Carrot Salad**
Preparation Time: 5 minutes
Cooking Time: 0 minutes
Servings: 4
Ingredients:

- Juice of 1 lime
- 2 tbsps. olive oil
- 1 tsp. ginger, grated
- 1 tbsp. balsamic vinegar
- 8 carrots, peeled and roughly grated
- Salt and black pepper to the taste
- ½ cup almonds, toasted and sliced
- ½ cup mint, chopped
- 1 tbsp. sumac, ground

Directions:
In a bowl, mix the carrots with the almonds, mint, sumac, and the rest of the ingredients, toss and serve cold.
Nutrition: Calories 100, Fat: 4g, Fiber: 4g, Carbs: 1g, Protein: 4g

SNACKS

300.   **Tzatziki**

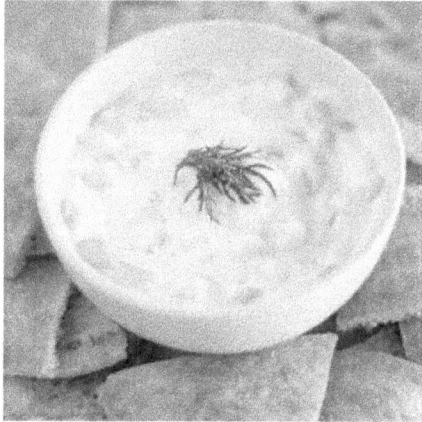

Preparation Time: 10 minutes
Cooking Time: 0 minutes
Servings: 4
Ingredients:

- 1 large cucumber, trimmed
- 3 oz Greek yogurt
- 1 tsp. olive oil
- 3 tbsps. fresh dill, chopped
- 1 tbsp. lime juice
- ¾ tsp salt
- 1 garlic clove, minced

Directions:
Grate the cucumber and squeeze the juice from it.
Then place the squeezed cucumber in the bowl.
Add Greek yogurt, olive oil, dill, lime juice, salt, and minced garlic.
Mix up the mixture until homogenous.
Store tzatziki in the fridge up to 2 days.
Nutrition: Calories 44, Fat: 1.8g, Fiber: 0.7g, Carbs: 5.1g, Protein: 3.2g

301.   **Kale Wraps with Apple and Chicken**

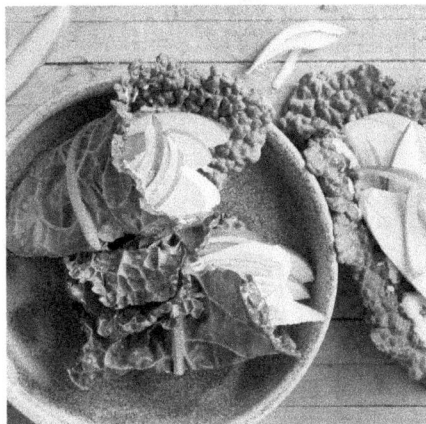

Preparation Time: 10 minutes
Cooking Time: 10 minutes
Servings: 4
Ingredients:

- 4 kale leaves
- 4 oz chicken fillet
- ½ apple
- 1 tbsp. butter
- ¼ tsp chili pepper
- ¾ tsp salt
- 1 tbsp. lemon juice
- ¾ tsp dried thyme

Directions:
Chop the chicken fillet into the small cubes. Then mix up together chicken with chili pepper and salt.

Heat up butter in the skillet. Add chicken cubes. Roast them for 4 minutes.

Meanwhile, chop the apple into small cubes and add it in the chicken.

Mix up well.

Sprinkle the ingredients with lemon juice and dried thyme.

Cook them for 5 minutes over the medium-high heat.

Fill the kale leaves with the hot chicken mixture and wrap.

Nutrition: Calories 106, Fat: 5.1g, Fiber: 1.1g, Carbs: 6.3g, Protein: 9g

302.   **Bell Pepper Muffins**

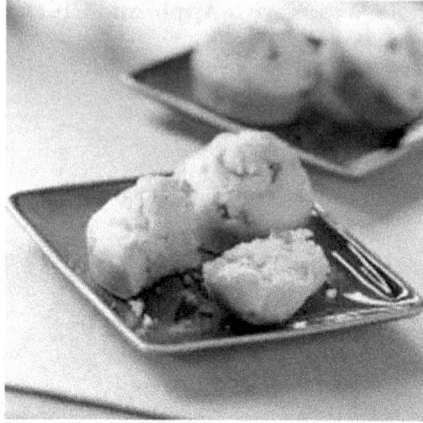

Preparation Time: 15 minutes
Cooking Time: 15 minutes
Servings: 4
Ingredients:

- 4 eggs, beaten
- 4 tsps. butter, softened
- 1 tsp. baking powder
- 2 bell peppers, chopped
- 4 tbsps. wheat flour, whole grain
- ½ tsp ground black pepper
- ½ tsp salt

Directions:
Mix up together eggs, butter, baking powder, wheat flour, ground black pepper, and salt.

When the batter is smooth, add chopped bell pepper. Stir well.

Fill ½ part of every muffin mold with bell pepper batter.

Bake the muffins for 15 minutes at 365°F.

Nutrition: Calories 146, Fat: 8.4g, Fiber: 1.1g, Carbs: 11.6g, Protein: 7g

303. **Whole-Grain Lavash Chips**

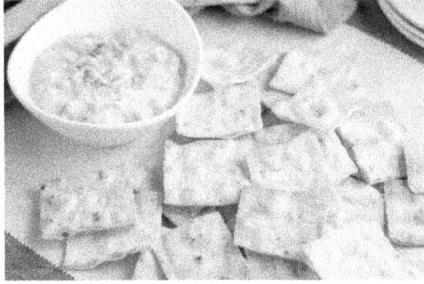

Preparation Time: 8 minutes
Cooking Time: 10 minutes
Servings: 4
Ingredients:

- 1 lavash sheet, whole grain
- 1 tbsp. canola oil
- 1 tsp. paprika
- ½ tsp chili pepper
- ½ tsp salt

Directions:
In the shallow bowl whisk together canola oil, paprika, chili pepper, and salt.

Then chop lavash sheet roughly (in the shape of chips).

Sprinkle lavash chips with oil mixture and arrange in the tray to get one thin layer.

Bake the lavash chips for 10 minutes at 365°F. Flip them on another side from time to time to avoid burning.

Cool the cooked chips well.

Nutrition: Calories 73, Fat: 4g, Fiber: 0.7g, Carbs: 8.4g, Protein: 1.6g

304.   **Quinoa Granola**
Preparation Time: 10 minutes
Cooking Time: 25 minutes
Servings: 15
Ingredients:

- 1 cup rolled oats
- 6 oz quinoa
- 7 oz almonds, chopped
- 5 tbsps. maple syrup
- 3 tbsps. peanut butter
- 1 tsp. ground cinnamon
- 1 tbsp. coconut flakes

Directions:
In the bog bowl mix up together rolled oats, quinoa, almonds, and coconut flakes.

Then add peanut butter and maple syrup.

Stir the mixture carefully with the help of the spoon.

Line the baking tray with parchment.

Transfer the quinoa mixture in the tray and flatten it well.

Bake granola for 25 minutes at 355°F.

Chill the cooked granola well and crack on the Servings.

Nutrition: Calories 177, Fat: 9.4g, Fiber: 3.3g, Carbs: 19.1g, Protein: 5.9g

305.   **Cheesy Artichoke Dip**

Preparation Time: 10 minutes

Cooking Time: 10 minutes

Servings: 6

Ingredients:

- 1 cup sour cream
- 1 cup fresh spinach
- 4 oz artichoke hearts, drained
- 1 cup Mozzarella cheese, shredded
- 1 tsp. chili flakes

Directions:
Chop the artichoke hearts on the tiny pieces.

Put spinach in a blender and blend until smooth.

Mix up together spinach with artichokes. Add sour cream, Mozzarella cheese, and chili flakes. Stir well.

Transfer the mixture in the mold/pan and flatten it.

Bake the dip for 10 minutes at 360°F.

Nutrition: Calories 105, Fat: 8.9g, Fiber: 1.1g, Carbs: 4g, Protein: 3.3g

306.   **Date and Fig Smoothie**

Preparation Time: 5 minutes

Cooking Time: 0 minutes

Servings: 1

Ingredients:

- 1 date, pitted
- 1 fig, chopped
- 1 oz Greek yogurt
- ⅓ cup organic almond milk
- ⅓ tsp ground cardamom
- 1 tsp. honey

Directions:

Place all ingredients in the food processor.

Blend the mixture until smooth.

After this, pour the cooked smoothie in the Servings glass.

Nutrition: Calories 146, Fat: 3.1g, Fiber: 2.7g, Carbs: 27.7g, Protein: 4.3g

307. **Cucumber Bites with Creamy Avocado**

Preparation Time: 10 minutes

Cooking Time: 0 minutes

Servings: 5

Ingredients:

- 1 cucumber
- 5 cherry tomatoes
- 2 oz avocado, pitted
- ¼ tsp minced garlic
- ¼ tsp dried basil
- ¾ tsp sour cream
- ¾ tsp lemon juice

Directions:

Trim the cucumber and slice it on 5 thick slices.

After this, churn avocado until you get cream mass.

Add minced garlic, dried basil, sour cream, and lemon juice. Mix up well.

Spread the avocado mass over the cucumber slices and top it with cherry tomatoes.

Nutrition: Calories 56, Fat: 2.7g, Fiber: 2.5g, Carbs: 8.1g, Protein: 1.7g

308. **Tomato Finger Sandwich**

Preparation Time: 10 minutes

Cooking Time: 0 minutes

Servings: 6

Ingredients:

- 6 corn tortillas
- 1 tbsp. cream cheese
- 1 tbsp. ricotta cheese
- ½ tsp minced garlic
- 1 tbsp. fresh dill, chopped
- 2 tomatoes, sliced

Directions:

Cut every tortilla into 2 triangles.

Then mix up together cream cheese, ricotta cheese, minced garlic, and dill.

Spread 6 triangles with cream cheese mixture.

Then place sliced tomato on them and cover with remaining tortilla triangles.

Nutrition: Calories 71, Fat: 1.6g, Fiber: 2.1g, Carbs: 12.8g, Protein: 2.3g

309.   Parsley Cheese Balls

Preparation Time: 10 minutes

Cooking Time: 1 minute

Servings: 6

Ingredients:

- ⅓ cup Cheddar cheese, shredded
- 1 tbsp. dried dill
- 1 egg, beaten
- ½ tsp salt
- 2 tbsps. coconut flakes
- 3 tbsps. sunflower oil

Directions:

Mix up together shredded cheese with dried dill, salt, and coconut flakes.

Then add egg and stir carefully until homogenous.

After this make small balls from the cheese mixture.

Heat up sunflower oil in the skillet.

Place cheese balls in the hot oil and roast them for 10 seconds from each side.

Dry the cooked cheese balls with the help of the paper towel.

Nutrition: Calories 105, Fat: 10.4g, Fiber: 0.2g, Carbs: 0.7g, Protein: 2.6g

310.   Layered Dip

Preparation Time: 10 minutes

Cooking Time: 0 minutes

Servings: 12

Ingredients:

- ½ cup hummus
- 8 tbsps. tzatziki
- 1 cup tomatoes, chopped
- 1 cup cucumbers, chopped
- 1 tsp. olive oil
- 1 tbsp. lemon juice
- ⅓ cup fresh parsley, chopped
- 1 jalapeno pepper, chopped

Directions:

In the mixing bowl mix up together fresh parsley, lemon juice, olive oil, cucumbers, tomatoes, and chopped jalapeno pepper.

Then make the layer of ½ part of tomato mixture in the casserole mold or glass mold.

Top it with the layer of hummus.

Then add remaining tomato mixture and flatten it well.

Top it with tzatziki and flatten well.

Store the dip in the fridge for up to 3 hours.

Nutrition: Calories 49, Fat: 3.6g, Fiber: 1g, Carbs: 3.3g, Protein: 1.1g

311.   **Grilled Tempeh Sticks**
Preparation Time: 5 minutes
Cooking Time: 8 minutes
Servings: 6
Ingredients:

- 11 oz soy tempeh
- 1 tsp. olive oil
- ½ tsp ground black pepper
- ¼ tsp garlic powder

Directions:
Cut soy tempeh into the sticks.

Sprinkle every tempeh stick with ground black pepper, garlic powder, and olive oil.

Preheat the grill to 375°F.

Place the tempeh sticks in the grill and cook them for 4 minutes from each side. The time of cooking depends on the tempeh sticks size.

The cooked tempeh sticks will have a light brown color.

Nutrition: Calories 88, Fat: 2.5g, Fiber: 3.6g, Carbs: 10.2g, Protein: 6.5g

312.   **Sweet Potato Fries**
Preparation Time: 10 minutes
Cooking Time: 35 minutes
Servings: 5
Ingredients:

- 1 tsp. Zaatar spices
- 3 sweet potatoes
- 1 tbsp. dried dill
- 1 tsp. salt
- 3 tsps. sunflower oil
- ½ tsp paprika

Directions:
Pour water in the crockpot. Peel the sweet potatoes and cut them into the fries.

Line the baking tray with parchment.

Place the layer of the sweet potato in the tray.

Sprinkle the vegetables with dried dill, salt, and paprika.

Then sprinkle sweet potatoes with Zaatar and mix up well with the help of the fingertips.

Sprinkle the sweet potato fries with sunflower oil.

Preheat the oven to 375°F.

Bake the sweet potato fries for 35 minutes. Stir the fries every 10 minutes.

Nutrition: Calories 28, Fat: 2.9g, Fiber: 0.2g, Carbs: 0.6g, Protein: 0.2g

313.   Italian Style Potato Fries

Preparation Time: 10 minutes

Cooking Time: 40 minutes

Servings: 4

Ingredients:

- ⅓ cup baby red potatoes
- 1 tbsp. Italian seasoning
- 3 tbsps. canola oil
- 1 tsp. turmeric
- ½ tsp of sea salt
- ½ tsp dried rosemary
- 1 tbsp. dried dill

Directions:

Cut the red potatoes into the wedges and transfer in the big bowl.

After this, sprinkle the vegetables with Italian seasoning, canola oil, turmeric, sea salt, dried rosemary, and dried dill.

Shake the potato wedges carefully.

Line the baking tray with baking paper.

Place the potatoes wedges in the tray. Flatten it well to make one layer.

Preheat the oven to 375F.

Place the tray with potatoes in the oven and bake for 40 minutes. Stir the potatoes with the help of the spatula from time to time.

The potato fries are cooked when they have crunchy edges.

Nutrition: Calories 122, Fat: 11.6g, Fiber: 0.5g, Carbs: 4.5g, Protein: 0.6g

314.   Lemon Cauliflower Florets

Preparation Time: 15 minutes

Cooking Time: 12 minutes

Servings: 6

Ingredients:

- 1-pound cauliflower head, trimmed
- 3 tbsps. lemon juice
- 3 eggs, beaten
- 1 tsp. salt

- 1 tsp. ground black pepper
- 2 cups water, for cooking
- 3 tbsps. almond butter
- 1 tsp. turmeric

Directions:
Place the cauliflower head in the pan.
Add water.
Boil the cauliflower for 8 minutes or until it is tender.
Then cool the vegetable well and separate it onto the florets.
Whisk together beaten eggs, salt, ground black pepper, and turmeric.
Dip every cauliflower floret in the egg mixture.
Toss the almond butter in the skillet and heat it up.
Roast the cauliflower florets for 2 minutes from each side over the medium heat.
When the cauliflower florets are golden brown, they are cooked.
Sprinkle the cooked florets with lemon juice.
Nutrition: Calories 103, Fat: 6.9g, Fiber: 2.9g, Carbs: 6.3g, Protein: 6.1g

315. **Greek Style Nachos**
Preparation Time: 7 minutes
Cooking Time: 0 minutes
Servings: 3
Ingredients:

- 3 oz tortilla chips
- ¼ cup Greek yogurt
- 1 tbsp. fresh parsley, chopped
- ¼ tsp minced garlic
- 2 kalamata olives, chopped
- 1 tsp. paprika
- ¼ tsp ground thyme

Directions:
In the mixing bowl mix up together Greek yogurt, parsley, minced garlic, olives, paprika, and thyme.
Then add tortilla chips and mix up gently.
The snack should be served immediately.
Nutrition: Calories 81, Fat: 1.6g, Fiber: 2.2g, Carbs: 14.1g, Protein: 3.5g

316. **Cheesy Phyllo Bites**
Preparation Time: 10 minutes
Cooking Time: 15 minutes
Servings: 8
Ingredients:

- 3 Phyllo sheets
- ½ cup Cheddar cheese
- 2 eggs, beaten
- 1 tbsp. butter

Directions:
Mix up together Cheddar cheese with eggs.
Spread the round springform pan with butter.
Place 2 Phyllo sheets inside the springform pan.
Place Cheddar cheese mixture over the Phyllo sheets and cover it with the remaining Phyllo dough sheet.
Preheat the oven to 365°F.
Cut the Phyllo dough pie onto 8 pieces and bake for 15 minutes.
Nutrition: Calories 113, Fat: 5.4g, Fiber: 0.4g, Carbs: 11.4g, Protein: 5g

317.   Cheddar Hot Pepper Dip
Preparation Time: 5 minutes
Cooking Time: 10 minutes
Servings: 6
Ingredients:

- 1 cup Cheddar cheese
- ¼ cup cilantro, chopped
- 1 chili pepper, chopped
- 1 tsp. garlic powder
- ¼ cup milk

Directions:
Bring the milk to boil.
Then add Cheddar cheese in the milk and simmer the mixture for 2 minutes. Stir it constantly.
After this, add cilantro, chili pepper, and garlic powder. Mix up the mixture well. If it doesn't get a smooth texture, use the hand blender to blend the mass.
It is recommended to serve the dip when it gets the room temperature.
Nutrition: Calories 83, Fat: 6.5g, Fiber: 0.1g, Carbs: 1.2g, Protein: 5.1g

318.   Traditional Mediterranean Hummus
Preparation Time: 10 minutes
Cooking Time: 45 minutes
Servings: 7
Ingredients:

- 1 cup chickpeas, soaked
- 6 cups of water
- ½ cup lemon juice

- 3 tbsp olive oil
- 1 tsp. salt
- ⅓ tsp harissa

Directions:
Combine chickpeas and water and boil for 45 minutes or until chickpeas are tender.

Then transfer chickpeas in the food processor.

Add 1 cup of chickpeas water and lemon juice.

After this, add salt and harissa.

Blend the hummus until it is smooth and fluffy.

Add olive oil and pulse it for 10 seconds more.

Transfer the cooked hummus in the bowl and store it in the fridge up to 2 days.

Nutrition: Calories 160, Fat: 7.9g, Fiber: 5g, Carbs: 17.8g, Protein: 5.7g

319. **Tuna Salad in Lettuce Cups**
Preparation Time: 10 minutes
Cooking Time: 10 minutes
Servings: 6
Ingredients:

- 4 Romaine lettuce leaves
- 8 oz tuna fillet
- 1 tsp. balsamic vinegar
- ½ tsp olive oil
- 1 tbsp. fresh dill, chopped
- ¼ tsp salt
- ¾ tsp chili pepper
- 1 tomato, chopped
- ¾ cup Plain yogurt

Directions:
Rub the tuna fillet with salt and chili pepper.

Then drizzle the fish with olive oil.

Bake tuna for 10 minutes at 365°F.

Then chill it little and chop.

In the bowl combine chopped tuna, Plain yogurt, tomato, fresh dill, and balsamic vinegar. Mix up well.

Fill the lettuce leaves with the tuna mixture.

Nutrition: Calories 152, Fat: 11.2g, Fiber: 0.3g, Carbs: 3.4g, Protein: 9g

320. **Rice Burgers**
Preparation Time: 10 minutes
Cooking Time: 30 minutes
Servings: 4

Ingredients:

- ⅓ cup rice
- 1 cup of water
- ½ tsp salt
- 2 tbsps. ricotta cheese
- 1 egg
- ¼ cup yellow onion, diced
- 1 tsp. sunflower oil
- ½ tsp ground black pepper
- 1 tbsp. wheat flour, whole grain

Directions:

Pour water in a pan. Add rice and salt.

Close the lid and boil rice for 15 minutes or until it will soak all liquid and will be done.

Meanwhile, heat up oil in the skillet.

Add diced onion and roast it until golden brown.

Combine cooked rice with onion.

Add ground black pepper, wheat flour, and egg.

Mix up the mixture. It should smooth but not liquid.

Then make medium size burgers.

Bake the burgers for 10 minutes at 355°F.

Top the cooked appetizer with ricotta cheese.

Nutrition: Calories 104, Fat: 3g, Fiber: 0.5g, Carbs: 15.1g, Protein: 3.7g

321. **Wheatberry Burgers**

Preparation Time: 25 minutes

Cooking Time: 15 minutes

Servings: 6

Ingredients:

- 1 cup wheatberry, cooked
- 2 eggs
- ¼ cup ground chicken
- 1 tbsp. wheat flour, whole grain
- 1 tsp. Italian seasoning
- 1 tbsp. olive oil
- 1 tsp. salt

Directions:

In the mixing bowl mix up together wheatberry and ground chicken.

Crack eggs in the mixture.

Then add wheat flour, Italian seasoning, and salt.

Mix up the mass with the help of the spoon until homogenous.

Then make burgers and freeze them in the freezer for 20 minutes.

Heat up olive oil in the skillet.

Place frozen burgers in the hot oil and roast them for 4 minutes from each side over the high heat.

Then cook burgers for 10 minutes more over the medium heat. Flip them onto another side from time to time.

Nutrition: Calories 97, Fat: 5.7g, Fiber: 1.5g, Carbs: 9.2g, Protein: 5.2g

322. **Easy Nachos**
Preparation Time: 10 minutes
Cooking Time: 10 minutes
Servings: 7
Ingredients:

- 1 cup nachos
- ⅓ cup Monterey Jack cheese, shredded
- 2 oz black olives, sliced
- 2 tomatoes, chopped

Directions:
Crash the nachos gently and arrange them in the casserole mold in one layer.

Make the layer of black olives and tomatoes over the nachos. Flatten the ingredients with the help of spatula if needed.

Then make the layer of cheese and cover casserole mold with foil. Secure the edges.

Bake the nachos for 10 minutes at 365°F.

Then remove the foil from the mold and serve nachos in the casserole mold.

Nutrition: Calories 133, Fat: 8g, Fiber: 2.3g, Carbs: 10.6g, Protein: 5.4g

323. **Salty Almonds**
Preparation Time: 1 hour 10 minutes
Cooking Time: 15 minutes
Servings: 5
Ingredients:

- 1 cup almonds
- 3 tbsps. salt
- 2 cups of water

Directions:
Bring water to boil.

After this, add 2 tbsps. of salt in water and stir it.

When salt is dissolved, add almonds, and let them soak for at least 1 hour.

Meanwhile, line the tray with baking paper and preheat oven to 350°F.

Dry the soaked almonds with a paper towel well and arrange them in one layer in the tray.

Sprinkle buts with remaining salt.

Bake the snack for 15 minutes. Mix it from time to time with the help of the spatula or spoon.

Nutrition: Calories 110, Fat: 9.5g, Fiber: 2.4g, Carbs: 4.1g, Protein: 4g

324.   Zucchini Chips
Preparation Time: 15 minutes
Cooking Time: 20 minutes
Servings: 4
Ingredients:

- 1 zucchini
- 2 oz Parmesan, grated
- ½ tsp paprika
- 1 tsp. olive oil

Directions:
Trim zucchini and slice it into the chips with the help of the vegetable slices.

Then mix up together Parmesan and paprika.

Sprinkle the zucchini chips with olive oil.

After this, dip every zucchini slice in the cheese mixture.

Place the zucchini chips in the lined baking tray and bake for 20 minutes at 375°F.

Flip the zucchini sliced onto another side after 10 minutes of cooking.

Chill the cooked chips well.

Nutrition: Calories 64, Fat: 4.3g, Fiber: 0.6g, Carbs: 2.3g, Protein: 5.2g

325.   Chili Chicken Wings
Preparation Time: 10 minutes
Cooking Time: 20 minutes
Servings: 3
Ingredients:

- 3 chicken wings, boneless
- 1 tsp. chili pepper, minced
- 1 tbsp olive oil
- 1 tsp. minced garlic
- 2 tbsps. balsamic vinegar
- ½ tsp salt

Directions:
Make the chicken sauce: whisk together minced chili pepper, olive oil, minced garlic, balsamic vinegar, and salt.

Preheat the oven to 360°F.

Line the baking tray with parchment.

Rub the chicken wings with chicken sauce generously and transfer in the tray.

Bake the poultry for 20 minutes. Flip them onto another side after 10 minutes of cooking.

Nutrition: Calories 138, Fat: 11g, Fiber: 0.2g, Carbs: 3.8g, Protein: 5.9g

326.   **Radish Flatbread Bites**

Preparation Time: 10 minutes

Cooking Time: 10 minutes

Servings: 8

Ingredients:

- 2 tbsps. butter
- ⅓ cup milk
- 1 ½ cup wheat flour, whole grain
- 1 tsp. salt
- 1 tsp. avocado oil
- 1 cup radish
- 1 tbsp. cream cheese

Directions:

Melt butter and combine it together with milk. Stir the liquid.

Then mix up together flour with butter mixture.

Knead the soft and non-sticky dough.

Cut the dough into 8 pieces.

Roll up every dough piece into the circle (flatbread).

Pour avocado oil in the skillet.

Roast the flatbreads for 1 minute from each side over the medium heat.

After this, slice the radish and mix it up with cream cheese and salt.

Top cooked flatbreads with radish.

Nutrition: Calories 123, Fat: 3.8g, Fiber: 0.9g, Carbs: 18.9g, Protein: 3g

327.   **Endive Bites**

Preparation Time: 10 minutes

Cooking Time: 0 minutes

Servings:10

Ingredients:

- 6 oz. endive
- 2 pears, chopped
- 4 oz Blue cheese, crumbled
- 1 tsp. olive oil
- 1 tsp. lemon juice
- ¾ tsp ground cinnamon

Directions:
Separate endive into the spears (10 spears).
In the bowl combine chopped pears, olive oil, lemon juice, ground cinnamon, and Blue cheese.
Fill the endive spears with cheese mixture.
Nutrition: Calories 72, Fat: 3.8g, Fiber: 1.9g, Carbs: 7.4g, Protein: 2.8g
328.   **Eggplant Bites**
Preparation Time: 15 minutes
Cooking Time: 30 minutes
Servings: 8
Ingredients:

- 2 eggs, beaten
- 3 oz Parmesan, grated
- 1 tbsp. coconut flakes
- ½ tsp ground paprika
- 1 tsp. salt
- 2 eggplants, trimmed

Directions:
Slice the eggplants into the thin circles. Use the vegetable slicer for this step.
After this, sprinkle the vegetables with salt and mix up. Leave them for 5-10 minutes.
Then drain eggplant juice and sprinkle them with ground paprika.
Mix up together coconut flakes and Parmesan.
Dip every eggplant circle in the egg and then coat in Parmesan mixture.
Line the baking tray with parchment and place eggplants on it.
Bake the vegetables for 30 minutes at 360°F. Flip the eggplants into another side after 12 minutes of cooking.
Nutrition: Calories 87, Fat: 3.9g, Fiber: 5g, Carbs: 8.7g, Protein: 6.2g
329.   **Peanut Butter Yogurt Dip**
Preparation Time: 10 minutes
Cooking Time: 0 minutes
Servings: 4
Ingredients:

- 2 tbsps. peanut butter
- 1 oz Greek Yogurt
- 1 tsp. sesame seeds
- ½ tsp vanilla extract
- 1 tbsp. honey

Directions:

Put peanut butter and Greek yogurt in the big bowl.

With the help of the mixer mix up the mixture until fluffy.

After this, add sesame seeds, vanilla extract, and honey.

Stir it carefully.

Store the dip in the fridge.

Nutrition: Calories 74, Fat: 4.5g, Fiber: 0.6g, Carbs: 6.5g, Protein: 2.9g

330. **Roasted Chickpeas**

Preparation Time: 10 minutes

Cooking Time: 3 hours

Servings: 8

Ingredients:

- 1 cup chickpeas, canned
- 1 tsp. salt
- ½ tsp ground coriander
- ½ tsp ground paprika
- ½ tsp dried thyme
- ¾ tsp cayenne pepper
- 2 tbsps. olive oil

Directions:

Drain the chickpeas and dry them carefully with the help of the towel.

After this, place them in the baking tray.

Mix up together salt, ground coriander, ground paprika, dried thyme, and cayenne pepper.

Sprinkle the chickpeas with spices and shake well.

After this, drizzle them with olive oil. Give a good shake again.

Preheat the oven to 375°F.

Place the tray with chickpeas in the preheated oven and cook them for 35 minutes.

Flip the chickpeas on another side from time to time.

Nutrition: Calories 122, Fat: 5.1g, Fiber: 4.5g, Carbs: 15.4g, Protein: 4.9g

331. **Beetroot Chips**

Preparation Time: 10 minutes

Cooking Time: 15 minutes

Servings: 4

Ingredients:

- 1 beetroot, peeled
- 1 tsp. salt
- 1 tbsp. sunflower oil

Directions:

Thinly slice the beetroot and sprinkle with salt.

Add the sunflower oil and stir gently with the help of the spatula.

Arrange the beetroot chips in the tray one-by-one and bake for 12 minutes at 370°F.

Then flip chips on another side and bake for 3 minutes more.

Nutrition: Calories 42, Fat: 3.6g, Fiber: 0.5g, Carbs: 2.5g, Protein: 0.4g

DESSERTS

332.   **Compote Dipped Berries Mix**
Preparation Time: 20 minutes
Servings: 8
Ingredients:

- 2 cups fresh strawberries, hulled and halved lengthwise
- 4 sprigs fresh mint
- 2 cups fresh blackberries
- 1 cup pomegranate juice
- 2 tsps. vanilla
- 6 orange pekoe tea bags
- 2 cups fresh red raspberries
- 1 cup water
- 2 cups fresh golden raspberries
- 2 cups fresh sweet cherries, pitted and halved
- 2 cups fresh blueberries
- 2 ml bottle Sauvignon Blanc

Directions:
Preheat the oven to 290°F and lightly grease a baking dish.

Soak mint sprigs and tea bags in boiled water for about 10 minutes in a covered bowl.

Mix all the berries and cherries in another bowl and keep aside.

Cook wine with pomegranate juice in a saucepan and add strained tea liquid.

Toss in the mixed berries to serve and enjoy.

Nutrition: Calories 356, Fat: 0.8g, Carbs: 89.9g, Fiber: 9.4g, Protein: 2.2g

333.   **Greek Almond Rounds Shortbread**

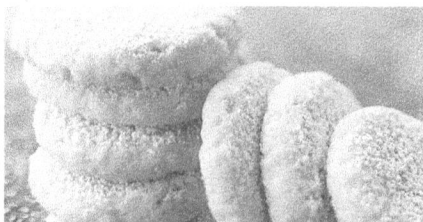

Preparation Time: 45 minutes, plus 1hr chilling
Cooking Time: 12 minutes
Servings: 84
Ingredients:

- 1 ½ cups butter, softened
- 1 cup blanched almonds, lightly toasted and finely ground
- 1 cup powdered sugar
- 2 egg yolks
- 2 tbsps. brandy or orange juice
- 2 tbsps. rose flower water, (optional)
- 2 tsps. vanilla
- 3 ½ cups cake flour
- Powdered sugar

Directions:
Using an electric mixer, beat the butter on MEDIUM or HIGH speed for about 30 seconds in a large sized bowl. Add the 1 cup powdered sugar; beat until the mixture is light in color and fluffy, occasionally scraping the bowl as needed.

Beat in the yolks, vanilla, and the brandy until combined.

With a wooden spoon, stir in the flour and almonds until well incorporated. Cover and refrigerate for about 1 hour or until chilled and the dough is easy to handle.

Preheat the oven to 325°F.

Shape the dough into 1-inch balls. Place the balls 2 inches apart int an ungreased cookie sheet. Dip a glass in the additional powdered sugar and use it to flatten each ball into ¼ -inch thickness, dipping the bottom of the glass every time you flatten a ball into cookies.

Place the cookie sheet into the preheated oven; bake for about 12-14 minutes or until the cookies are set.

When the cookies are baked, transfer them on wire racks. While they are still warm, brush with the rose water, if desired. Sprinkle with more powdered sugar. Let cool completely on the wire racks.

Notes: If using rose water, make sure that you use the edible kind. To store, layer the cookies with waxed paper between each cookie and keep on airtight containers. Close the container tightly and store at room temperature for up to 3 days or freeze for up to 3 months.

Nutrition: Calories 62, Fat: 4g, Carbs: 5.7g, Protein: 0.9g

334.   **Tiny Orange Cardamom Cookies**

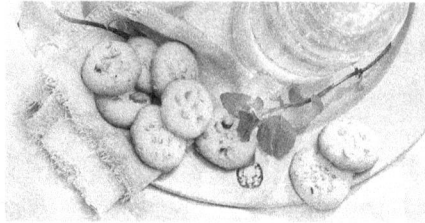

Preparation Time: 48 minutes
Cooking Time: 12 minutes
Servings: 80 cookies (5 cookies per Servings)
Ingredients:

- ½ cup whole-wheat flour
- ½ cup all-purpose flour
- 1 large egg
- 1 tbsp. sesame seeds, toasted, optional (salted roasted pistachios, chopped)
- 1 tsp. orange zest
- 1 tsp. vanilla extract
- ½ cup butter, softened
- ½ cup sugar
- ¼ tsp ground cardamom

Directions:
Preheat the oven to 375°F.

In a medium bowl, blend the orange zest and the sugar thoroughly, and then blend in the cardamom. Add the butter and with a mixer, beat until the mixture is fluffy and light. Beat in the egg and the vanilla into the mixture. With the mixer on low speed, mix in the flours into the mixture.

Line 3 baking sheets with parchment paper. Using a level tsp measure, drop batter of the cookie mixture onto the sheets. Top each cookie with a pinch of sesame seeds or nuts, if desired; bake for 1bout 10-12 minutes or until the cookies are brown at the edges and crisp. When baked, transfer the cookies on a cooling rack and let them cool completely.

Nutrition: Calories 113, Protein: 1.4g, Fat: 6.5g, Carbs: 12g, Fiber: 0.3g

335.   **Hazelnut-Orange Olive Oil Cookies**

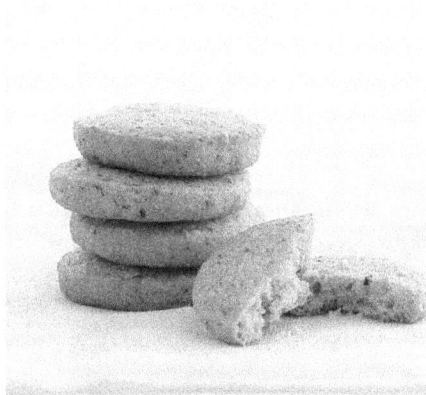

Preparation Time: 30 minutes, plus 1-hour firming
Cooking Time: 20 minutes
Servings: 6 dozen cookies
Ingredients:

- 5 oz. (1-⅛ cups) whole-wheat flour
- 5 oz. (1-⅛ cups) unbleached all-purpose flour
- ¾ cup plus 2 tbsps. granulated sugar
- 2 large eggs
- 2 cups toasted and skinned hazelnuts
- ¼ tsp table salt
- ½ cup olive oil, extra-virgin
- 1 tsp. vanilla extract, pure
- 1 tsp. of baking powder
- Finely grated zest of 2 medium-sized oranges (about 1 ½ packed tbsp)

Directions:
Put the hazelnuts in a food processor; process until finely ground. In a medium bowl, whisk the ground hazelnuts, flours, baking powder, and salt until blended. With a stand or a hand mixer fitted with a paddle attachment, beat the eggs, oil, sugar, orange zest, and vanilla on LOW speed for about 15 seconds or until the sugar is moistened. Increase the speed to HIGH; mix for 15 minutes more or until well combined, the sugar will be dissolved at this point. Add the hazelnut mixture; mix on LOW speed for about 30 to 60 seconds or until the dough has just pulled together.

Divide the dough into 2 portions. Pile one of the doughs on a piece of parchment paper. With the aid of the parchment paper, shape the dough into a 2-inch diameter 11-inch long log. Wrap the parchment around the log, twisting the ends to secure it. Repeat the process with the remaining dough. Refrigerate and chill for about 1 hour or until firm.

Position the oven racks in the lower thirds and the upper position in the oven; preheat the oven to 350°F. Line 4 pieces cookie sheets with nonstick baking liners or parchment paper.

Unwrap the logs. Cut the logs into ¼ -inch thick slices. Set them 1-inch apart from each other on the prepared sheets. Place 2 baking sheets in the oven; bake the cookies for about 10 minutes or until the cookies are light golden around the edges and on the bottoms, swapping and rotating the sheets halfway through the baking. Let the cookies cool completely on racks. These can be kept in an airtight container at normal room temperature for up to 7 days.

Notes: you can make the dough logs ahead of time. Freeze them for up to 1 month.

Nutrition: Calories 60, Fat: 4g, Carbs: 6g, Fiber: 0g

336.   **Greek Cheesecake**
Preparation Time: 1 hour, 20 minutes
Cooking Time: 30 minutes
Servings: 8-10
Ingredients:

- 4 eggs
- 250g whole-wheat digestive cookies
- 125g butter, melted
- ½ tsp cinnamon
- ½ cup sugar
- ½ cup honey
- 1 tsp. vanilla extract
- 1 tsp. lemon zest
- 1 kilo white mizithra cheese, fresh or anything similar like ricotta

For the topping:

- 750g black cherries, pitted
- 2 leaves gelatin
- 300g sugar

Directions:
Process the digestive biscuits in a food processor until crumbled. Add the butter and cinnamon, process again until the mixture is like wet sand in texture. Press the mixture into a 20-cm spring-form tin, pressing some of the mixture up the sides of the tin to make a ridge. Refrigerate until ready to use.

Preheat the oven to 180°C.

With an electric mixer, beat the sugar and the cheese together until creamy. One by one, add in the eggs, the lemon zest, the vanilla extract, and honey. Pour the cheese mixture over the refrigerated biscuit base.

Place the spring-form tin in the oven and with the oven door ajar, bake for 30 minutes or until firm. Remove the cake from the oven and let cool.

Meanwhile prepare the cherries. Place the gelatin leaves in a bowl with cold water, soak until soft. Put the sugar and the pitted cherries into a frying pan, heat over high flame or hear; stew for about 6 minutes or until the cherries release their juices. Add in the softened gelatins; stir well until well mixed. Remove the pan from the heat and let cool for a bit. When slightly cool, pour over the cooled cheesecake.

Refrigerate until the cherry topping set. Serve cold. If desired, serve with vanilla ice cream.

Nutrition: Calories 561, Fat: 19.9g, Carbs: 80.5g, Fiber: 0.6g, Protein: 18.8g

337. Phyllo Cups

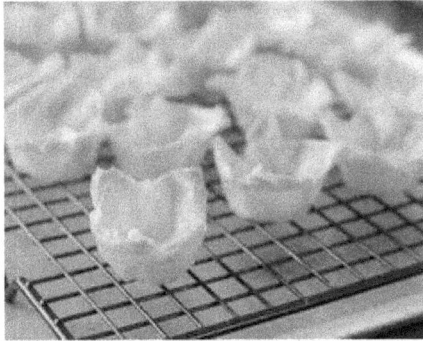

Preparation Time: 25 minutes
Cooking Time: 8 minutes
Servings: 12
Ingredients:

- 8 sheets (14 x 9-inch) frozen phyllo dough, thawed
- Nonstick cooking spray
- 4 tsps. sugar
- For the lemon cheesecake filling:
- 1 package (8 ounce) cream cheese, softened
- 3 tbsps. lemon curd
- ⅓ cup sugar

For the berry-honey filling:

- 3 oz. cream cheese, softened

- ½ cup whipping cream
- ½ tsp vanilla
- 2 tbsps. honey
- Fresh strawberries, sliced (or other berries)
- For thee macadamia espresso coconut filling:
- 1 package (8 ounce) cream cheese, softened
- ⅓ cup sugar
- ½ cup whipping cream
- 1 tsp. espresso powder, instant
- ½ cup toasted coconut
- ¼ cup macadamia nuts, finely chopped

Directions:

For the phyllo cups:

Preheat the oven to 350°F.

Lightly grease 12 pieces of 2 ½-inch muffin cups with the cooking spray; set aside.

Lay out 1 phyllo sheet, lightly grease with the cooking spray, sprinkle with some sugar, and then top with another 1 phyllo sheet. Repeat the process until 4 phyllo sheets are stacked, lightly greasing with the cooking spray, sprinkling with the sugar in the process. Repeat the procedure to make 2 stacks of 4-pieces phyllo sheets. Cut each stack lengthwise into halves. Then cut crosswise into thirds, making 12 rectangles.

Press 1 rectangle into each greased muffin cup, pleating the phyllo to form a cup, as necessary. Put the muffin cups in the oven and bake for about 8 minutes or until the phyllo cups are golden. When baked, remove the muffin tins from the oven and let cool in the pan for about 5 minutes. Remove the phyllo cups from the muffin tins and let cool completely. Fill each cup with desire filling. They can be filled for up to 1 hour before Servings.

For the lemon cheesecake filling:

Put the cream cheese and the sugar into a bowl; beat until the mixture is smooth. Beat in the lemon curd until mixed. Spoon the mixture into phyllo cups. If desired, garnish with lemon peel twists.

For the berry-honey filling:

Put the cream cheese in a bowl; beat until smooth. Beat in the vanilla and the honey. Add in the whipping cream; beat until stiff peaks form. Spoon the mixture into phyllo cups. Top with sliced strawberries or with preferred berry. Drizzle with more honey, if desired.

For thee macadamia espresso coconut filling:

Put the cream cheese, sugar, and the espresso powder in a bowl; beat. Add in the whipping cream until stiff peaks form Stir in the nuts and toasted coconut. Spoon the mixture into phyllo cups. If desired, garnish with additional toasted coconut and nuts.

Nutrition: Calories 161, Fat: 8g, Carbs: 20g, Fiber: 1g, Protein: 3g

338.   **Poached Cherries**
Preparation Time: 10 minutes
Cooking Time: 10 minutes
Servings: 5 (½ cup each)
Ingredients:

- 1 lb. fresh and sweet cherries, rinsed, pitted
- 3 strips (1 x 3 inches each) orange zest,
- 3 strips (1 x 3 inches each) lemon zest,
- ⅔ cup sugar
- 15 peppercorns
- ¼ vanilla bean, split but not scraped
- 1 ¾ cups water

Directions:

In a saucepan, mix the water, citrus zest, sugar, peppercorns, and vanilla bean; bring to a boil, stirring until the sugar is dissolved. Add the cherries; simmer for about 10 minutes until the cherries are soft, but not falling apart. Skim any foam from the surface and let the poached cherries cool. Refrigerate with the poaching liquid. Before Servings, strain the cherries.

Nutrition: Calories 170, Fat: 1g, Carbs: 42g, Fiber: 2g

339.   **Watermelon-Strawberry Rosewater Yogurt Panna Cotta**

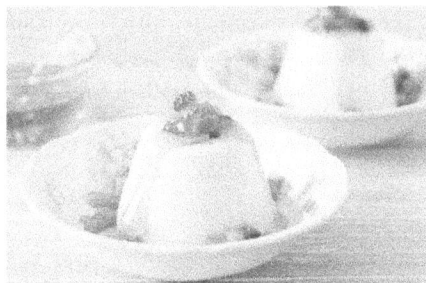

Preparation Time: 20 minutes
Cooking Time: 5 minutes
Servings: 4
Ingredients:

- 500 g seedless watermelon, peeled, and cut into 5-mm pieces
- 3 tsps. rosewater
- 250 ml honey-flavored yogurt
- 250 ml (1 cup) thickened cream
- 2 tsps. gelatin powder

- 2 tbsps. caster sugar
- 10 strawberries, washed, hulled, and cut into 5-mm pieces
- 1 tbsp. hot water
- Honey, to serve
- Vegetable oil, to grease

Directions:
Brush 4 pieces of 125 ml or ½ cup sprinkle molds with vegetable oil to grease.

Put the yogurt into a large-sized heat-safe bowl.

Place the sugar and the cream into a small-sized saucepan and heat over medium heat; stir until the sugar is heated through and the sugar is dissolved.

Place the hot water into a small-sized heat-safe bowl. Sprinkle the gelatin over the hot water. Place the bowl into a small-sized saucepan. Add enough boiling water to fill the saucepan about ¾ deep on the side of the bowl. With a fork, whisk the mixture until the gelatin is dissolved.

Add the gelatin mixture and the cream mixture into the yogurt, whisking until well combined. Strain the mixture through a fine sieve over a large-sized jug. Pour the strained mixture into the prepared molds. Cover each mold with a plastic wrap. Refrigerate for at least 6 hours or overnight until set.

In a medium bowl, combine the strawberry, watermelon, and rosewater.

Turn the panna cottas into Servings bowl. Spoon the strawberry-watermelon over each panna cotta. Drizzle with honey and serve.

Notes: For a different version, you can omit the rosewater, strawberries, and the honey. Combine the watermelon with ⅓ cup of fresh passion fruit pulp, and spoon over the panna cottas.

Nutrition: Calories 364.96, Fat: 26g, Carbs: 26g, Fiber: 1g, Protein: 7g

340.   **Mascarpone and Ricotta Stuffed Dates**

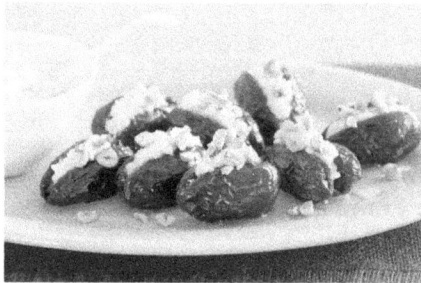

Preparation Time: 20 minutes
Cooking Time: 10 minutes
Servings: 5
Ingredients:

- 125 g fresh ricotta
- 125 g mascarpone
- 2 tsps. finely grated orange rind
- 30 pieces fresh dates
- 45 g (¼ cup) dry roasted hazelnuts, coarsely chopped, for sprinkling
- 45 g (¼ cup) icing sugar mixture

For the Frangelico syrup:

- 80 ml (⅓ cup) Frangelico liqueur
- 125 ml (½ cup) water
- 215 g (1 cup) caster sugar

Directions:
With an electric beater, beat the mascarpone, icing sugar, ricotta, and orange rind into a large-sized bowl until the mixture is smooth.

With a sharp knife, cut a slit in each date. Remove the stones and discard. Spoon 1 heaped tsp of the ricotta mixture into each date.

To make the Frangelico syrup:
Put the water and the sugar into a medium-sized saucepan. Heat over low heat: cook for about 2 to 3 minutes, stirring until the sugar is dissolved. Increase the heat to high and bring the mixture to a boil. Cook for 5 minutes without stirring or until the syrup is slightly thick. Stir the Frangelico liqueur. Remove from saucepan from the heat, set aside for 30 minutes to cool.

Put the dates into a Servings platter. Pour the Frangelico syrup over the dates. Sprinkle with hazelnuts and then serve.

Nutrition: Calories 115.92, Fat: 3.5g, Carbs: 26g, Fiber: 1g, Protein: 1.5g

341. **Glazed Mediterranean Puffy Fig**
Preparation Time: 5 minutes
Cooking Time: 25 minutes
Servings: 8
Ingredients:

- 2 sheets (from 1 pack of 4 sheets) puff pastry
- 20 figs or dry figs (dry or fresh)
- 8 oz. mascarpone cheese
- 2 tbsps. butter
- ½ cup (or 8 tbsps.) honey
- ½ tsp cinnamon
- ½ tsp nutmeg
- ¼ tsp salt
- 4 mint leaves, for garnish

Directions:

Preheat the oven 400°F.

Slice the puff pastry into triangle and place into a nonstick baking sheet; bake for about 15-20 minutes or until golden brown. When bakes, remove from the oven and allow to cool.

If using dry figs, rehydrate for 1 hour and then cut into half. Put the butter into a nonstick pan over medium flame or heat. Add the figs; cook for about 3 to 5 minutes. Add the honey, salt, cinnamon, and nutmeg; cook, stirring, for about 3 minutes. Remove the skillet from hat and allow to cool for about 5 to 10 minutes.

Place a baked pastry slice in a serving plate, top with 1 tbsp. of cheese, some figs, and then drizzle with the glaze. Repeat the topping, if desired. Garnish with the mint leaves and serve.

Nutrition: Calories 486, Fat: 22.8g, Carbs: 67.4g, Fiber: 5.4g, Protein: 7.9g

342. Mediterranean Stuffed Custard Pancakes

Preparation Time: 60 minutes
Cooking Time: 20 minutes
Servings: 10
Ingredients:
For the batter:

- 2 cups flour
- ½ cup whole-wheat flour
- 2 cups milk
- 1 cup water
- 1 tsp. yeast
- 1 tsp. baking powder
- 1 tsp. sugar
- For the custard:
- 2 cups whole milk
- 2 cups fat-free milk or 2 % milk
- 1 cup heavy cream
- 3 tbsps. sugar
- ½ cup cornstarch
- ½ cup water
- 7 pieces medium-sized white bread, crust removed
- 1 tbsp. rose water
- 1 tbsp. orange blossom water
- For the topping:
- 1 cup pistachio
- 1 tbsp. honey or simple syrup

Directions:
For the custard:

In a medium-sized pot, pour in the milks, heavy cream, cornstarch, and sugar; heat the mixture, stirring.

Cut the bread into pieces and add into the pot; stir until the mixture starts to thicken. Add the orange and rose water; stir until the custard is very thick. Remove from the heat and then pour into a bowl; let cool for 1 hour, stirring every 15 minutes. Cover with saran wrap and then refrigerate to completely cool.

For the batter:

Mix all the batter ingredients in a mixing bowl, stirring until well combined; let sit for 20 minutes.

Over medium-low flame or heat, heat a nonstick pan. Pour ¼ cup-worth of the batter to make a 3-inch diameter pancake; cook for about 30 seconds or until the top of the batter is bubbly and no longer wet and the bottom is golden brown. Transfer into a dish to cool. Repeat the process with the remaining batter.

To assemble:

Take out the bowl of custard from the refrigerator. Transfer the chilled custard into a piping bag.

Fold a pancake together, pinching the edges to make a pocket. Pipe the custard into the pancake pocket, filling it. Repeat the process with the remaining pancakes and custard. Top each filled pocket with the ground pistachio. Refrigerate until ready to serve. To serve, transfer the custard-filled pancakes into a serving plate, drizzle with honey or simple syrup.

Nutrition: Calories 450, Fat: 19g, Carbs: 60g, Fiber: 2.8g, Protein: 13g

343. **Mediterranean Cheesecake**
Preparation Time: 15 minutes
Cooking Time: 20 minutes
Servings: 8
Ingredients:

- 1 package (8 oz.) cream cheese
- ¼ cup sour cream
- ½ cup condensed milk, sweetened
- 5 tbsps. sugar, divided
- 1 tbsp. vanilla
- 1 tbsp. orange blossom
- 1 tbsp. rose water
- 1 tbsp. orange zest
- 1 egg
- ½ cup butter
- 2 cups phyllo dough or kadaifi
- ½ cup toasted coconut
- ½ cup pistachios
- ½ cup simple syrup

Directions:
Preheat the oven to 325°F.

With a hand mixer, mix the condensed milk, cream cheese, and the sour cream in a large bowl until well blended. Alternatively, you can blend them until well blended.

Add the orange zest, orange blossom, rose water, vanilla, and sugar, blend for 1 minute. Add in the egg and blend for 30 seconds.

In another bowl, break the kadaifi into pieces. Add 3 tbsps. of the sugar, and the butter, mix until well combined.

Line the bottom and the sides of a cheesecake pan or a muffin tin with the kadaifi mixture.

Pour the cheesecake mixture into the cheesecake pan or muffin tin, filling 80% of the container. Place into the oven and bake for 20 minutes. Remove from the oven and let completely cool before Servings.

When completely cool, slice the cake into 8 portions, top with the syrup, pistachio and/or coconut, and glaze with more simple syrup. Serve.

Nutrition: Calories 742, Fat: 43g, Carbs: 78g, Fiber: 2.6g, Protein: 12g

344. **Mediterranean Bread Pudding**
Preparation Time: 10 minutes, plus 6 hr. chilling
Cooking Time: 20 minutes
Servings: 6
Ingredients:

- ¼ of a large-sized lemon, juiced
- ½ cup sugar
- 8 white bread slices, edges removed, toasted, or more as needed
- 2 cups Ashta or Lebanese cream, or more as needed
- 1 ½ cup simple syrup
- ½ cup shredded coconut, toasted
- ½ cup pine nuts

Directions:
Put the sugar, lemon juice, and water into a thick-bottomed pan. Place the pan on the stove and heat over high flame or heat; bring to a boil, continuously stirring. When boiling, let simmer for 5 minutes, continuously stirring, until the mixture is amber in color, being careful it does not burn and turn bitter.

Choose a metal pan according to your desired size. Immediately pour the caramel into the pan, swirling the pan to spread the caramel evenly.

In a single layer, arrange the toasted bread on top of the caramel layer. Generously pour the simple syrup over the bread and spread with the Ashta. If you are using a small metal pan, repeat the layer of bread, drizzle of caramel, and Ashta. Generously sprinkle with the coconut and the pine nuts. Cover the pan and refrigerate for at least 6 hours or overnight. When chilled, slice into 6 portion sand serve.

Notes: you can decorate this dessert with your preferred choice of topping, such as pistachios, almonds, strawberries, candied orange, etc. You can even layer the ingredients in glasses and ramekins for a fancy presentation.

Nutrition: Calories 619, Fat: 10g, Carbs: 130g, Fiber: 5.3g, Protein: 5g

345.   **Banana Shake Bowls**
Preparation Time: 5 minutes
Cooking Time: 0 minutes
Servings: 4
Ingredients:

- 4 medium bananas, peeled
- 1 avocado, peeled, pitted and mashed
- ¾ cup almond milk
- ½ tsp vanilla extract

Directions:
In a blender, combine the bananas with the avocado and the other ingredients, pulse, divide into bowls and keep in the fridge until serving.

Nutrition: Calories 185, Fat: 4.3g, Fiber: 4g, Carbs: 6g, Protein: 6.45g

346.   **Mediterranean Biscotti**
Preparation Time: 25 minutes
Cooking Time: 1 hour
Servings: 3 dozen
Ingredients:

- 2 eggs
- 1 cup whole-wheat flour
- 1 cup all-purpose flour
- ¾ cup parmesan cheese, grated
- 2 tsps. baking powder
- 2 tbsps. sugar
- ¼ cup sun-dried tomato, finely chopped
- ¼ cup Kalamata olive, finely chopped
- ⅓ cup olive oil
- ½ tsp salt
- ½ tsp black pepper, cracked
- 1 tsp. dried oregano (preferably Greek)
- 1 tsp. dried basil

Directions:
Into a large-sized bowl, beat the eggs and the sugar together. Pour in the olive; beat until smooth.

In another bowl, combine the flours, baking powder, pepper, salt, oregano, and basil. Stir the flour mix into the egg mixture, stirring until blended.

Stir in the cheese, tomatoes, and olives; stirring until thoroughly combined.

Divide the dough into 2 portions: shape each into 10-inch long logs. Place the logs into a parchment-lined cookie sheet; flatten the log tops slightly.

Bake for about 30 minutes in a preheated 375°F oven or until the logs are pale golden and not quite firm to the touch.

Remove from the oven; let cool on the baking sheet for 3 minutes. Transfer the logs into a cutting board; slice each log into ½-inch diagonal slices using a serrated knife.

Place the biscotti slices on the baking sheet, return into the 325°F oven, and bake for about 20 to 25 minutes until dry and firm. Flip the slices halfway through baking. Remove from the oven, transfer on a wire rack, and let cool.

Notes: Store the biscotti slices into airtight containers.

Nutrition: Calories 731.6, Fat: 36.5g, Carbs: 77.8g, Fiber: 3.5g, Protein: 23.3g

347.   Chocolate Baklava
Preparation Time: 46 minutes
Cooking Time: 35 minutes
Servings: 24(1 piece)
Ingredients:

- 24 sheets (14 x 9-inch) frozen whole-wheat phyllo (filo) dough, thawed
- ⅛ tsp salt
- ⅓ cup toasted walnuts, chopped coarsely
- ⅓ cup almonds, blanched toasted, chopped coarsely
- ½ tsp ground cinnamon
- ½ cup water
- ½ cup hazelnuts, toasted, chopped coarsely
- ½ cup pistachios, roasted, chopped coarsely
- ¾ cup honey
- ½ cup of butter, melted
- 1 cup chocolate-hazelnut spread (I used Nutella)
- 1-piece (3-inch) cinnamon stick
- Cooking spray

Directions:
Into medium-sized saucepan, combine the water, honey, and the cinnamon stick; stir until the honey is dissolved. Increase the heat/flame to medium; continue cooking for about 10 minutes without stirring. A candy thermometer should read 230°F. Remove the saucepan from the heat and then keep warm. Remove and discard the cinnamon stick.

Preheat the oven to 350°F.

Put the chocolate-hazelnut spread into microwavable bowl; microwave the spread for about 30 seconds on HIGH or until the spread is melted.

In a bowl, combine the hazelnuts, pistachios, almonds, walnuts, ground cinnamon, and the salt.

Lightly grease with the cooking spray a 9 x 13-inch ceramic or glass baking dish.

Put 1 sheet lengthwise into the bottom of the prepared baking dish, extending the ends of the sheet over the edges of the dish. Lightly brush the sheet with the butter. Repeat the process with 5 sheets phyllo and a light brush of butter. Drizzle ⅓ cup of the melted chocolate-hazelnut spread over the buttered phyllo sheets. Sprinkle about ⅓ of the nut mixture (½ cup) over the spread. Repeat the process, layering phyllo sheet, brush of butter, spread, and with nut mixture. For the last, nut mixture top layer, top with 6 phyllo sheets, pressing each phyllo gently into the dish and brushing each sheet with butter.

Slice the layers into 24 portions by making 3 cuts lengthwise and then 5 cuts crosswise with a sharp knife; bake for about 35 minutes at 350°F or until the phyllo sheets are golden. Remove the dish from the oven, drizzle the honey sauce over the baklava. Pace the dish on a wire rack and let cool. Cover and store the baklavas at normal room temperature if not serving right away.

Notes: The sheets of phyllo are delicately thin so handle them with care to avoid tearing them. Cover the sheets with damp cloth so they won't dry out while you are working.

Nutrition: Calories 238, Fat: 13.4g, Carbs: 27.8g, Fiber: 1.6g, Protein: 4g

348. **Orange-Glazed Fruit and Ouzo Whipped Cream**

Preparation Time: 20 minutes, plus 30 minutes chilling

Cooking Time: 10 minutes

Servings: 4

Ingredients:

3 cups fruit (such as tangerine wedges, quartered apricots or plums, or strips of mango)

1 tbsp. olive oil spread/butter divided (I Can't Believe It's Not Butter! ®), melted

Chopped almonds, optional (or pistachios)

For the ouzo whipped cream:

- 1 tsp. sugar
- 1 tsp. ouzo liqueur (anise-flavored), orange juice, orange liqueur, or several drops of anise extract
- ½ cup whipping cream

For the sauce:

- 2 tbsps. sugar
- 2 tbsps. honey
- ¼ cup orange juice

Directions:
For the syrup:
Mix the syrup ingredients inside a small-sized saucepan. Bring the mixture to a boil, stirring, until the honey and the sugar are dissolved and reduce the heat. Simmer the mixture, without cover, for 10 minutes and set aside.
For the ouzo whipped cream:
In a medium-sized chilled bowl, beat the ouzo whipped cream ingredients using electric mixer on medium speed until soft peaks form with the tips curled. Cover and refrigerate for about 30 minutes to chill.
For the grilled fruit:
Toss the melted olive oil butter and the fruit in a mixing bowl. Transfer the fruit into a foil pan (see notes) or grill pan.

If using charcoal grill, put pan with fruits on the uncovered grill rack over medium coals; grill for about 10-12 minutes, stirring occasionally, until the fruits are heated through.

If using gas grill, first, preheat the grill, then reduce to medium heat. Put the grill rack on the grill rack. Cover the grill and grill for about 10-12 minutes, stirring occasionally, until the fruits are heated through.

Divide the fruits between 4 pieces dessert plates and drizzle with the honey syrup. If desired, sprinkle with the almonds. Serve with the ouzo whipped cream.

Notes: I Can't Believe It's Not Butter! ® is a great butter alternative made with oil blends, water, and salt. It's a simple and delicious spread that's all-natural. To make the foil pan, fold a heavy foil into double thickness. Fold the sides up to create a pan and then cut slits in the bottom.

Nutrition: Calories 267, Fat: 15g, Carbs: 36g, Fiber: 2g, Protein: 2g
349.   Lemon Curd Filled Almond-Lemon Cake
Preparation Time: 30 minutes
Cooking Time: 35 minutes
Servings: 8 (1 wedge)
Ingredients:

- 4 large egg yolks
- 4 large egg whites
- 2 tsps. matzo cake meal
- 2 cups fresh raspberries
- ¼ tsp of salt
- ¼ cup matzo cake meal
- ¼ cup blanched almonds, ground
- ½ tsp grated lemon rind

- 1 tsp. lemon juice, fresh
- 1 cup sugar
- 1 cup Lemon Curd
- 1 ½ tsps. water
- Cooking spray

Directions:
Preheat the oven to 350°F.

Coat a 9-inch spring-form pan with the cooking spray. Dust the pan with the 2 tsps. of matzo cake meal.

Place the yolks into a large-sized bowl; beat with a mixer at high speed for about 2 minutes. Gradually add the sugar and beat the mixture until pale and thick, about 1 minute. Add the ¼ cup matzo cake meal, water, lemon rind, lemon juice, and salt; beat until the mixture is just blended. Fold in the almonds.

Place the egg whites into a large-sized bowl. With clean, dry beaters, beat the egg whites using a mixer at high speed until stiff peaks form. Gently stir in ¼ of the egg whites into the yolk mixture; gently fold in the remaining of the egg whites. Spoon the batter into prepared spring-form pan.

Bake for about 35 minutes at 350°F or until the cake is set and brown; remove the pan from the oven, place in a wire rack, and let cool for 10 minutes. Run a knife around the edge of the cake, remove the cake from the pan, place in the wire rack and let cool completely. The cake will sink as it cools.

Spread about 1 cup of lemon curd in the center of the cake. Top with the raspberries. Cut the cake into 8 wedges with a serrated knife. Serve immediately.

Notes: You can prepare the curd 1 or 2 days ahead of time. You can enjoy leftovers on fruit or ice cream. You can also bake the cake earlier in the day and let it cool on a wire rack.

Decorate the cake with the curd and the berries just before serving.

Nutrition: Calories 238, Fat: 6.6g, Protein: 5.9g, Carbs: 41.4g, Fiber: 2.7g

350. **Cold Lemon Squares**
Preparation Time: 30 minutes
Cooking Time: 0 minutes
Servings: 4
Ingredients:

- 1 cup avocado oil + a drizzle
- 2 bananas, peeled and chopped
- 1 tbsp. honey
- ¼ cup lemon juice
- A pinch of lemon zest, grated

Directions:
In your food processor, mix the bananas with the rest of the ingredients, pulse well and spread on the bottom of a pan greased with a drizzle of oil.

Introduce in the fridge for 30 minutes, slice into squares and serve.

Nutrition: Calories 136, Fat: 11.2g, Fiber: 0.2g, Carbs: 7g, Protein: 1.1g

351.   Blackberry and Apples Cobbler
Preparation Time: 10 minutes
Cooking Time: 30 minutes
Servings: 6
Ingredients:

- ¾ cup stevia
- 6 cups blackberries
- ¼ cup apples, cored and cubed
- ¼ tsp baking powder
- 1 tbsp. lime juice
- ½ cup almond flour
- ½ cup water
- 3 and ½ tbsp avocado oil
- Cooking spray

Directions:
In a bowl, mix the berries with half of the stevia and lemon juice, sprinkle some flour all over, whisk and pour into a baking dish greased with cooking spray.

In another bowl, mix flour with the rest of the sugar, baking powder, the water and the oil, and stir the whole thing with your hands.

Spread over the berries, introduce in the oven at 375°F and bake for 30 minutes.

Serve warm.

Nutrition: Calories 221, Fat: 6.3g, Fiber: 3.3g, Carbs: 6g, Protein: 9g

352.   Black Tea Cake
Preparation Time: 10 minutes
Cooking Time: 35 minutes
Servings: 8
Ingredients:

- 6 tbsps. black tea powder
- 2 cups almond milk, warmed up
- 1 cup avocado oil
- 2 cups stevia
- 4 eggs
- 2 tsps. vanilla extract
- 3 ½ cups almond flour

- 1 tsp. baking soda
- 3 tsps. baking powder

Directions:
In a bowl, combine the almond milk with the oil, stevia and the rest of the ingredients and whisk well.

Pour this into a cake pan lined with parchment paper, introduce in the oven at 350°F and bake for 35 minutes.

Leave the cake to cool down, slice and serve.

Nutrition: Calories 200, Fat: 6.4g, Fiber: 4g, Carbs: 6.5g, Protein: 5.4g

353. **Green Tea and Vanilla Cream**
Preparation Time: 2 hours
Cooking Time: 0 minutes
Servings: 4
Ingredients:

- 14 oz. almond milk, hot
- 2 tbsps. green tea powder
- 14 oz. heavy cream
- 3 tbsps. stevia
- 1 tsp. vanilla extract
- 1 tsp. gelatin powder

Directions:
In a bowl, combine the almond milk with the green tea powder and the rest of the ingredients, whisk well, cool down, divide into cups, and keep in the fridge for 2 hours before Servings.

Nutrition: Calories 120, Fat: 3g, Fiber: 3g, Carbs: 7g, Protein: 4g

354. **Figs Pie**
Preparation Time: 10 minutes
Cooking Time: 1 hour
Servings: 8
Ingredients:

- ½ cup stevia
- 6 figs, cut into quarters
- ½ tsp vanilla extract
- 1 cup almond flour
- 4 eggs, whisked

Directions:
Spread the figs on the bottom of a springform pan lined with parchment paper.

In a bowl, combine the other ingredients, whisk, and pour over the figs,

Bake at 375°F for 1 hour, flip the pie upside down when it's done and serve.
Nutrition: Calories 200, Fat: 4.4g, Fiber: 3g, Carbs: 7.6g, Protein: 8g
355.   Cherry Cream
Preparation Time: 2 hours
Cooking Time: 0 minutes
Servings: 4
Ingredients:

- 2 cups cherries, pitted and chopped
- 1 cup almond milk
- ½ cup whipping cream
- 3 eggs, whisked
- ⅓ cup stevia
- 1 tsp. lemon juice
- ½ tsp vanilla extract

Directions:
In your food processor, combine the cherries with the milk and the rest of the ingredients, pulse well, divide into cups and keep in the fridge for 2 hours before Servings.
Nutrition: Calories 200, Fat: 4.5g, Fiber: 3.3g, Carbs: 5.6g, Protein: 3.4g
356.   Strawberries Cream
Preparation Time: 10 minutes
Cooking Time: 20 minutes
Servings: 4
Ingredients:

- ½ cup stevia
- 2 pounds strawberries, chopped
- 1 cup almond milk
- Zest of 1 lemon, grated
- ½ cup heavy cream
- 3 egg yolks, whisked

Directions:
Heat up a pan with the milk over medium-high heat, add the stevia and the rest of the ingredients, whisk well, simmer for 20 minutes, divide into cups and serve cold.
Nutrition: Calories 152, Fat: 4.4g, Fiber: 5.5g, Carbs: 5.1g, Protein: 0.8g
357.   Apples and Plum Cake
Preparation Time: 10 minutes
Cooking Time: 40 minutes
Servings: 4
Ingredients:

- 7 oz. almond flour
- 1 egg, whisked
- 5 tbsps. stevia
- 3 oz. warm almond milk
- 2 pounds plums, pitted and cut into quarters
- 2 apples, cored and chopped
- Zest of 1 lemon, grated
- 1 tsp. baking powder

Directions:
In a bowl, mix the almond milk with the egg, stevia, and the rest of the ingredients except the cooking spray and whisk well.

Grease a cake pan with the oil, pour the cake mix inside, introduce in the oven, and bake at 350°F for 40 minutes.

Cool down, slice, and serve.

Nutrition: Calories 209, Fat: 6.4g, Fiber: 6g, Carbs: 8g, Protein: 6.6g

358.   Cinnamon Chickpeas Cookies
Preparation Time: 10 minutes
Cooking Time: 20 minutes
Servings: 12
Ingredients:

- 1 cup canned chickpeas, drained, rinsed, and mashed
- 2 cups almond flour
- 1 tsp. cinnamon powder
- 1 tsp. baking powder
- 1 cup avocado oil
- ½ cup stevia
- 1 egg, whisked
- 2 tsps. almond extract
- 1 cup raisins
- 1 cup coconut, unsweetened and shredded

Directions:
In a bowl, combine the chickpeas with the flour, cinnamon, and the other ingredients, and whisk well until you obtain a dough.

Scoop tbsps. of dough on a baking sheet lined with parchment paper, introduce them in the oven at 350°F and bake for 20 minutes.

Leave them to cool down for a few minutes and serve.

Nutrition: Calories 200, Fat: 4.5g, Fiber: 3.4g, Carbs: 9.5g, Protein: 2.4g

359.   Cocoa Brownies
Preparation Time: 10 minutes
Cooking Time: 20 minutes
Servings: 8

Ingredients:

- 30 oz. canned lentils, rinsed and drained
- 1 tbsp. honey
- 1 banana, peeled and chopped
- ½ tsp baking soda
- 4 tbsps. almond butter
- 2 tbsps. cocoa powder
- Cooking spray

Directions:

In a food processor, combine the lentils with the honey and the other ingredients except the cooking spray and pulse well.

Pour this into a pan greased with cooking spray, spread evenly, introduce in the oven at 375°F and bake for 20 minutes.

Cut the brownies and serve cold.

Nutrition: Calories 200, Fat: 4.5g, Fiber: 2.4g, Carbs: 8.7g, Protein: 4.3g

360.   Grapes Stew
Preparation Time: 10 minutes
Cooking Time: 10 minutes
Servings: 4
Ingredients:

- ⅔ cup stevia
- 1 tbsp. olive oil
- ⅓ cup coconut water
- 1 tsp. vanilla extract
- 1 tsp. lemon zest, grated
- 2 cup red grapes, halved

Directions:

Heat up a pan with the water over medium heat, add the oil, stevia and the rest of the ingredients, toss, simmer for 10 minutes, divide into cups and serve.

Nutrition: Calories 122, Fat: 3.7g, Fiber: 1.2g, Carbs: 2.3g, Protein: 0.4g

361.   Cocoa Sweet Cherry Cream
Preparation Time: 2 hours
Cooking Time: 0 minutes
Servings: 4
Ingredients:

- ½ cup cocoa powder
- ¾ cup red cherry jam
- ¼ cup stevia
- 2 cups water

- 1 lb. cherries, pitted and halved

Directions:

In a blender, mix the cherries with the water and the rest of the ingredients, pulse well, divide into cups and keep in the fridge for 2 hours before serving.

Nutrition: Calories 162, Fat: 3.4g, Fiber: 2.4g, Carbs: 5g, Protein: 1g

362.   Apple Couscous Pudding

Preparation Time: 10 minutes

Cooking Time: 25 minutes

Servings: 4

Ingredients:

- ½ cup couscous
- 1 ½ cups milk
- ¼ cup apple, cored and chopped
- 3 tbsps. stevia
- ½ tsp rose water
- 1 tbsp. orange zest, grated

Directions:

Heat up a pan with the milk over medium heat, add the couscous and the rest of the ingredients, whisk, simmer for 25 minutes, divide into bowls and serve.

Nutrition: Calories 150, Fat: 4.5g, Fiber: 5.5g, Carbs: 7.5g, Protein: 4g

363.   Ricotta Ramekins

Preparation Time: 10 minutes

Cooking Time: 1 hour

Servings: 4

Ingredients:

- 6 eggs, whisked
- 1 ½ pounds ricotta cheese, soft
- ½ pound stevia
- 1 tsp. vanilla extract
- ½ tsp baking powder
- Cooking spray

Directions:

In a bowl, mix the eggs with the ricotta and the other ingredients except the cooking spray and whisk well.

Grease 4 ramekins with the cooking spray, pour the ricotta cream in each and bake at 360°F for 1 hour.

Serve cold.

Nutrition: Calories 180, Fat: 5.3g, Fiber: 5.4g, Carbs: 11.5g, Protein: 4g

364.   **Papaya Cream**
Preparation Time: 10 minutes
Cooking Time: 0 minutes
Servings: 2
Ingredients:

- 1 cup papaya, peeled and chopped
- 1 cup heavy cream
- 1 tbsp. stevia
- ½ tsp vanilla extract

Directions:

In a blender, combine the cream with the papaya and the other ingredients, pulse well, divide into cups and serve cold.

Nutrition: Calories 182, Fat: 3.1g, Fiber: 2.3g, Carbs: 3.5g, Protein: 2g

365.   **Orange Cake**
Preparation Time: 20 minutes
Cooking Time: 60 minutes
Servings: 8
Ingredients:

- 4 oranges
- ⅓ cup water
- ½ cup Erythritol
- ½ tsp ground cinnamon
- 4 eggs, beaten
- 3 tbsps. stevia powder
- 10 oz. Phyllo pastry
- ½ tsp baking powder
- ½ cup Plain yogurt
- 3 tbsps. olive oil

Directions:

Squeeze the juice from 1 orange and pour it in the saucepan.

Add water, squeezed oranges, water, ground cinnamon, and Erythritol. Bring the liquid to boil.

Simmer the liquid for 5 minutes over the medium heat. When the time is over, cool it.

Grease the baking mold with 1 tbsp. of olive oil. Chop the phyllo dough and place it in the baking mold.

Slice ½ of orange for decorating the cake. Slice it. Squeeze juice from remaining oranges.

Then mix up together, squeeze orange juice, Plain yogurt, baking powder, stevia powder, and eggs. Add remaining olive oil

Mix up the mixture with the help of the hand mixer.

Pour the liquid over the chopped Phyllo dough. Stir to evenly distribute.

Top the cake with sliced orange (that one which you leave for decorating).

Bake the dessert for 50 minutes at 370°F.

Pour the baked cake with cooled orange juice syrup. Leave it for 10 minutes to let the cake soaks the syrup.

Cut it into servings.

Nutrition: Calories 237, Fat: 4.4 g, Fiber: 1.4 g, Carbs: 36.9 g, Protein: 1.9 g

366.   Cardamom Almond Cream

Preparation Time: 30 minutes

Cooking Time: 0 minutes

Servings: 4

Ingredients:

- Juice of 1 lime
- ½ cup stevia
- 1 ½ cups water
- 3 cups almond milk
- ½ cup honey
- 2 tsps. cardamom, ground
- 1 tsp. rose water
- 1 tsp. vanilla extract

Directions:

In a blender, combine the almond milk with the cardamom and the rest of the ingredients, pulse well, divide into cups and keep in the fridge for 30 minutes before Servings.

Nutrition: Calories 283, Fat: 11.8g, Fiber: 0.3g, Carbs: 4.7g, Protein: 7.1g

367.   Banana Cinnamon Cupcakes

Preparation Time: 10 minutes

Cooking Time: 20 minutes

Servings: 4

Ingredients:

- 4 tbsps. avocado oil
- 4 eggs
- ½ cup orange juice
- 2 tsps. cinnamon powder
- 1 tsp. vanilla extract
- 2 bananas, peeled and chopped
- ¾ cup almond flour
- ½ tsp baking powder

- Cooking spray

Directions:
In a bowl, combine the oil with the eggs, orange juice and the other ingredients except the cooking spray, whisk well, pour in a cupcake pan greased with the cooking spray, introduce in the oven at 350°F and bake for 20 minutes.

Cool the cupcakes down and serve.

Nutrition: Calories 142, Fat: 5.8g, Fiber: 4.2g, Carbs: 5.7g, Protein: 1.6g

368.   Rhubarb and Apples Cream
Preparation Time: 10 minutes
Cooking Time: 0 minutes
Servings: 6
Ingredients:

- 3 cups rhubarb, chopped
- 1 ½ cups stevia
- 2 eggs, whisked
- ½ tsp nutmeg, ground
- 1 tbsp. avocado oil
- ⅓ cup almond milk

Directions:
In a blender, combine the rhubarb with the stevia and the rest of the ingredients, pulse well, divide into cups and serve cold.

Nutrition: Calories 200, Fat: 5.2g, Fiber: 3.4g, Carbs: 7.6g, Protein: 2.5g

369.   Almond Rice Dessert
Preparation Time: 10 minutes
Cooking Time: 20 minutes
Servings: 4
Ingredients:

- 1 cup white rice
- 2 cups almond milk
- 1 cup almonds, chopped
- ½ cup stevia
- 1 tbsp. cinnamon powder
- ½ cup pomegranate seeds

Directions:
In a pot, mix the rice with the milk and stevia, bring to a simmer, and cook for 20 minutes, stirring often.

Add the rest of the ingredients, stir, divide into bowls, and serve.

Nutrition: Calories 234, Fat: 9.5g, Fiber: 3.4g, Carbs: 12.4g, Protein: 6.5g

370.   **Peach Sorbet**
Preparation Time: 2 hours
Cooking Time: 10 minutes
Servings: 4
Ingredients:

- 2 cups apple juice
- 1 cup stevia
- 2 tbsps. lemon zest, grated
- 2 pounds peaches, pitted and quartered

Directions:
Heat up a pan over medium heat, add the apple juice and the rest of the ingredients, simmer for 10 minutes, transfer to a blender, pulse, divide into cups and keep in the freezer for 2 hours before Servings.
Nutrition: Calories 182, Fat: 5.4g, Fiber: 3.4g, Carbs: 12g, Protein: 5.4g

371.   **Cranberries and Pears Pie**
Preparation Time: 10 minutes
Cooking Time: 40 minutes
Servings: 4
Ingredients:

- 2 cup cranberries
- 3 cups pears, cubed
- A drizzle of olive oil
- 1 cup stevia
- ⅓ cup almond flour
- 1 cup rolled oats
- ¼ avocado oil

Directions:
In a bowl, mix the cranberries with the pears and the other ingredients except the olive oil and the oats, and stir well.

Grease a cake pan with a drizzle of olive oil, pour the pears mix inside, sprinkle the oats all over and bake at 350°F for 40 minutes.

Cool the mix down and serve.
Nutrition: Calories 172, Fat: 3.4g, Fiber: 4.3g, Carbs: 11.5g, Protein: 4.5g

372.   **Lemon Cream**
Preparation Time: 1 hour
Cooking Time: 10 minutes
Servings: 6
Ingredients:

- 2 eggs, whisked

- 1 ¼ cup stevia
- 10 tbsps. avocado oil
- 1 cup heavy cream
- Juice of 2 lemons
- Zest of 2 lemons, grated

Directions:
In a pan, combine the cream with the lemon juice and the other ingredients, whisk well, cook for 10 minutes, divide into cups, and keep in the fridge for 1 hour before Servings.
Nutrition: Calories 200, Fat: 8.5g, Fiber: 4.5g, Carbs: 8.6g, Protein: 4.5g
373.   **Blueberries Stew**
Preparation Time: 10 minutes
Cooking Time: 10 minutes
Servings: 4
Ingredients:

- 2 cups blueberries
- 3 tbsps. stevia
- 1 ½ cups pure apple juice
- 1 tsp. vanilla extract

Directions:
In a pan, combine the blueberries with stevia and the other ingredients, bring to a simmer and cook over medium-low heat for 10 minutes.
Divide into cups and serve cold.
Nutrition: Calories 192, Fat: 5.4g, Fiber: 3.4g, Carbs: 9.4g, Protein: 4.5g
374.   **Mandarin Cream**
Preparation Time: 20 minutes
Cooking Time: 0 minutes
Servings: 8
Ingredients:

- 2 mandarins, peeled and cut into segments
- Juice of 2 mandarins
- 2 tbsps. stevia
- 4 eggs, whisked
- ¾ cup stevia
- ¾ cup almonds, ground

Directions:
In a blender, combine the mandarins with the juice and the other ingredients, whisk well, divide into cups and keep in the fridge for 20 minutes before Servings.

Nutrition: Calories 106, Fat: 3.4g, Fiber: 0g, Carbs: 2.4g, Protein: 4g

375.   **Creamy Mint Strawberry Mix**

Preparation Time: 10 minutes

Cooking Time: 30 minutes

Servings: 6

Ingredients:

- Cooking spray
- ¼ cup stevia
- 1 ½ cup almond flour
- 1 tsp. baking powder
- 1 cup almond milk
- 1 egg, whisked
- 2 cups strawberries, sliced
- 1 tbsp. mint, chopped
- 1 tsp. lime zest, grated
- ½ cup whipping cream

Directions:

In a bowl, combine the almond with the strawberries, mint and the other ingredients except the cooking spray and whisk well.

Grease 6 ramekins with the cooking spray, pour the strawberry mix inside, introduce in the oven and bake at 350°F for 30 minutes.

Cool down and serve.

Nutrition: Calories 200, Fat: 6.3g, Fiber: 2g, Carbs: 6.5g, Protein: 8g

376.   **Vanilla Cake**

Preparation Time: 10 minutes

Cooking Time: 25 minutes

Servings: 10

Ingredients:

- 3 cups almond flour
- 3 tsps. baking powder
- 1 cup olive oil
- 1 and ½ cup almond milk
- 1 and 2/3 cup stevia
- 2 cups water
- 1 tbsp. lime juice
- 2 tsps. vanilla extract
- Cooking spray

Directions:

In a bowl, mix the almond flour with the baking powder, the oil, and the rest of the ingredients except the cooking spray and whisk well.

Pour the mix into a cake pan greased with the cooking spray, introduce in the oven, and bake at 370°F for 25 minutes.

Leave the cake to cool down, cut and serve!

Nutrition: Calories 200, Fat: 7.6g, Fiber: 2.5g, Carbs: 5.5g, Protein: 4.5g

377.   Pumpkin Cream
Preparation Time: 5 minutes
Cooking Time: 5 minutes
Servings: 2
Ingredients:

- 2 cups canned pumpkin flesh
- 2 tbsps. stevia
- 1 tsp. vanilla extract
- 2 tbsps. water
- A pinch of pumpkin spice

Directions:

In a pan, combine the pumpkin flesh with the other ingredients, simmer for 5 minutes, divide into cups and serve cold.

Nutrition: Calories 192, Fat: 3.4g, Fiber: 4.5g, Carbs: 7.6g, Protein: 3.5g

378.   Chia and Berries Smoothie Bowl
Preparation Time: 5 minutes
Cooking Time: 0 minutes
Servings: 2
Ingredients:

- 1 ½ cup almond milk
- 1 cup blackberries
- ¼ cup strawberries, chopped
- 1 ½ tbsps. chia seeds
- 1 tsp. cinnamon powder

Directions:

In a blender, combine the blackberries with the strawberries and the rest of the ingredients, pulse well, divide into small bowls and serve cold.

Nutrition: Calories 182, Fat: 3.4g, Fiber: 3.4g, Carbs: 8.4g, Protein: 3g

379.   Minty Coconut Cream
Preparation Time: 4 minutes
Cooking Time: 0 minutes
Servings: 2
Ingredients:

- 1 banana, peeled
- 2 cups coconut flesh, shredded

- 3 tbsps. mint, chopped
- 1 and ½ cups coconut water
- 2 tbsps. stevia
- ½ avocado, pitted and peeled

Directions:
In a blender, combine the coconut with the banana and the rest of the ingredients, pulse well, divide into cups and serve cold.

Nutrition: Calories 193, Fat: 5.4g, Fiber: 3.4g, Carbs: 7.6g, Protein: 3g

380.   **Watermelon Cream**
Preparation Time: 15 minutes
Cooking Time: 0 minutes
Servings: 2
Ingredients:

- 1 lb. watermelon, peeled and chopped
- 1 tsp. vanilla extract
- 1 cup heavy cream
- 1 tsp. lime juice
- 2 tbsps. stevia

Directions:
In a blender, combine the watermelon with the cream and the rest of the ingredients, pulse well, divide into cups and keep in the fridge for 15 minutes before Servings.

Nutrition: Calories 122, Fat: 5.7g, Fiber: 3.2g, Carbs: 5.3g, Protein: 0.4g

Chapter Six

MEDITERRANEAN RECIPES

*S*tart your morning with a portion of goodness. With a healthy and nutritious start, you are not just physically ready to face the da, but mentally charged as well.

On that note, let us dive into some delicious Mediterranean breakfast recipes.

1. Eggs Caprese

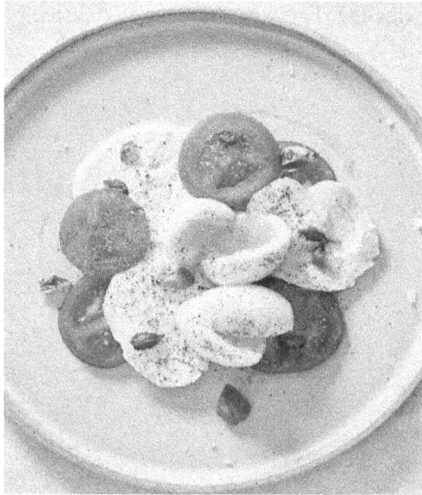

Eggs are just perfect for breakfast, and this caprese is going to add a fine twist to a typical poached eggs recipe.

Servings: 2
Prep Time: 10 minutes
Cook time: 10 minutes
Energy Value Per Serving: 2,025 kj
Calories: 484 calories
Protein: 33.3 g
Total Fat: 24.9 g
Carbohydrate: 31.7 g

Ingredients

- 1 tablespoon distilled white vinegar
- 2 teaspoons salt
- 4 eggs
- 2 English muffin, split
- 4 (1 ounce) slices mozzarella cheese
- 1 tomato, thickly sliced
- 4 teaspoons pesto
- salt to taste

Instructions

- Fill a large saucepan with about 2 to 3 inches of water. Place the saucepan over high heat and bring the water to a boil.
- When the water starts boiling, bring the heat to medium-low. Add in the vinegar and about 2 teaspoons of salt (you can adjust salt content as needed). Bring the water down to a gentle simmer.
- As the water simmers, add the slice of tomato and mozzarella cheese to each half of the English muffin. Place them into the toaster oven until you notice the muffin has toasted and the cheese has softened. This should usually take around 5 minutes.
- Take a small bowl and crack an egg into it. Gently add the egg into the simmering water. Using the same procedure, add the remaining eggs into the water as well.
- Allow the eggs to poach until you notice the yolks have thickened but are not hard and the whites are firm. This should take you about 3 minutes.
- Use a slotted spoon (or any other spoon that will help you with the job) and remove the eggs from the water. Use a kitchen towel to gently dab the eggs to remove any excess water.
- Finally, the presentation. Place one poached egg on each muffin. Take one teaspoon of pesto sauce and spread it on each egg.
- You can sprinkle a little salt to taste, or you can skip this step.

2. Mediterranean Style Quinoa

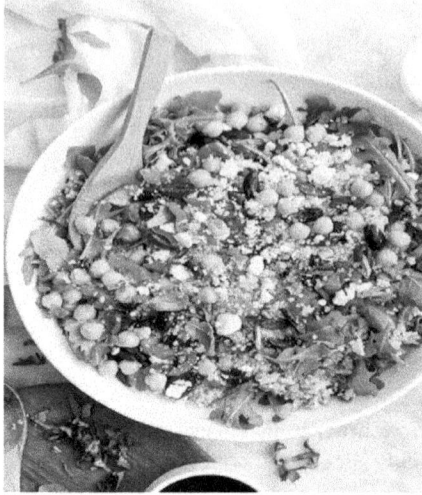

Quinoa has taken the world by storm. and for good reason. This breakfast is going to make your quinoa wishes come true with a lot of flavor and nutrition.

Servings: 4

Prep Time: 10 minutes

Cook time: 15 minutes

Energy Value Per Serving: 1,368 kj

Calories: 327 calories

Protein: 11.5 g

Total Fat: 7.9 g

Carbohydrate: 53.9 g

Ingredients

- 1/4 cup chopped raw almonds
- 1 teaspoon ground cinnamon
- 1 cup quinoa
- 2 cups almond milk
- 1 teaspoon sea salt
- 1 teaspoon vanilla extract
- 2 tablespoons honey
- 2 dried pitted dates, finely chopped
- 5 dried apricots, finely chopped

Instructions

- Take out a skillet and place it over medium heat. Add the almonds into it and toast them for about 3 to 5 minutes, or until they turn just a mild shade of golden. Place the skillet aside.
- Lower the heat to medium high. Take out a saucepan and add both the quinoa and cinnamon. Heat the mixture until they are warmed properly.

- Add the sea salt and milk into the saucepan. Stir the ingredients properly.
- Reduce the heat to low and place a cover over the saucepan. Allow the ingredients to simmer for about 15 minutes.
- Open the cover and add the honey, vanilla, honey, apricots, and about half the toasted almonds into the saucepan.
- Serve using the remaining almonds as toppings.

3. Spinach, Egg, and Feta Wrap

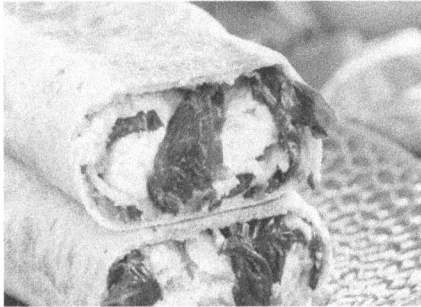

When you are craving some spinach and eggs, you can simply toss them into this hearty wrap.

Servings: 1

Prep Time: 10 minutes

Cook time: 5 minutes

Energy Value Per Serving: 2,929 kj

Calories: 700 calories

Protein: 36.6 g

Total Fat: 36.8 g

Carbohydrate: 78 g

Ingredients

- 1 large whole-wheat tortilla
- 1 teaspoon olive oil
- 1 cup chopped baby spinach leaves
- 1 sun-dried tomato, chopped
- 2 eggs, beaten
- 1/3 cup feta cheese
- 1 tomato, diced

Instructions

- Place a skillet over medium heat. Add the tortilla into the skillet and allow it to warm.
- Meanwhile, take another skillet and place it over medium-high heat. Add the olive oil into it.
- Add the tomato and spinach. Saute the vegetables.

- Toss in the eggs and scramble them for about 2 minutes, or until they are set.
- Sprinkle feta cheese on the mixture. Continue cooking for about 1 minute or until the cheese melts.
- Keep the tortilla in the skillet. Add the egg mixture into it. Add the diced tomato on top. Roll the tortilla and keep in the skillet for about 30 seconds, or until you notice the wrap can hold its shape.

4. Zucchini Noodles and Baked Egg with Avocado

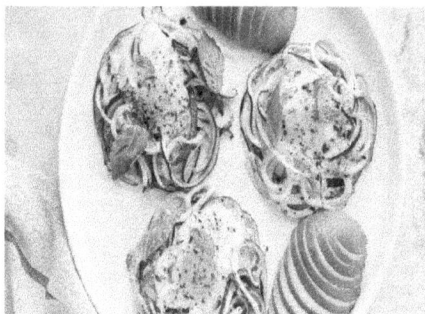

Zucchini noodles are just heart and delicious. Combine them with egg and avocado, and you are probably going to have so much energy, you might just run a marathon.

Servings: 2

Prep Time: 10 minutes

Cook time: 10 minutes

Energy Value Per Serving: 2,644 kj

Calories: 633 calories

Protein: 20 g

Total Fat: 53 g

Carbohydrate: 27 g

Ingredients

- 2 tablespoons extra-virgin olive oil
- 3 zucchinis, spiralized into noodles
- nonstick spray
- 4 large eggs
- 2 avocados, halved and thinly sliced
- fresh basil, for garnishing
- red-pepper flakes, for garnishing
- salt and freshly ground black pepper, to taste

Instructions

- Begin by preheating the oven to 350° F. Take out a baking tray and line it with a baking sheet. Lightly grease the sheet with nonstick spray.
- Take out a large bowl and then add in the zucchini noodles. Pour the olive oil and mix them together.

- Season with salt and pepper. Divide the zucchini mixture into 4 portions and place them on the baking sheet. Create a hollow in the center of each mixture in such a way, that it looks like a nest.
- Crack an egg into the hollow of each mixture. Pop the tray into the oven and then bake for about 10 minutes, or until the eggs are set.
- Take out the tray. You can season with a little more salt and pepper if you like. Top each zucchini mixture with basil and red pepper flakes. Serve them with the avocado slices.

5. Banana and Mocha Oats

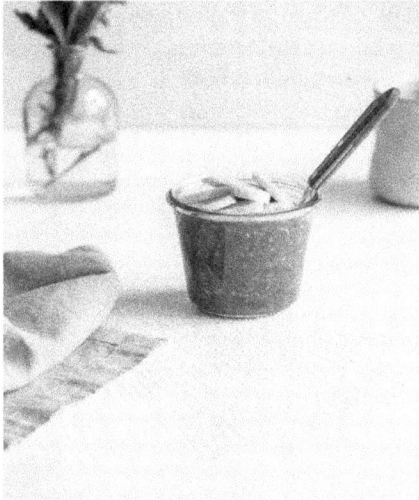

Here is an example of how the Mediterranean diet avoids added sugar and makes use of the natural sweetness found in fruits. Do note that you have to place the dish in the refrigerator overnight, which is perfect for those times you just want to quickly grab a healthy breakfast before heading out.

Servings: 2

Prep Time: 10 minutes

Cook time: None

Energy Value Per Serving: 1,537 kj

Calories: 369 calories

Protein: 11 g

Total Fat: 12 g

Carbohydrate: 61 g

Ingredients

- 1 banana
- 1 cup rolled oats
- One 1/2 tablespoons chia seeds
- 2 tablespoons cocoa powder

- 2 pitted dates, blended
- 3/4 cup almond milk
- 1/2 cup strong coffee
- pinch of sea salt

Instructions

- Take out a blender and add the almond milk, dates, banana, coffee, cocoa powder, and sea salt. Pulse them together until the mixture turns smooth.
- Add the chia seeds and oats in an airtight container. Take the blended mixture and pour them over the chia seeds and oats. Mix all the ingredients well, cover them, and place them in the refrigerator.
- When you take out the container in the morning, simply stir the mixture and add a little more almond milk, if you prefer.
- Top with fresh fruits of your choice.

6. Healthy Steel Cut Oatmeal

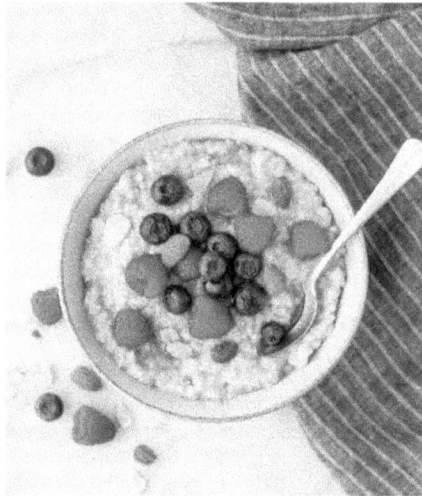

More oatmeal? Sure, why not. Do note that this meal takes around 45 minutes to complete. If you are in a hurry, then try the other recipes in this chapter.

Servings: 4

Prep Time: 10 minutes

Cook time: 35 minutes

Energy Value Per Serving: 1,236 kj

Calories: 295 calories

Protein: 13.7 g

Total Fat: 13.4 g

Carbohydrate: 13.4 g

Ingredients

- 3 cups water
- 1 cup almond milks
- 1 tablespoon unsalted butter
- 1 cup steel-cut oats
- ¼ teaspoon salt, to taste
- freshly ground black pepper, to taste

Instructions

- Take out a large saucepan and place it over medium heat. Add the milk and water. Bring the mixture to a simmer.
- Take out a skillet and place it over medium heat. Add the butter and allow it to melt. When you notice the butter sizzling, add the oats.
- Cook the oats, stirring occasionally for about 2 minutes, or until the oats turn fragrant and golden.
- Add the oats into the saucepan with milk and water. Bring down the heat to medium low and then stir the ingredients for about 20 minutes, or until the mixture turns thick.
- Add the salt and continue to stir for 10 minutes more. Reduce the heat if you think that the oats might become scorched.
- Remove the oatmeal from the heat and allow it to cool for about 5 minutes.

7. Tahini Toast

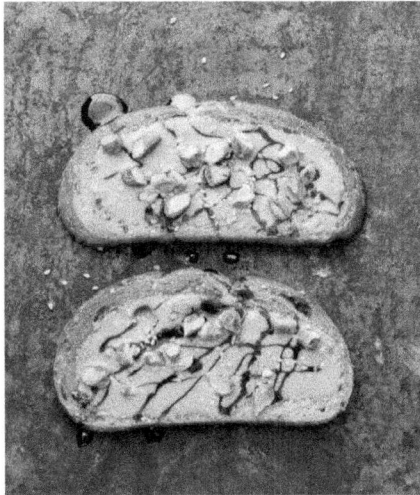

Want to make something healthy and filling quickly? Then why not this tahini toast recipe that can be made in under 5 minutes!

Servings: 2

Prep Time: 5 minutes

Cook time: None

Energy Value Per Serving: 745 kj
Calories: 178 calories
Protein: 5.1 g
Total Fat: 16.13 g
Carbohydrate: 6.36 g
Ingredients
- 2 slices whole wheat bread
- 2 teaspoons of pine nuts
- 1 teaspoon of water
- 2 teaspoons of crumbled feta
- 1 tablespoon tahini
- juice of 1/2 lemon
- pepper, to taste

Instructions
- Take out a small bowl and mix lemon juice, water, and tahini together. You are looking for a consistency that is not too thick. How thin should it be? Ideally, the mixture should be as thin as peanut butter. If you think you need to add more water to get the right consistency, then go ahead and add it. Just be careful that the mixture does not become too smooth.
- Toast the bread according to your preference.
- Once done, place the toast on a plate, spread the tahini sauce over it. Complete the dish by sprinkling pine nuts and feta.
- Add pepper for additional flavor.

8. Tuna and Avocado Tapas

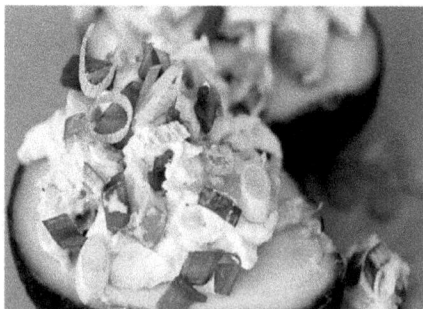

How about a little seafood in the morning? Adding tuna makes it easier (and quicker) to grab a seafood bite at the start of your day.
Servings: 2
Prep Time: 20 minutes
Cook time: None
Energy Value Per Serving: 1,237 kj
Calories: 294 calories
Protein: 23.9 g

Total Fat: 18.2 g

Carbohydrate: 11 g

Ingredients

- 1/2 red bell pepper, chopped
- 1 tablespoon low-fat mayonnaise
- 1 (12 ounce) can solid white tuna packed in water, drained
- 1 dash balsamic vinegar
- 3 green onions, thinly sliced, plus additional for garnish
- 2 ripe avocados, halved and pitted
- salt and pepper to taste

Instructions

- Take out a large bowl and add in mayonnaise, tuna, red pepper, green onions, and balsamic vinegar.
- Mix all the ingredients well and season them with salt. A pinch of salt would do, but add based on your preference.
- Take out the avocado halves and pack them with the tuna mixture.
- Garnish with black pepper and onions before serving.

9. Greek Yogurt Pancakes

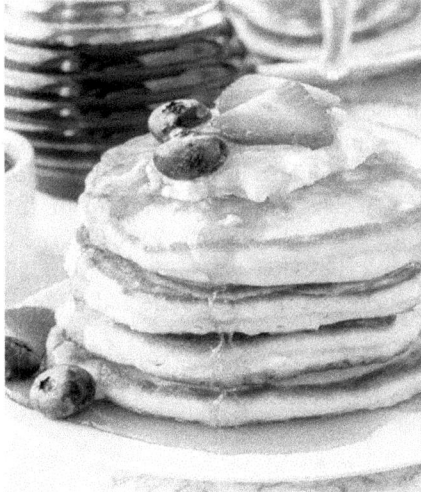

Can't get rid of your craving for pancakes? Then you might want to try this healthy version.

Servings: 6

Prep Time: 15 minutes

Cook time: 15 minutes

Energy Value Per Serving: 1,072 kj

Calories: 258 calories

Protein: 11 g

Total Fat: 8 g

Carbohydrate: 33 g

Ingredients

- One 1/2 cups Greek yogurt plain, non-fat
- One 1/4 cup all-purpose flour
- 1/2 cup milk
- 2 teaspoons baking powder
- 1 teaspoon baking soda
- 1/4 cup sugar
- 3 tablespoons butter unsalted, melted
- 3 eggs
- 1/4 teaspoon salt
- ½ cup blackberries (or you can choose raspberries or blueberries)

Instructions

- Take out a large bowl and then add salt, flour, baking powder and baking soda. Whisk them together well.
- Take out a separate bowl and add the butter, sugar, Greek yogurt, eggs, and milk. Whisk them well until the mixture turns smooth.
- Allow the Greek yogurt mixture to sit for about 15 minutes. Pour the Greek yogurt mixture into the bowl with baking soda. Mix them well to combine.
- Heat up the pancake griddle and spray it with a non-stick butter spray. Alternatively, you can use a brush to apply a thin layer of butter on the griddle.
- Pour the batter into the griddle in ¼ cup portions. For each portion, allow the pancake batter to cook until you see bubbles on the top of the pancake burst open. Check whether the bottom of the pancake is golden brown by lifting it using a spatula. If the color has turned golden brown, then flip the pancake and cook the other side until it turns a light brown color.
- Remove the pancakes from the griddle and serve them hot.
- Top each of the pancakes with Greek yogurt and the cup of your choice of berries.

10. Spinach and parmesan Cakes

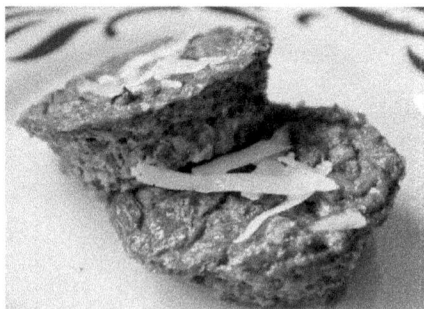

Cakes in the morning? That's an unhealthy way to start the day, isn't it? Not with these delicious, cheesy, and healthy cakes.

Servings: 4

Prep Time: 20 minutes

Cook time: 20 minutes

Energy Value Per Serving: 619 kj

Calories: 148 calories

Protein: 12.9 g

Total Fat: 7.9 g

Carbohydrate: 5.5 g

Ingredients

- 1 ½ cup (12 ounces) fresh spinach
- 1 clove garlic, minced
- 2 large eggs, beaten
- ½ cup finely shredded parmesan cheese, plus more for garnish
- 1/2 cup part-skim ricotta cheese
- ¼ teaspoon salt
- ¼ teaspoon freshly ground pepper

Instructions

- Begin by preheating the oven to around 400° F.
- Take out your blender and add the spinach into it. Pulse the spinach until it is finely chopped. For best results, add the spinach in small batches.
- Transfer all the spinach to a medium-sized bowl. Add parmesan, ricotta, garlic, eggs, salt, and pepper (you can lower the salt and pepper content to your preference). Mix all the ingredients well.
- Take out a muffin tray and then spray 8 cups in the pan with low-calorie cooking spray.
- Add the spinach mixture equally into each of the 8 cups. Place the tray into the oven.
- Bake the spinach for about 20 minutes, or until the cakes are set. Take out the tray and allow the cakes to set for about 5 minutes in the pan before serving.
- When serving, you can sprinkle the cakes with more parmesan if you like.

11. Orange Polentina

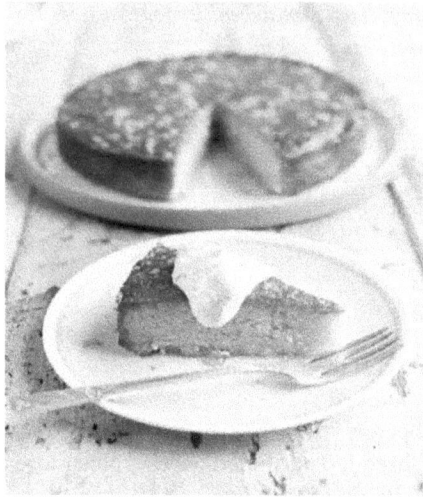

Italians love polentina and create it in such unique ways. This is a creamy and wholesome twist to the classic recipe. Be prepared to wolf it down!

Servings: 4

Prep Time: 10 minutes

Cook time: 10 minutes

Energy Value Per Serving: 1,464 kj

Calories: 350 calories

Protein: 8.9 g

Total Fat: 13.9 g

Carbohydrate: 50.3 g

Ingredients

- 1 medium orange
- 4 tablespoons honey, divided
- ¼ cup mascarpone
- 1 ½ cups low-fat milk
- ¼ cup nonfat Greek-style yogurt
- ¾ cup instant polenta
- 2 cups water
- ¼ teaspoon salt
- 1 teaspoon finely chopped fresh tarragon

Instructions

- Take out the orange and zest it. You should aim to get about 1 ½ teaspoons of orange zest. Once done, you can remove the rest of the peel.
- Take out a large bowl and cut the orange into their individual segments.
- Place a saucepan over medium-high heat. Add water, milk, and salt into the saucepan and bring the mixture to a boil. Reduce the heat to medium.

- Gently add in the polenta in small batches into the saucepan, whisking as you do so. Increase the heat back to medium-high and allow the mixture to boil again. When it starts boiling, bring the heat down to medium-low. Keep the polenta at this heat for about 5 minutes, or until it thickens. You might notice bubbles form gently on the polenta. Don't worry, that's completely normal.

- Once the polenta thickens, remove the saucepan from the heat and set it aside. Take out a small bowl and add yogurt, mascarpone, 1 tablespoon honey, and 1/2 teaspoon of orange zest. Mix the ingredients well.

- Add the remaining zest and honey into the polenta and mix them well.

12. Lemon Cream Blueberries

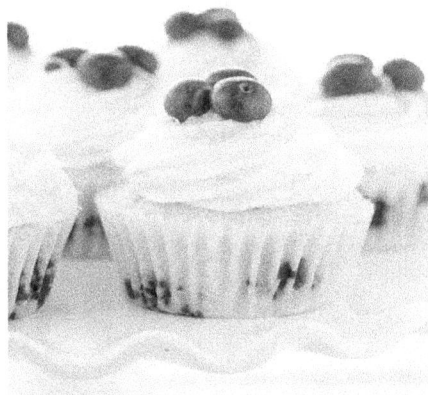

A breakfast that is quick to make, but hearty and filled with flavors. Plus, it is going to bring a smile to your face in the morning.

Servings: 4

Prep Time: 10 minutes

Cook time: None

Energy Value Per Serving: 602 kj

Calories: 144 calories

Protein: 5.1 g

Total Fat: 5.2 g

Carbohydrate: 21 g

Ingredients

- 2 cups fresh blueberries
- ¾ cup low-fat vanilla yogurt
- ½ cup (4 ounces) reduced-fat cream cheese
- 1 teaspoon honey

- 2 teaspoons freshly grated lemon zest

Instructions

- Take out a medium bowl and add cream cheese to it. Break it up using a fork. Add in honey and then the yogurt (make sure that you drain any water). Use an electric mixer and beat the mixture until it is creamy and light. Use the high speed setting for best results.
- Once done, add the lemon zest and stir the mixture well.
- Add the lemon cream into a small bowl or dish. Top it with blueberries.

MEDITERRANEAN SALADS

Fancy a salad? Then why not make it healthy with a whole lot of unique flavors. You can have the salads for breakfast or lunch.

1. Courgette, Fennel, and Orange Salad

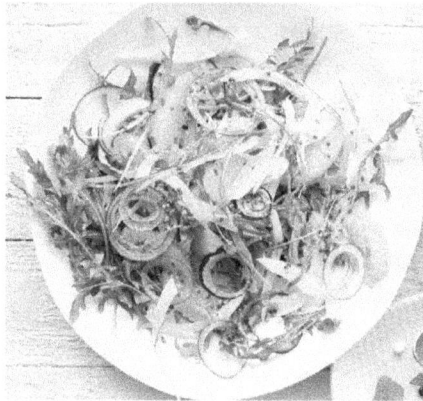

This salad combines the zestiness of the orange with the tang of fennel. The courgette gives the salad the crunch.

Servings: 4

Prep Time: 15 minutes

Cook time: None

Energy Value Per Serving: 711 kj

Calories: 170 calories

Protein: 3 g

Total Fat: 12 g

Carbohydrate: 10 g

Ingredients

- 1 orange
- 2 small courgettes (green or yellow)
- 2 small fennel bulbs

- 2 teaspoon sherry vinegar
- 4 tablespoon olive oil
- 1 Baby Gem lettuce, washed and leaves separated
- juice ½ lemon

Instructions

- Cut the peel off the orange. Remove any pith. Slice the orange and halve each slice. Ideally, you should be cutting the orange on a plate or the chopping board since we are going to collect the juice left over from the cutting.
- Take the fennel and remove any outer leaves that are tough. Cut the cores into halves and then slice them as thinly as you can.
- Remove the ends of the courgettes and shave thin and long slices using a vegetable peeler. You can toss away the watery and seedy centers.
- Take a small bowl and mix together olive oil, vinegar, and the orange juice left over on the plate or chopping board.
- Take out another bowl and mix the courgette, fennel, orange slices, and lettuce leaves.
- Serve the fennel mixture and top it with the orange juice dressing.

2. Potato Salad

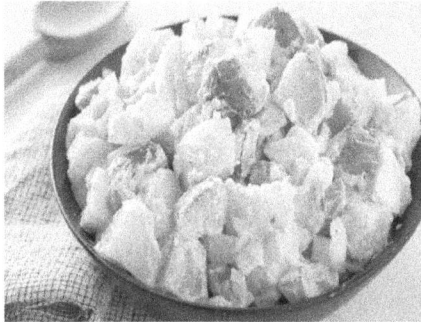

A low-fat salad with potatoes?

Servings: 4

Prep Time: 10 minutes

Cook time: 15 minutes

Energy Value Per Serving: 464 kj

Calories: 111 calories

Protein: 3 g

Total Fat: 4 g

Carbohydrate: 16 g

Ingredients

- 1 small onion, thinly sliced
- 1 tablespoon olive oil

- 1 garlic clove, crushed
- 100 g roasted red pepper sliced
- 25 g black olive, sliced
- 1 teaspoon fresh oregano
- 200 g canned cherry tomatoes
- 300 g new potato, halved if large
- handful basil leaves, torn

Instructions

- Take out a saucepan and place it over medium heat. Pour the olive oil into it and allow it to heat. Add the onions and cook for about 10 minutes, or until the onions have become soft.
- Add oregano and garlic. Cook for another 1 minute.
- Add the peppers and tomato. Let the mixture simmer for about 10 minutes.
- Use a pan and place it over medium-high heat. Bring it to a boil and then add the potatoes into the water. Cook the potatoes for about 15 minutes, or until they turn tender. Drain the potatoes.
- Take out a small bowl and add the pepper and tomato sauce into it. Toss in the potatoes and mix well.
- Serve your salad with a sprinkle of basil and olives.

3. Tuna Salad

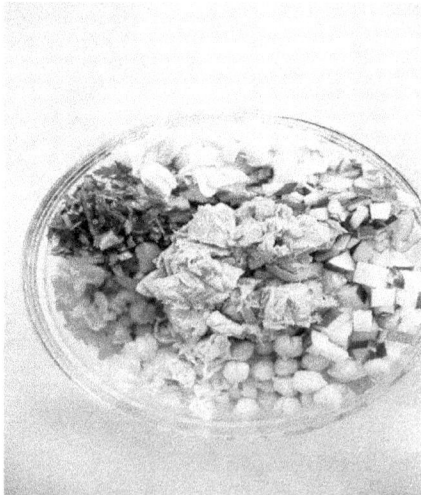

This tuna salad is packed with a little bit of crunch and a whole lot of delights. Perfect for a summer day.

Servings: 4

Prep Time: 10 minutes

Cook time: None

Energy Value Per Serving: 833 kj
Calories: 199 calories
Protein: 16.5 g
Total Fat: 8.8 g
Carbohydrate: 19.8 g

Ingredients

- 10 cherry tomatoes, quartered
- 4 scallions, trimmed and sliced
- 2 tablespoons extra-virgin olive oil
- 2 6-ounce cans chunk light tuna, drained
- 2 tablespoons lemon juice
- One 15-ounce can cannellini white beans, rinsed
- ¼ teaspoon salt, to taste
- freshly ground pepper, to taste

Instructions

- Take out a medium bowl and combine tomatoes, tuna, beans, lemon juice, scallions, oil, salt and pepper.
- Mix them well and serve.
- Refrigerate if you are planning to serve later.

4. Tomato, Cucumber, and Feta Salad

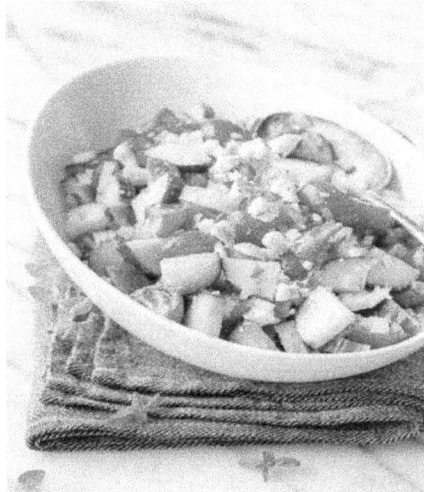

The coolness of the cucumber with the sweetness of the tomato. Oh, and let's not forget the VIP: feta cheese.

Servings: 4
Prep Time: 10 minutes
Cook time: None
Energy Value Per Serving: 640 kj

Calories: 153 calories

Protein: 3 g

Total Fat: 13.1 g

Carbohydrate: 6.1 g

Ingredients

- 3 tablespoons extra-virgin olive oil
- ½ teaspoon Dijon mustard
- 4 medium Persian cucumbers, thinly sliced crosswise
- 1 teaspoon chopped fresh oregano, plus extra for garnish
- 1 ½ tablespoons red-wine vinegar
- 1 cup (8 ounces) tomatoes, cut into wedges
- ¼ teaspoon salt
- 1 ½ ounces feta cheese, crumbled

Instructions

- Take out a medium bowl and combine oregano, vinegar, mustard, and salt.
- Drizzle the oil on top. Add tomatoes, cucumbers, and feta.
- Mix them well and serve with oregano leaves toppings, if you prefer.
- Refrigerate if you are planning to serve later.

5. Goat Cheese Stuffed Tomatoes

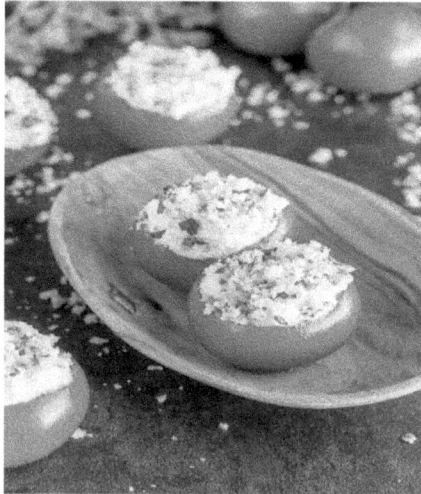

Goat cheese has an earth and a tart flavor. When you combine it with an earth fruit like tomato, the flavors are like a match made in earthy heaven.

Servings: 4

Prep Time: 10 minutes

Cook time: None

Energy Value Per Serving: 594 kj

Calories: 142 calories

Protein: 7 g

Total Fat: 13.1 g

Carbohydrate: 7 g

Ingredients

- 6-8 arugula leaves
- 3 ounces crumbled feta cheese
- 2 medium ripe tomatoes
- extra-virgin olive oil to drizzle
- balsamic vinegar to drizzle
- 1 red onion, very thinly sliced for garnish
- fresh chopped parsley for garnish
- salt and freshly ground pepper to taste

Instructions

- Arrange the arugula leaves in the center of a plate.
- Remove the tops and the core of the tomatoes. Ideally, you should remove the top first and scoop out the core.
- Fill the tomatoes with feta cheese. Add salt and pepper, to taste
- Drizzle with olive oil and balsamic vinegar.
- Garnish with chopped parsley and red onion.
- Serve at room temperature.

6. Classic Tabbouleh

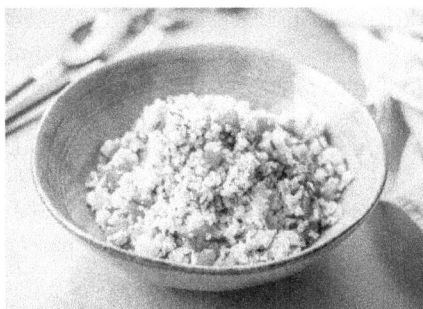

There is a reason why this dish is so popular in Middle Eastern countries. It is healthy, delicious, and wholesome. Often, people eat only the salad for dinner, since it can be quite filling.

Servings: 4

Prep Time: 10 minutes

Cook time: 10 minutes (Additional 5-10 minutes if you decide to roast the pine nuts)

Energy Value Per Serving: 741 kj

Calories: 177 calories

Protein: 12 g

Total Fat: 11 g

Carbohydrate: 28 g

Ingredients

- ¾ cup bulgur
- 2 cups freshly chopped parsley
- 1½ cups water
- ½ cup fresh lemon juice
- ½ cup extra-virgin olive oil
- ½ red bell pepper, diced
- 3 ripe plum tomatoes, peeled, seeded, and diced
- 1 large cucumber, peeled, seeded, and diced
- ¾ cup chopped scallions, white and green parts
- ½ green bell pepper, diced
- ½ cup finely chopped fresh mint
- handful of greens for serving
- seasoned pita wedges
- sea salt and freshly ground pepper to taste

Instructions

- Preheat the oven to around 375° F.
- Take a medium-sized bowl and add the asparagus with 2 tablespoons of salt and olive oil.
- Take out a baking dish and add the asparagus. Place the tray in the oven and roast for about 10 minutes, or until the asparagus becomes tender.
- Take out the asparagus and set aside.
- Use another medium-sized bowl and add garlic, lime juice, orange juice, and remaining 2 tablespoons of olive oil. Whisk all the ingredients together. Add salt and pepper to taste.
- Take the lettuce and split it into 6 plates. Take out the asparagus and place it on top of the lettuce.
- Pour the dressing over the asparagus and lettuce salad. Top the salad with basil and pine nuts. Add a small amount of Romano cheese for garnish, if you prefer.

You can also toast the pine nuts in the oven. Use the method below:

- Take out a baking tray and line it with a non-stick baking sheet. Add the pine nuts on top.
- Bake at 375 degrees for about 5-10 minutes, or until the nuts are lightly browned.
- Remove from the oven and set aside to cool.
- Add the nuts to the salad as a topping.

7. Mediterranean Greens

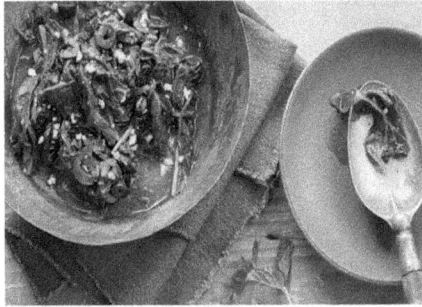

Going green does not have to be so boring, especially when you combine feta cheese and cranberries to pack this salad with some unique flavors.

Servings: 4

Prep Time: 10 minutes

Cook time: None

Energy Value Per Serving: 586 kj

Calories: 140 calories

Protein: 2 g

Total Fat: 12 g

Carbohydrate: 6 g

Ingredients

- 6 cups assorted fresh mixed greens (such as radicchio, arugula, watercress, baby spinach, and romaine)
- 1 small red onion, thinly sliced
- 20 cherry tomatoes, halved
- ¼ cup dried cranberries
- ¼ cup chopped walnuts
- crumbled feta cheese
- freshly ground pepper to taste
- 2 tablespoons balsamic vinegar
- 2 cloves fresh garlic, finely minced
- 4 tablespoons extra-virgin olive oil
- 1 tablespoon water
- ½ teaspoon crushed dried oregano

Instructions

- Take out a large salad bowl, combine walnuts, greens, tomatoes, onion, and cranberries. Gently toss.
- For the dressing, combine water, vinegar, oregano, olive oil, and garlic. Mix the ingredients well. Pour over the salad and lightly toss.
- Add feta cheese as garnish, if preferred.
- Add pepper to taste.

8. North African Zucchini Salad

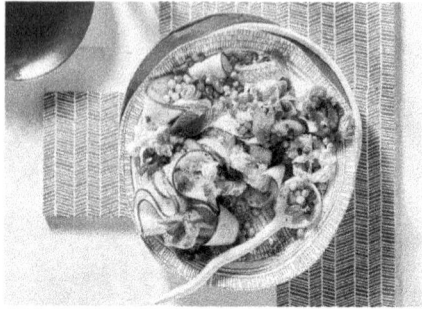

This lovely zucchini salad is combined with a popular North African spice: cumin. The result is a spectacular feast.

Servings: 4

Prep Time: 10 minutes

Cook time: None

Energy Value Per Serving: 586 kj

Calories: 140 calories

Protein: 2 g

Total Fat: 12 g

Carbohydrate: 6 g

Ingredients

- 1 pound firm green zucchini, thinly sliced
- ½ teaspoon ground cumin
- 2 cloves fresh garlic, finely minced
- juice from 1 large lemon
- 1 tablespoon extra-virgin olive oil
- 1½ tablespoons plain low-fat yogurt
- crumbled feta cheese
- finely chopped parsley for garnish
- salt and freshly ground pepper to taste

Instructions

- Add the zucchini into a large saucepan and steam it for about 2-5 minutes, or until it becomes tender and crispy. Place the zucchini under cold water and drain well.
- Take out a large bowl and mix cumin, olive oil, lemon juice, garlic, and yogurt. Add salt and pepper to taste.
- Add the zucchini into the mixture in the bowl and toss gently.
- Serve with feta cheese and parsley as garnish.

9. Avocado Salad

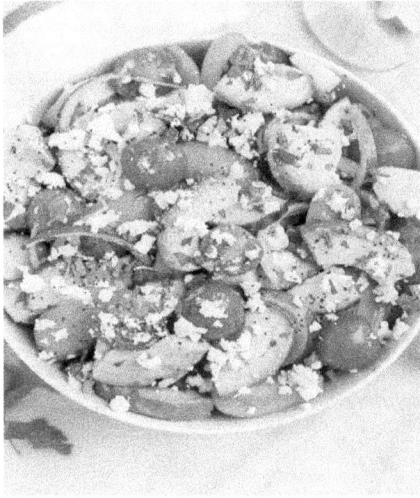

When your avocado cravings also wake up in the morning with you, then you can make this simple salad.

Servings: 3

Prep Time: 10 minutes

Cook time: None

Energy Value Per Serving: 544 kj

Calories: 130 calories

Protein: 2 g

Total Fat: 10 g

Carbohydrate: 10 g

Ingredients

- 1 small onion, finely chopped
- 1 large ripe avocado, pitted and peeled
- 2 tablespoons chopped fresh parsley
- 2 teaspoons fresh lime juice
- ½ small hot pepper, finely chopped (optional)
- 1 cup halved cherry tomatoes
- salt and freshly ground pepper to taste

Instructions

- Start with the avocado and cut it into bite-sized pieces.
- Add parsley, lime juice, tomatoes, onion, and hot pepper. Mix all the ingredients well. Add salt and pepper to taste.
- Finally, add the avocado into the mixture and mix them well.

10. Tunisian Style Carrot Salad

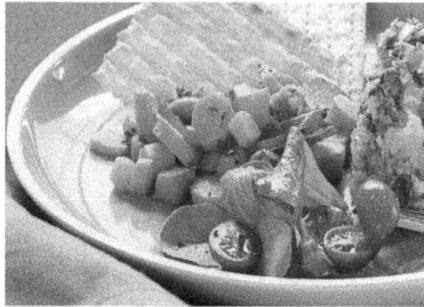

From the land of the North African country of Tunisia comes this mildly sweet, little spicy (or more spicy, depending on the heat level if the sauce), and cheesy carrot salad.

Servings: 6

Prep Time: 15 minutes

Cook time: None

Energy Value Per Serving: 577 kj

Calories: 138 calories

Protein: 7 g

Total Fat: 5 g

Carbohydrate: 13 g

Ingredients

- 10 medium carrots, peeled and sliced
- 1 cup crumbled feta cheese, divided
- 2 teaspoons caraway seed
- ¼ cup extra-virgin olive oil
- 6 tablespoons apple cider vinegar
- 5 teaspoons freshly minced garlic
- 1 tablespoon Harissa paste (choose the level of heat based on your preference)
- 20 pitted Kalamata olives, reserving some for garnish
- salt to taste

Instructions

- Take out a medium saucepan and place it on medium heat. Fill it with water and add the carrots. Cook carrots until tender. Drain and cool the carrots under cold water. Drain again to remove any excess water.
- Take out a large bowl and place the carrots in them.
- Take out a mortar and combine salt, garlic, and caraway seeds. Grind them until they form a paste. Otherwise, you can also use a small bowl, preferably one not made out of glass for grind. The final option would be to toss the ingredients into a blender and pulse them.
- Add vinegar and Harissa into the bowl with the carrots and mix them well.
- Use a large spoon and mash the carrots. Add the garlic mixture into the

carrot and mix again until they have all blended well. Add the olive oil and mix again.

- Finally, add about ½ the feta cheese and all the olives and mix well again.
- Take out a large bowl and add the salad to it. Top it with the remaining feta cheese.

11. Classic Greek Salad

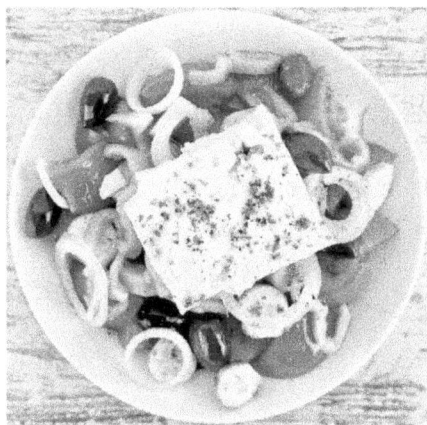

No Mediterranean salad list is complete without the popular and classic Greek salad. The only thing required to complete the recipe list is a Caesar salad. Oh wait, we have that too.

Servings: 6

Prep Time: 15 minutes

Cook time: None

Energy Value Per Serving: 1,121 kj

Calories: 268 calories

Protein: 23 g

Total Fat: 17 g

Carbohydrate: 44 g

Ingredients

- 6 large firm tomatoes, quartered
- 20 Greek black olives
- ½ pound Greek feta cheese, cut into small cubes
- ½ head of escarole, shredded
- 3 tablespoons red wine vinegar
- ¼ cup extra-virgin olive oil
- 1 tablespoon dried oregano
- ½ English cucumber, peeled, seeded, and thinly sliced
- 2 cloves fresh garlic, finely minced

- ½ red onion, sliced
- 1 medium red bell pepper, seeded and sliced
- ¼ cup freshly chopped Italian parsley
- salt and freshly ground pepper to taste

Instructions

- Take out a large bowl and add vinegar, oregano, olive oil, and garlic. Add salt and pepper to taste. Set aside the bowl.
- In another large bowl, add onion, tomatoes, escarole, cucumber, bell pepper, and cheese and mix them well.
- Take the vinegar mixture and pour it over the salad in the second bowl.
- Top the salad with olives and parsley.

12. Caesar Salad

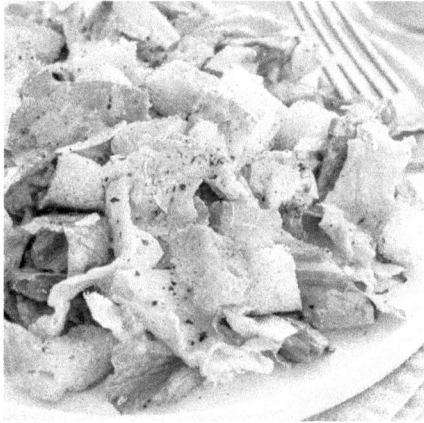

Presenting, the only and only – Caesar Salad. The salad is light and is perfect if you would like to have something to stave off hunger.

Servings: 6
Prep Time: 5 minutes
Cook time: None

Energy Value Per Serving: 205 kj
Calories: 49 calories
Protein: 4 g
Total Fat: 1 g
Carbohydrate: 4 g

Ingredients

- 10 small pitted black olives, chopped
- 1-2 bunches romaine lettuce, cleaned and torn in pieces
- 2 teaspoons lemon juice
- 2½ teaspoons balsamic vinegar
- ½ cup grated parmesan cheese

- ½ cup nonfat plain yogurt
- 1 teaspoon worcestershire sauce
- ½ teaspoon anchovy paste
- 2 cloves freshly minced garlic

Instructions

- Take out a large bowl and place romaine lettuce in it.
- Take out your blended and add mix lemon juice, yogurt, garlic, anchovy paste, vinegar, worcestershire sauce, and ¼ cup parmesan cheese. Mix all the ingredients well until they are smooth.
- Pour the yogurt mixture over the lettuce and toss lightly.
- Top the salad with the remaining parmesan cheese.

13. Spanish Salad

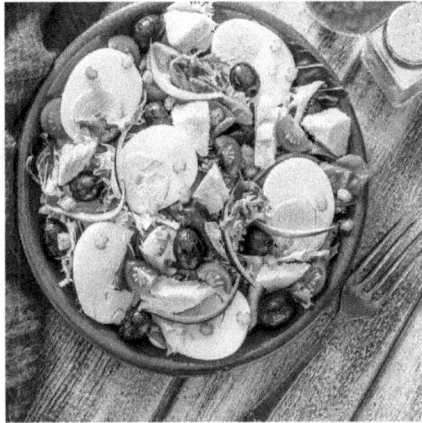

Another salad that does not take a lot of time to prepare but has a nice kick to it because of the bell peppers.

Servings: 6

Prep Time: 10 minutes

Cook time: None

Energy Value Per Serving: 448 kj

Calories: 107 calories

Protein: 2 g

Total Fat: 9 g

Carbohydrate: 6 g

Ingredients

- 2 bunches romaine lettuce, cleaned and trimmed
- 1 large sweet onion, thinly sliced
- 3 medium ripe tomatoes, chopped
- 3 tablespoons balsamic vinegar
- ¼ cup extra-virgin olive oil

- 1 red bell pepper, seeded and thinly sliced
- 1 green bell pepper, seeded and thinly sliced
- ¼ cup chopped and pitted black olives
- ¼ cup chopped and pitted marinated green olives
- salt and freshly ground pepper to taste

Instructions

- Take out 6 plates and place romaine lettuce on them to form a base.
- Add peppers, tomatoes, onion, and olives on top of each of the lettuce bases.
- In a small bowl, combine olive oil and vinegar together. Add the dressing over the salad.
- Add salt and pepper to taste, if preferred.

14. Parsley Couscous Salad

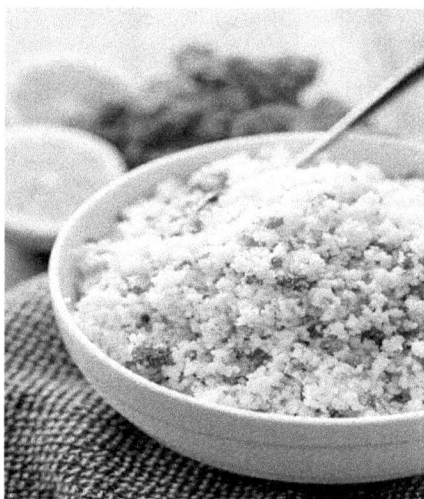

Parsley is a refreshing herb to use in food. Combine it with couscous and you have a wonderful flavor profile. However, because of the preparation time, you can either choose to make it in the morning, or the previous night if you don't get too much time.

Servings: 4

Prep Time: 2 hours (refrigerate overnight if you are having in the morning)

Cook time: None

Energy Value Per Serving: 502 kj

Calories: 120 calories

Protein: 5 g

Total Fat: 2 g

Carbohydrate: 18 g

Ingredients

- ¼ cup couscous

- 2 teaspoons extra-virgin olive oil
- ¼ cup water
- 2 teaspoons lemon zest
- 1 medium ripe tomato, peeled, seeded, and diced
- 2 tablespoons pine nuts
- 2 tablespoons fresh lemon juice
- ¼ cup finely chopped fresh flat parsley leaves
- 2 tablespoons finely chopped fresh mint leaves
- 2 heads Belgian endive, leaves for scooping
- whole wheat pita rounds, cut into wedges and toasted until crispy
- salt and freshly ground pepper to taste

Instructions

- Take out a medium bowl and then combine lemon juice and water. All the mixture to stand for about 1 hour.
- After the hour, add mint, parsley, lemon zest, olive oil, and pine nuts. Mix the ingredients well.
- Add in the couscous to the mixture. Allow it to stand for about 1 hour. After 1 hour, add salt and pepper to taste.
- Place couscous mixture in the center of a plate and top it with tomato. You can surround the couscous salad with toasted pita wedges and endive leaves, which makes for a wonderful presentation.
- Refrigerator overnight so that you can have it the next day.

15. Cress and Tangerine Salad

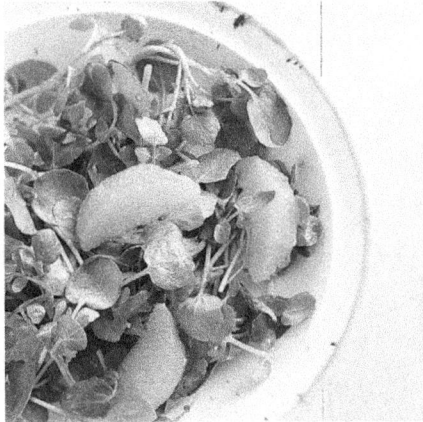

The healthy addition of a watercress combines well with the tangy flavors of tangerine. With some lemon juice added into the mix, you have a salad that might just make you lick your fork dry.

Servings: 4

Prep Time: 15 minutes

Cook time: None

Energy Value Per Serving: 816 kj

Calories: 195 calories

Protein: 3 g

Total Fat: 16 g

Carbohydrate: 14 g

Ingredients

- 4 large sweet tangerines
- ¼ cup extra-virgin olive oil
- 2 large bunches watercress, washed and stems removed
- juice from 1 fresh lemon
- 10 cherry tomatoes, halved
- 16 pitted Kalamata olives
- Sea salt and freshly ground pepper to taste

Instructions

- Take the tangerines and peel them into a medium-sized bowl. Make sure that you remove any pits and squeeze the sections. You should have around ¼ cup of tangerine juice. Set sections aside.
- Take a large bowl and add lemon juice, tangerine juice, and olive oil. Mix them together and add salt and pepper for flavor, if you prefer.
- Use paper towels to pat the cress dry. Add watercress, tomatoes, and olives to the bowl containing the tangerine sections (not to be confused with the bowl containing tangerine juice). Toss them lightly.
- Pour the tangerine juice mixture on top. Mix well and serve.

16. Prosciutto and Figs Salad

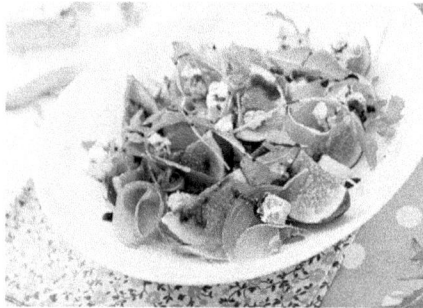

Figs are such an earthy delight. What makes this salad earthier is the presence of crunchy walnuts.

Servings: 4

Prep Time: 10 minutes

Cook time: None

Energy Value Per Serving: 795 kj

Calories: 190 calories

Protein: 26 g

Total Fat: 9 g

Carbohydrate: 17 g

Ingredients

- One 10-12-ounce package fresh baby spinach
- 1 small hot red chili pepper, finely diced
- 1 carton figs, stems removed and quartered
- ½ cup walnuts, coarsely chopped
- 1 tablespoon fresh orange juice
- 1 tablespoon honey
- 4 slices prosciutto, cut into strips
- shaved parmesan cheese for garnish

Instructions

- Take your spinach and divide them into 4 equal portions. Each portion should be on a separate plate and will act as a base. Add quartered prosciutto, figs, and walnuts on each spinach as toppings.
- For the dressing, take a small bowl and add honey, orange juice, and diced pepper. Add the mixture over the salad.
- Finally, toss the salad lightly and use parmesan cheese for the garnish.

17. Garden Vegetables and Chickpeas Salad

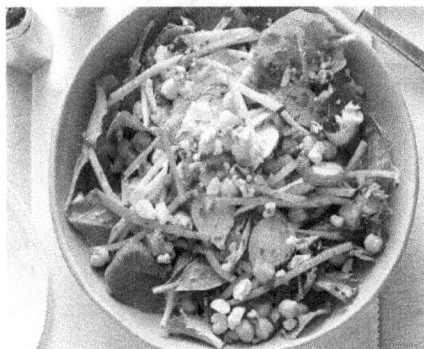

Your healthy variety tomatoes and carrots along with some greens are used as garden vegetables. The chickpeas give the smooth texture that goes well with the vegetables.

Servings: 4

Prep Time: 10 minutes (or you can refrigerate it overnight)

Cook time: None

Energy Value Per Serving: 816 kj

Calories: 195 calories

Protein: 16 g

Total Fat: 7 g

Carbohydrate: 24 g

Ingredients

- 2 tablespoons freshly squeezed lemon juice
- ⅛ teaspoon freshly ground pepper
- 1 cup cubed part-skim mozzarella cheese
- 1 tablespoon fresh basil leaf, snipped
- 1 (15-ounce) can chickpeas, rinsed and well drained
- 2 cups coarsely chopped fresh broccoli
- 2 cloves fresh garlic, finely minced
- ½ cup sliced fresh carrots
- 1 7½-ounce can diced tomatoes, undrained

Instructions

- Use a large bowl and add garlic, basil, lemon juice, and ground pepper. Mix them well.
- Add the chickpeas, carrots, tomatoes with juice, broccoli, and mozzarella cheese. Toos all the ingredients well.
- You can serve immediately, or you can keep it refrigerated overnight.

18. Peppered Watercress Salad

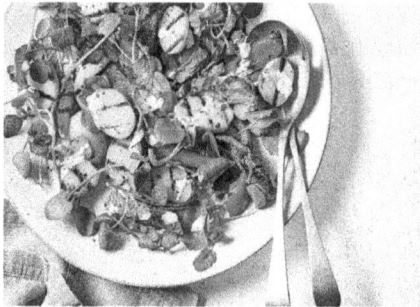

This salad is so simple to make that we are not sure you will require not even 5 minutes. When you are in a hurry and you want to grab a quick bite, then perhaps this dish might help. Or you could prepare it in advance for lunch if you know you are going to have a busy day.

Servings: 4

Prep Time: 5 minutes (or less)

Cook time: None

Energy Value Per Serving: 280 kj

Calories: 67 calories

Protein: 4 g

Total Fat: 7 g

Carbohydrate: 1 g

Ingredients

- 2 teaspoons champagne vinegar
- 2 bunches (about 8 cups) watercress, rinsed and rough stems removed
- 2 tablespoons extra-virgin olive oil

- salt and freshly ground pepper to taste

Instructions
- Drain the watercress properly.
- Take out a small bowl and then add salt, pepper, vinegar, and olive oil. Mix them well together.
- Transfer the watercress to a bowl. Add the vinegar mixture into it and toss well.
- Serve immediately.

19. Watermelon Salad

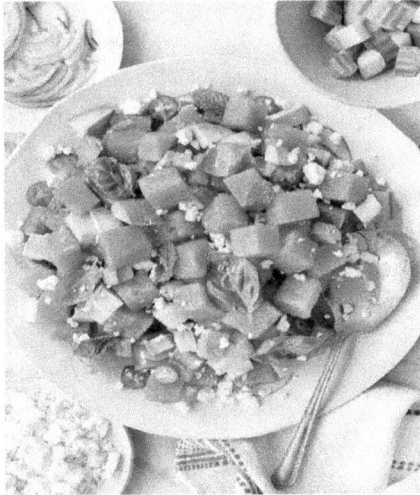

The sweetness of watermelon combined with the flavor of pepper. A summer treat!

Servings: 4

Prep Time: 5 minutes

Cook time: None

Energy Value Per Serving: 393 kj

Calories: 94 calories

Protein: 5 g

Total Fat: 7 g

Carbohydrate: 7 g

Ingredients
- 2 cups cubed seedless watermelon
- 2 cups arugula
- 1 cup sliced cucumber, with skin on
- 3 tablespoons extra virgin olive oil
- 2 teaspoons white balsamic vinegar
- 4 ounces fresh feta cheese, cut into bite-sized pieces
- salt and freshly ground pepper to taste

Instructions

- Take a small bowl and add watermelon, arugula, salt and pepper, cucumber, vinegar, feta, and olive oil.
- Mix them well and serve immediately.

20. Watercress and Pear Salad

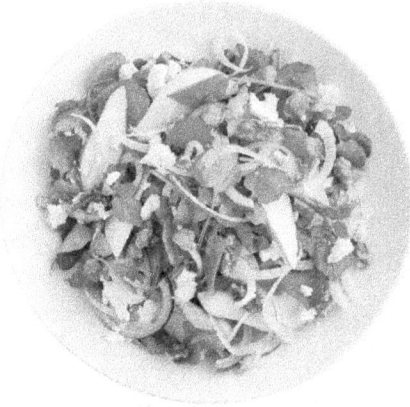

Two wonderful fruits get together to make this salad a fruity sensation.

Servings: 4

Prep Time: 5 minutes

Cook time: None

Energy Value Per Serving: 393 kj

Calories: 94 calories

Protein: 5 g

Total Fat: 7 g

Carbohydrate: 7 g

Ingredients

- 4 ripe-but-firm smooth-skin pears
- 2 tablespoons toasted pecan halves
- 2 ounces crumbled blue cheese
- 2 cups watercress
- juice from 1 lemon
- honey to drizzle
- ¼ cup vinaigrette dressing

Instructions

- Take each pear and core it. Leave the stem intact.
- Take a medium sized bowl and add watercress, pecans, blue cheese, and vinaigrette. Mix all the ingredients well. Set aside.
- Slice each pear in 4 horizontal slices. Use lemon juice to brush the cut sides.

- For the next part, reassemble the pears into their original shape but with the salad mixture between each slice.
- Add honey as a topping.

MEDITTERANEAN SOUPS

Sometimes, all you need is a soup to warm your belly or satiate your hunger. For your soup requirements, we have these incredible recipes.

1. Lemon and Egg Pasta Soup

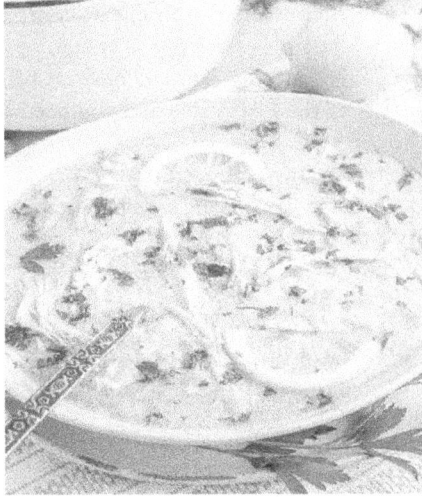

The lemon juice adds the acidic kick to the soup while then parsley brings its fresh fragrance to complete the dish. Aromatic, healthy, and filling - everything you need in a soup.

Servings: 4
Prep Time: 15 minutes
Cook time: None
Energy Value Per Serving: 674 kj
Calories: 161 calories
Protein: 10 g
Total Fat: 2 g
Carbohydrate: 65 g
Ingredients

- 4 ounces ditalini pasta
- 4 cups fat-free and low-sodium chicken broth
- 2 large whole eggs
- ½ cup fresh lemon juice
- 4 tablespoons chopped fresh parsley

- 1 lemon, thinly sliced for garnish
- salt and freshly ground pepper to taste

Instructions

- Place medium saucepan on medium-high heat. Add chicken broth to it and bring it to a boil, stirring it a couple of times.
- Bring down the heat to low and allow the broth to simmer for about 5 minutes. Take the saucepan off the heat.
- Take a bowl and add the eggs into it. Beat them well, add the lemon juice, and beat the eggs again.
- Use a ladle to transfer a single serving of the chicken broth into the egg bowl. Mix them well and then transfer the entire contents of the bowl into the saucepan.
- Heat the soup while ensuring that the heat is still at low. Keep an eye out on the eggs because they tend to curdle and you need to prevent that from happening by gently stirring the soup.
- Add salt and pepper to taste, if preferred.
- Serve hot and garnish with lemon slices and parsley.

2. Green Creamy Soup

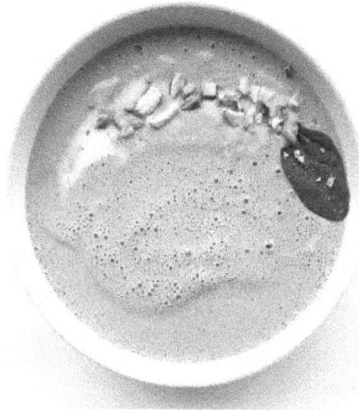

This soup is infused with plenty of greens. But that does not stop it from being creamy. The lemon juice adds that sour kick to the entire dish.

Servings: 6

Prep Time: 10 minutes

Cook time: 30 minutes

Energy Value Per Serving: 682 kj

Calories: 163 calories

Protein: 4 g

Total Fat: 8 g

Carbohydrate: 15 g

Ingredients
- 5 ounces fresh green beans, thinly sliced
- 8 ounces fresh Brussels sprouts, sliced
- 5 cups low-sodium, fat-free vegetable broth
- 1½ cups frozen peas, defrosted
- 4 tablespoons olive oil
- 1 white onion, chopped
- 1 tablespoon freshly squeezed lemon juice
- 4 cloves fresh garlic, minced
- 1 large leek, slice both white parts and sliced green parts thinly but keep them separate
- 1 teaspoon ground coriander
- 1 cup low-fat milk
- salt and freshly ground pepper to taste
- croutons for garnish

Instructions
- Take out a large skillet and place it over low heat. Add the olive oil and allow the oil to heat up slightly.
- Add onion and garlic. Cook them until they turn fragrant and soft. Make sure that you do not allow them to turn brown.
- Add the green parts of the Brussels sprouts, leek, and green beans to the skillet. Add the broth and mix the ingredients well. Bring the broth to a boil. When it starts boiling, lower the heat and let simmer for about 12 minutes.
- Add lemon juice, peas, and coriander. Let the broth continue to simmer for another 10 minutes, or until the vegetables become tender.
- Remove the broth mixture from heat and allow it to cool slightly. Transfer the mixture to a blender and pulse until they turn smooth.
- Take out a saucepan and add the white parts of leek. Add the blended mixture into the saucepan. Place the saucepan over medium high heat and allow the soup to boil. Reduce the heat to low and allow the soup to simmer for about 5 minutes.
- Take out another bowl and add flour and milk. Whisk them until they turn smooth.
- Add salt and pepper to taste, if preferred.

3. Orzo and Lemon Chicken Soup

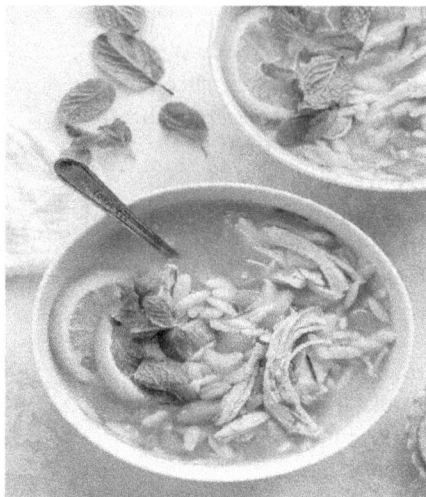

They say that warm chicken soup nourishes your body well. In that case, this chicken soup is packed with plenty of nutrients to supercharge you.

Servings: 6

Prep Time: 10 minutes

Cook time: 40 minutes

Energy Value Per Serving: 1,038 kj

Calories: 248 calories

Protein: 25 g

Total Fat: 4 g

Carbohydrate: 23 g

Ingredients

- 12 ounces skinless, boneless chicken breasts
- 1 tablespoon olive oil
- ½ cup chopped celery
- ½ cup chopped white onion
- 6 cups low-sodium, fat-free chicken broth
- ½ cup sliced carrot
- ½ cup orzo
- ¼ cup chopped fresh dill
- salt and freshly ground pepper to taste
- lemon halves

Instructions

- Take out a large pot and place it over medium heat. Add olive oil to it and allow it to heat.
- Add celery and onion. Cook them until the onions are fragrant and the celery is soft. Add chicken, chicken broth, and carrot to the mixture. Add salt and pepper to taste, if preferred.

- Increase the temperature to medium high heat and allow the broth to boil. When it starts boiling, reduce heat and allow the soup to simmer for about 20 minutes, or until the chicken is cooked.
- Take out the chicken from the pot, transfer it to a bowl and allow it to cool. Cover the pot so that the ingredients inside are simmering. When the chicken is sufficiently cool, shred the chicken into small pieces.
- Open the cover of the pot and add orzo. Increase the heat to medium high and allow the broth to boil for about 8 minutes. Make sure that the cover is back on the pot during the boiling process.
- Remove pot from heat and add dill and the shredded chicken broth.
- Squeeze lemon juice into the broth. Serve immediately.

4. Chilled Avocado Soup

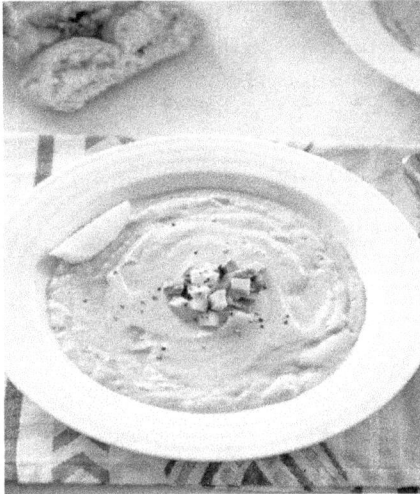

Avocado in a soup? And it's chilled as well? Yes indeed.

Servings: 6

Prep Time: 2.5 hours (including the time it takes to chill the bowls)

Cook time: None

Energy Value Per Serving: 1,067 kj

Calories: 255 calories

Protein: 4 g

Total Fat: 22 g

Carbohydrate: 15 g

Ingredients

- 3 medium ripe avocados, halved, seeded, peeled, and cut to chunks
- 2 cloves fresh garlic, minced
- 2 cups low-sodium, fat-free chicken broth, divided
- ½ cucumber, peeled and chopped

- ½ cup chopped white onion
- ¼ cup finely diced carrot
- thin avocado slices for garnish
- paprika to sprinkle
- salt and freshly ground pepper to taste
- hot red pepper sauce to taste

Instructions

- Place 6 bowls into the freezer and allow them to chill for half an hour.
- In the meantime, take out your blender and add garlic, cucumber, avocados, onion, carrot, and 1 cup broth. Blend all the ingredients together until they turn smooth.
- Add the remaining broth. Add the salt and pepper and hot sauce to taste, if preferred. Blend all the ingredients again until they are smooth.
- Take out the chilled bowls and pour the blended ingredients into them.
- This time, place the bowls in the refrigerator for another 1 hour.
- When you are ready to serve, top the soup with paprika and slices of avocado.
- Serve chilled.

5. Broccoli and Potato Soup

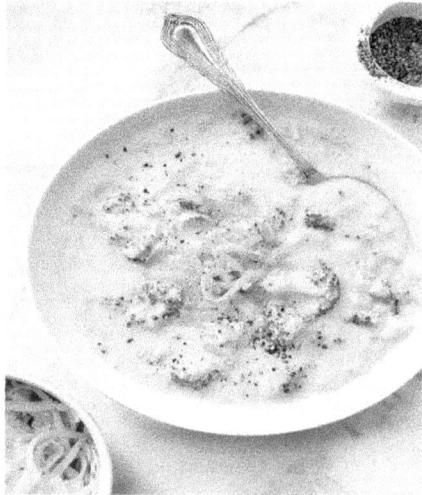

The potatoes are mashed and add a soft texture while the broccoli brings the crunchiness to the soup. The almond milk takes the dish to a whole new level.

Servings: 4

Prep Time: 10 minutes

Cook time: 25 minutes

Energy Value Per Serving: 1,464 kj

Calories: 350 calories

Protein: 17 g

Total Fat: 14 g

Carbohydrate: 42 g

Ingredients

- 2 cups escarole leaves, rinsed and drained
- 3 tablespoons all-purpose flour
- 3 cups fresh broccoli florets
- 3 scallions, sliced
- 2 cups smoked Gouda cheese, shredded and more for garnish
- 2 cups low-sodium, fat-free chicken broth
- 1 cups almond milk
- 3 medium red-gold potatoes, chopped
- 2 cloves fresh garlic, minced
- salt and freshly ground pepper to taste

Instructions

- Take out a large pot and place it over medium high heat. Add potatoes, garlic, and chicken broth. Bring the mixture to a boil and reduce the heat to low. Allow the mixture to simmer for a while until you notice the potatoes begin to soften.
- Use a fork and mash the potatoes slightly.
- Add broccoli, milk, and scallions. Continue to heat to a simmer until broccoli turns tender and crispy.
- Bring down the heat to low and then add the Gouda cheese. Continue stirring until the sauce thickens and the cheese melts.
- Add salt and pepper for seasoning, if preferred. Serve the soup in 4 equal portions.
- Add additional cheese and escarole as toppings.

6. Tortellini and Vegetable Soup

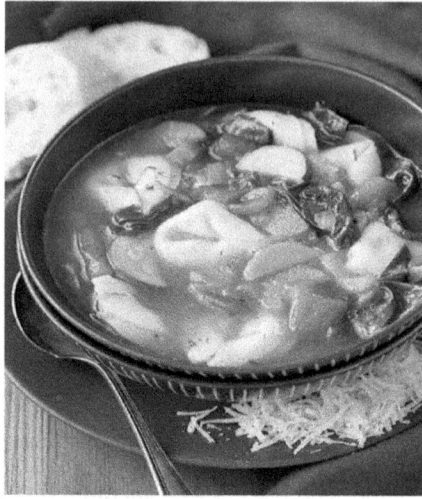

With plenty of vegetables put together, this soup will fill you up in no time. Plus, you can make a large portion that can serve around 8 people.

Servings: 8

Prep Time: 10 minutes

Cook time: 30 minutes

Energy Value Per Serving: 891 kj

Calories: 213 calories

Protein: 7 g

Total Fat: 7 g

Carbohydrate: 26 g

Ingredients

- 32 ounces low-sodium, fat-free chicken broth
- 3 cups fresh chicken-filled tortellini
- 1 large white onion, chopped
- 4 cloves fresh garlic, chopped
- 3 celery stalks, chopped
- 1 teaspoon minced chives
- 2 14.5-ounce cans diced tomatoes, undrained
- 2 tablespoons olive oil
- 1 teaspoon dried sweet basil
- 1 cup frozen corn
- 1 teaspoon dried thyme
- 1 cup chopped carrot
- 1 cup frozen cut green beans
- 1 cup diced raw potato

Instructions

- Take out a large pot and place it over medium heat. Add garlic, onion, celery, and olive oil. Saute until you notice the onion and garlic become fragrant and soft.

- Add potato, basil, carrot, beans, broth, thyme, corn, and chives. Increase the heat to medium high and then bring the broth to a boil.

- When it starts boiling, reduce the heat and cover the pot. Allow the mixture to simmer for about 15 minutes, or until the vegetables become tender.

- Add tortellini and tomatoes. Remove the cover and allow the soup to simmer uncovered for about 5 minutes.

- Serve hot.

7. Traditional Oyster Soup

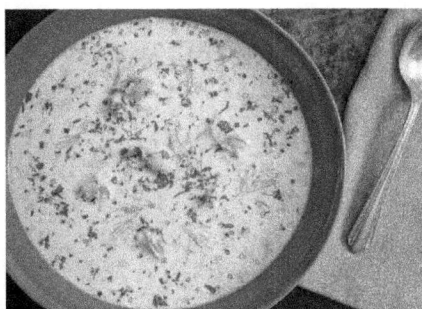

There are plenty of oyster soup recipes, but none of the others pack the incredible flavors and nutrition of the Mediterranean. In this version, we are going to spice things up with a little (or maybe more) cayenne pepper.

Servings: 6

Prep Time: 5 minutes

Cook time: 30 minutes

Energy Value Per Serving: 1,301 kj

Calories: 311 calories

Protein: 23 g

Total Fat: 11 g

Carbohydrate: 22 g

Ingredients

- 2 pints (about 32 ounces) fresh shucked oysters, undrained
- 4 tablespoons olive oil
- 1 cup finely chopped celery
- 3 (12-ounce) cans low-fat evaporated milk
- 6 tablespoons minced shallots
- 2 pinches of cayenne pepper (add more if you like more spice)
- toasted bread squares
- salt and freshly ground pepper to taste

Instructions

- Start with the oysters. Drain the liquid from them in a small bowl. Set the liquid aside since we are going to use it. Place the oysters separately.
- Run the liquid through a strainer to remove any solid materials.
- Take out a large pot and place it over medium heat. Add olive oil into it. Toss in oysters, celery, and shallots. Allow the ingredients to simmer for about 5 minutes, or until you notice the edges of the oysters begin to curl.
- Take a separate pot (or pan) and then heat the oyster liquid and milk. When the mixture is sufficiently warm, then pour it over the oysters. Stir all the ingredients together.
- Add salt and pepper,and cayenne pepper to taste.
- Serve soup warm with toasted bread squares as toppings or on the side.

8. Eggplant Soup

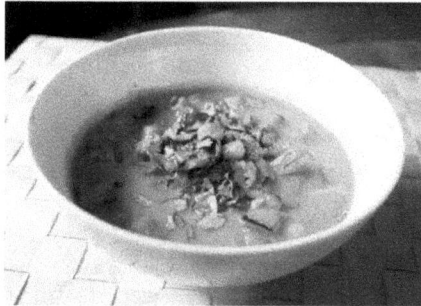

There are plenty of oyster soup recipes, but none of them pack the incredible flavors and nutrition of the Mediterranean. In this version, we are going to spice things up with a little (or maybe more) cayenne pepper.

Servings: 2
Prep Time: 10 minutes
Cook time: 30 minutes
Energy Value Per Serving: 1,146 kj
Calories: 274 calories
Protein: 9 g
Total Fat: 17 g
Carbohydrate: 23 g

Ingredients

- 3 tablespoons olive oil
- 1 (14-ounce) can low-sodium tomato and basil pasta sauce
- ½ cup chopped white onion
- 2 tablespoons Italian bread crumbs
- 2 cloves fresh garlic, minced
- 2 cups low sodium, fat-free chicken broth
- ½ cup shredded reduced-fat mozzarella cheese
- 1 small eggplant, halved and sliced thinly (about 2 cups)

- 2 tablespoons freshly grated parmesan cheese for garnish

Instructions

- Preheat the oven to 500° F. We are aiming for a broiling temperature. An oven's broiling temperature is anywhere from 500° F to 550° F. If you feel that you want to increase the temperature, feel free to do so when you place the dish in the oven.

- Take out a nonstick pan and place it over medium heat. Add olive oil into the pan and allow it to heat. Add the eggplant and cook for about 5 minutes, stirring occasionally.

- Add garlic and onion and continue cooking until you notice the eggplant turn into a golden brown color.

- Add broth and sauce. Increase the heat to medium high and then allow the mixture to boil. When it starts boiling, lower the heat to a simmer. Continue to cook until the soup thickens.

- Take out a baking tray and line it with tin foil. Use 2 oven-safe crock bowls and place them on the tray. Split the soup into equal portions and pour them into the bowls. Top with bread crumbs, mozzarella cheese, and a sprinkling of parmesan cheese.

- Allow the dish to broil for about 2 to 3 minutes, or until cheese has melted and turned golden.

- Serve hot.

9. Tortellini and Spinach Soup

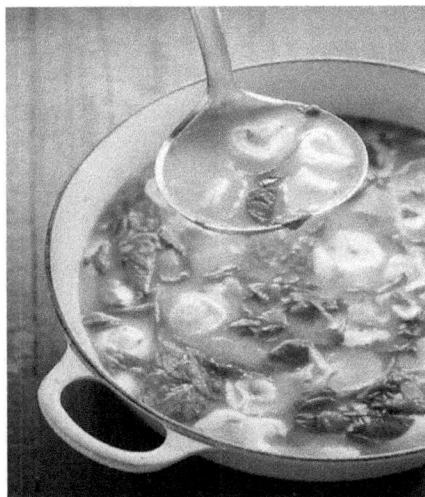

Prefer to make soup quickly? Here is a popular pasta soup that also includes spinach and a bit of pepper to raise the heat slightly.

Servings: 4

Prep Time: 5 minutes

Cook time: 20 minutes
Energy Value Per Serving: 406 kj
Calories: 97 calories
Protein: 6 g
Total Fat: 4 g
Carbohydrate: 14 g
Ingredients

- 4 cups low-sodium, fat-free chicken broth
- ¼ teaspoon ground pepper
- 2 cups coarsely chopped fresh spinach leaves
- 4 scallions, chopped
- 5 ounces fresh cheese-filled tortellini
- 2 cloves fresh garlic, minced
- freshly grated parmesan cheese

Instructions

- Take a large pot and place it on medium heat. Add broth and stir for half a minute. Add garlic, scallions, and pepper and increase the heat to medium high.
- Allow the broth to boil and when it starts boiling, bring the heat back to medium.
- Add the tortellini and cook for 10 minutes. Toss in the spinach and cook for an additional 5 minutes, or until the pasta becomes tender.
- Transfer the soup equally to 4 bowls. Top it with parmesan cheese, if preferred.

10. Spicy Vegetable Soup

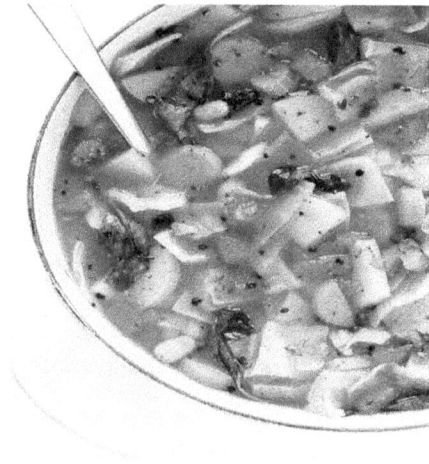

Lovers of all things spicy, we have a treat for you! And it's packed with nutritious vegetables.

Servings: 4
Prep Time: 10 minutes
Cook time: 20 minutes
Energy Value Per Serving: 954 kj
Calories: 228 calories
Protein: 12 g
Total Fat: 2 g
Carbohydrate: 43 g

Ingredients

- One 14-ounce can fiery roasted diced tomatoes, undrained
- 4 cups fresh cauliflower florets
- 1 cup frozen baby peas
- 2 teaspoons curry powder
- ½ teaspoon cumin
- 1 tablespoon finely chopped Serrano chili pepper
- 1 cup frozen corn
- cooked couscous
- 2 cloves fresh garlic, finely minced
- One 15-ounce can chickpeas, drained
- ¾ cup solid packed canned pumpkin mash
- ¾ cup water
- salt and freshly ground pepper to taste

Instructions

- Take a pot and place it over medium high heat. Cover it partially with water and add the cauliflower florets into it.
- Bring the water to a boil and then place the cover on the pot. Allow the florets to steam until they are tender.
- Remove the pot from the heat and drain the florets well. Cut them into small pieces and set aside.
- Take out a non-stick skillet and place it over medium heat. In a large, non-stick skillet over medium heat, add cumin and curry powder until fragrant. Add chili pepper, garlic, pumpkin, tomatoes with juices, chickpeas, and water.
- Allow the ingredients to reach a boil and then lower the heat. Let them simmer for about a minute before you add the salt and pepper to taste, if you prefer. Keep the ingredients simmering for another 15 minutes.
- Add the corn and peas and let the ingredients simmer for another 5 minutes.
- Remove from the heat and serve the soup separately with couscous or serve it over the couscous. You can also make use of brown rice instead of couscous.

11. Mediterranean Lentil Soup

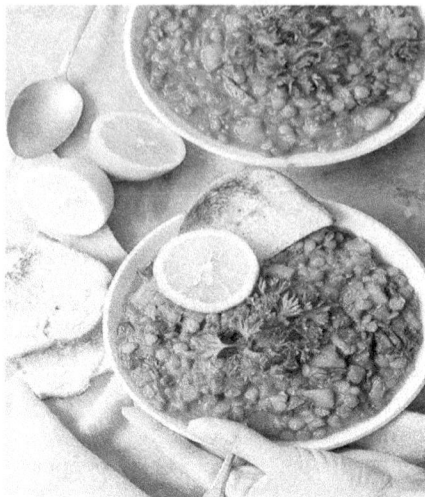

When you want to have a soup that is light on the stomach but packed with so much nutrition, then lentil soup is the choice for you.

Servings: 4

Prep Time: 10 minutes

Cook time: 50 minutes

Energy Value Per Serving: 1,054 kj

Calories: 252 calories

Protein: 15 g

Total Fat: 7 g

Carbohydrate: 31 g

Ingredients

- 1 cup red lentils
- 1 tablespoon olive oil
- 3 cups chicken broth, low sodium
- 1 chicken andouille sausage, sliced
- 1/3 cup onions, chopped
- 1/3 cup celery, chopped
- 1/3 cup carrots, chopped

Instructions

- Place your lentils in a colander and rinse them well. Drain them properly and set them aside.
- Place a pot over medium high heat and add olive oil into it.
- Add carrots, onions, and celery. Cook for about 4 minutes, or until the onions begin to caramelize.
- Add lentils and sausage and stir well. Reduce the heat to low.
- Add the chicken broth and cover the pot. Let the lentils simmer for about 45 minutes.

- Serve hot.

12. Mediterranean Bean Soup

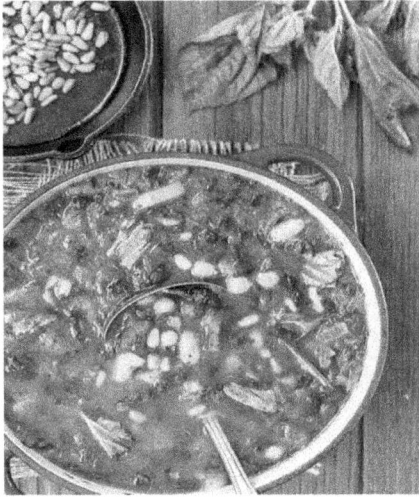

What if you could combine three different kinds of beans in one soup? You'd get this Mediterranean delight.

Servings: 4

Prep Time: 5 minutes

Cook time: 30 minutes

Energy Value Per Serving: 887 kj

Calories: 212 calories

Protein: 11 g

Total Fat: 1 g

Carbohydrate: 36 g

Ingredients

- 1 medium onion, chopped
- 3/4 cup red wine
- One 1/2 teaspoons dried thyme
- 2 bay leaves
- 4 cloves garlic, crushed
- 2 medium carrots, sliced
- 3 tablespoon dried parsley
- 1 teaspoon dried oregano
- One 15 ounces can tomato sauce
- One 15 ounces can garbanzo beans
- One 15 ounces can cannellini beans
- One 15 ounces can dark red kidney beans
- 6 cups vegetable broth

- salt and pepper

Instructions

- Take out a pot and place it over medium heat. Add olive oil.
- Add onions and carrots and saute them for 4 minutes, or until the onions have become semi-transparent and soft. Add the garlic and continue to saute until fragrant.
- Put in the remaining ingredients and raise the temperature to medium high. Bring the mixture to a boil.
- Once it starts boiling, reduce the heat to medium low and allow the soup to simmer for about 20 minutes.

13. Mediterranean Fish Soup

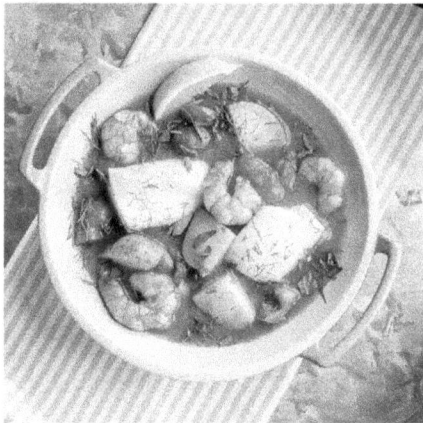

This soup is a seafood lover's dream!

Servings: 4

Prep Time: 5 minutes

Cook time: 30 minutes

Energy Value Per Serving: 887 kj

Calories: 212 calories

Protein: 11 g

Total Fat: 1 g

Carbohydrate: 36 g

Ingredients

- 2 tablespoons olive oil
- 1/4 cup dry white wine
- 1 large sweet onion, chopped
- 14.5 ounces diced tomatoes, undrained
- 192 ounces mussels, scrubbed and beards removed
- 1 pound cod fillets, cut into 1-inch pieces
- 1/2 pound large shrimp, peeled and deveined

- 4 cups vegetable broth
- fresh basil leaves (Shredded)
- salt and ground pepper, for taste

Instructions

- Place a pot over medium heat. Heat the oil in it and toss the onions. Cook the onions for about 4 minutes, or until they are tender.
- Pour the wine and continue cooking for another 1 minute, stirring a couple of times.
- Add the tomatoes and broth and increase the heat to medium high. Let the ingredients reach a boil and stir in all the ingredients properly.
- Lower the heat to low and add fish, mussels, and shrimp. Place the cover on the pot and cook until you notice the fish flaking easily when you use a fork, the mussels have opened up, and the shrimps are cooked properly.
- If you notice that some mussels have not opened, then discard them. Add salt and pepper for taste, if preferred.

14. Chicken and Lemon Soup

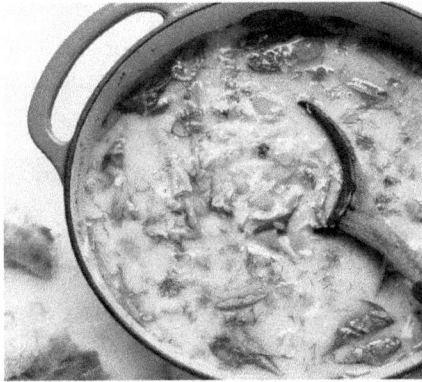

No points for guessing what the star ingredients of this hearty and healthy soup are. But what you might not know is that this dish features couscous as well.

Servings: 6

Prep Time: 10 minutes

Cook time: 20 minutes

Energy Value Per Serving: 895 kj

Calories: 214 calories

Protein: 11 g

Total Fat: 8 g

Carbohydrate: 23 g

Ingredients

- 2 boneless skinless chicken breasts
- 10 cups chicken broth
- 3 tablespoon olive oil

- 8 cloves garlic, minced
- 1 large lemon, zested
- 1 cup couscous
- 1/2 teaspoons crushed red pepper
- 2 ounces crumbled feta
- 1/3 cup chopped chive
- 1 sweet onion
- salt and pepper, to taste

Instructions

- Place a large pot over medium low heat. Add olive oil. Chop the onion into thin strips and add it into the pot once the oil is hot. Throw in the minced garlic and saute for about 4 minutes, or until the ingredients soften.
- Add the lemon zest, raw chicken breasts, chicken broth, and crushed red pepper to the pot. Increase the heat to high and place a cover on the pot. Bring the mixture to a boil and once it does, lower the heat to medium. Keep the cover on and let the ingredients simmer for about 5 minutes.
- Add the couscous. Add black pepper and 1 teaspoon salt to taste, if preferred. Let them simmer for another 5 minutes.
- Remove the chicken breasts from the pot and using a fork, shred them to small pieces. Put the pieces back into the pot. Add chopped chives and feta cheese. Mix them well.
- Add more salt and pepper to taste.

15. Cauliflower Soup

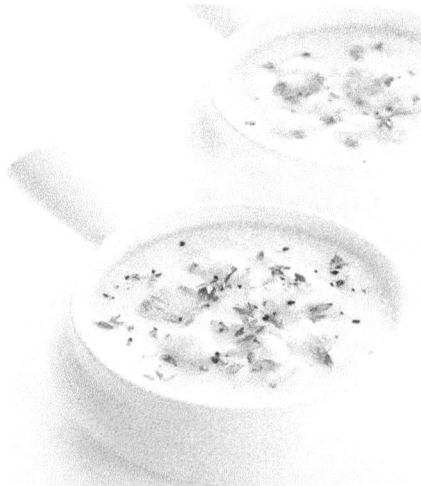

What many cauliflower soups get wrong is how to balance the flavor of cauliflower. This time, we are going to allow Mediterranean flavors to lead the way. Plus, this soup is so low on calories, so you can have it if you are feeling a bit calorie-conscious.

Servings: 6
Prep Time: 10 minutes
Cook time: 40 minutes
Energy Value Per Serving: 285 kj
Calories: 68 calories
Protein: 2 g
Total Fat: 5 g
Carbohydrate: 4 g

Ingredients

- 6 cups fresh cauliflower florets
- 2 tablespoons olive oil
- ½ cup chopped celery
- 1 bay leaf
- ½ teaspoon ground cumin
- ½ cup chopped carrot
- 1 large yellow onion, coarsely chopped
- 2 teaspoons finely chopped fresh garlic
- 1 small jalapeño pepper, seeds removed and diced
- 3½ cups low-sodium, fat free chicken broth
- One 14.5-ounce can diced tomatoes
- salt and freshly ground pepper to taste
- crumbled feta cheese for garnish

Instructions

- Place a large pot over medium heat. Pour olive oil in it, and when the oil is hot, add garlic and onion. Saute the ingredients until they are soft.
- Add cauliflower florets, carrot, celery, and jalapeño. Cook the ingredients until you notice the florets turn brown. Add broth, cumin, tomatoes, and bay leaf. Add salt and pepper for taste, if you prefer. Raise the heat to medium high and bring all the ingredients to a boil.
- Lower the heat and allow the ingredients to simmer for about 25 minutes while stirring occasionally, or until the cauliflower becomes tender.
- Remove the pot from the heat and take out the bay leaf.
- Serve with feta cheese as topping.

16. Garden Gazpacho Soup

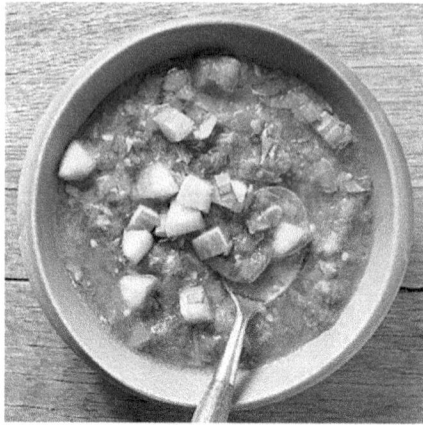

A taste of fresh vegetables with a wonderful and earthy twist.
Servings: 4
Prep Time: 6 hours
Cook time: 15 minutes
Energy Value Per Serving: 879 kj
Calories: 210 calories
Protein: 4 g
Total Fat: 14 g
Carbohydrate: 20 g

Ingredients
- 10 medium ripe tomatoes
- 5 cloves fresh garlic, minced
- 2 tablespoons chopped onion
- 2 cups low-sodium, fat-free chicken broth
- ½ tablespoon extra-virgin olive oil
- 2 teaspoons low-calorie baking sweetener
- ½ teaspoon chopped fresh basil
- salt and freshly ground pepper to taste

Instructions
- Place a large pot of water on medium high heat and bring it to a boil. without lowering the temperature, introduce tomatoes to the water. Allow the tomatoes to soften, which should take around 30 seconds.
- Transfer the tomatoes immediately to cold water. Allow them to cool until you can pick them up with your bare hands.
- Skin the tomatoes, cut them in a crosswise section and remove the seeds. Transfer the tomatoes to a blender and pulse them until they are smooth.
- Place a skillet over medium heat and add olive oil, garlic, and onions. Saute them until the onions are tender. Remove the skillet from the heat.

- Take a large bowl and add tomatoes (the ones you have pureed), chicken broth, sautéed onion mixture, sweetener, and basil. Add salt and pepper for taste, if you prefer.
- Keep the soup refrigerated for about 4 to 6 hours.
- When serving, top the soup with cucumbers, scallion, and zucchini.

17. Cabbage and Chicken Soup

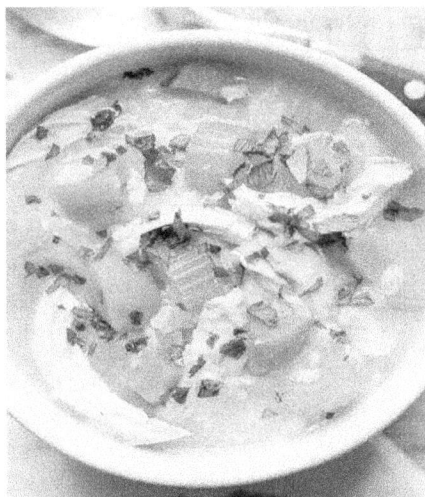

What do you get when you add a chunky cabbage with a chunky chicken? More chunky-ness!

Servings: 6

Prep Time: 10 minutes

Cook time: 1 hour

Energy Value Per Serving: 598 kj

Calories: 143 calories

Protein: 15 g

Total Fat: 2 g

Carbohydrate: 21 g

Ingredients

- 4 cups low-sodium, fat-free chicken broth
- 8 ounces skinless, boneless chicken, cubed
- 1 cup chopped celery
- 1 medium onion, chunked
- 3 cloves fresh garlic, chopped
- ¼ cup fresh parsley, finely chopped
- 1 small head of cabbage, torn
- 2 medium tomatoes, peeled and quartered
- 2 medium potatoes, peeled and cubed

- 1 cup chopped carrots
- 2 bay leaves
- 6 whole peppercorns
- 2 cups water
- ½ teaspoon cumin
- salt and freshly ground pepper to taste

Instructions

- Place a large pot over medium high heat. Add potatoes, chicken broth, water, bay leaves, chicken, carrots, peppercorns, and cumin. Bring the mixture to a boil.
- Reduce the heat to medium and allow the ingredients to simmer for about 30 to 40 minutes, or until the chicken is cooked. Add cabbage, garlic, celery, onion, tomatoes, and parsley. Cook for another 15 minutes, or until the vegetables are tender.
- Add salt and pepper to taste, if you like.

18. French Pistou Soup

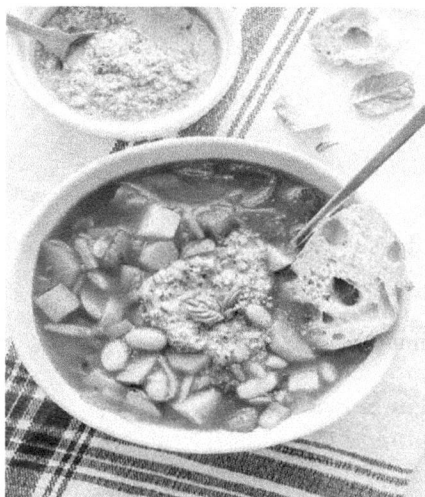

Bring the flavors of France with this delicious soup featuring potatoes and kidney beans. The soup can be quite filling too!

Servings: 6

Prep Time: 15 minutes

Cook time: 20 minutes

Energy Value Per Serving: 1,038 kj

Calories: 248 calories

Protein: 10 g

Total Fat: 9 g

Carbohydrate: 35 g

Ingredients
- 1 medium onion, finely chopped
- ½ cup dry kidney beans
- 2 medium tomatoes, peeled and chopped
- 1 tablespoon extra-virgin olive oil
- 3 cloves fresh garlic
- 2 cups fresh basil leaves
- 2 cups chopped carrots
- 8 cups water
- 8 ounces fresh green beans cut into 1-inch pieces
- 1 leek, green part only, thinly sliced
- 1 tablespoon hot liquid from soup (see directions below)
- 2 small zucchini cut into 1-inch cubes
- 1 cup whole wheat elbow macaroni
- freshly grated Gruyere cheese for garnish
- 2 medium potatoes, diced
- 1 stalk celery, chopped
- 3 tablespoons extra-virgin olive oil
- salt and freshly ground pepper to taste

Instructions
- Place a large saucepan over medium heat and add olive oil. Add onions and cook them until they become tender.
- Add potatoes, kidney beans, celery, carrots, and water. Bring the mixture to a boil and then reduce the heat to medium. Place a cover over the saucepan and allow the ingredients to simmer for about 15 minutes.
- Add tomatoes, green beans, zucchini, leek, and pasta. Cook the ingredients for another 10 minutes, or until the vegetables are tender.
- Add salt and pepper to taste.
- Bring the heat down to low and keep the soup warm. We are going to prepare the pistou.
- Add basil and garlic into a food processor and pulse them until they are smooth. Add soup liquid and olive oil. If you like, you can add in more salt and pepper to taste.
- To prepare the dish, serve soups equally into 6 bowls and then add the pistou into the soup. Top it with some cheese.

19. Fish Chowder with Saffron

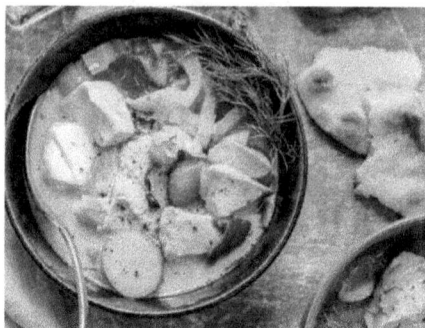

Saffron is a unique spice not only because it adds a wonderful flavor to the dish, but also because it has a sweet smell that simply transforms your dish.

Servings: 6

Prep Time: 15 minutes

Cook time: 30 minutes

Energy Value Per Serving: 1,238 kj

Calories: 296 calories

Protein: 35 g

Total Fat: 9 g

Carbohydrate: 11 g

Ingredients

- 8-10 diced scallions
- 1 pound fresh grouper fillets
- 1 pound fresh cod fillets
- 2 bay leaves
- ½ teaspoon fresh thyme
- 1 teaspoon turmeric
- ¼ teaspoon ground saffron
- 8 ounces bottled clam juice
- 4 cups water
- 1¼ cup dry white wine
- 1 small yellow bell pepper, diced
- 1 small red bell pepper, diced
- ¼ teaspoon crushed red hot pepper flakes
- ¾ cup small elbow macaroni
- 4 tablespoons chopped fresh parsley for garnish
- 2 tablespoons lemon juice
- 3 large cloves fresh garlic, crushed
- 2 tablespoons extra-virgin olive oil
- 1 cup chopped celery
- salt to taste

Instructions

- Wash your cod fillets and cut them into small cubes. Place them into the refrigerator to chill.
- Take a large skillet and place it over medium heat. Add olive oil, and when it is hot, add celery, garlic, scallions, and yellow and red bell peppers.
- Add in saffron and turmeric into the dish. Saute them until the vegetables become tender.
- Put the clam juice, wine, and water into the skillet and mix well.
- Add bay hot pepper flakes, leaves, thyme, and salt. Increase the skillet heat to medium high and bring the dish to a boil. When it starts boiling, reduce the heat back to medium and allow it to simmer for about 10 minutes.
- Toss in the pasta and cook until it is tender. Introduce the fish to the dish and continue simmering for another 10 minutes, or until the fish is cooked.
- When the fish is cooked, take the dish off the heat and remove bay leaves.
- Finish it off with lemon juice. Stir well and serve hot.

20. Eggplant Soup with Feta Cheese and Dry Sherry

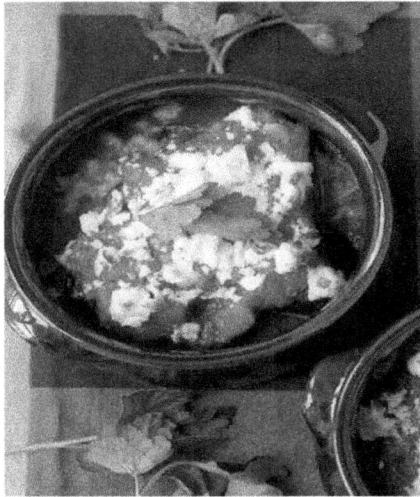

What does wine and eggplant have in common? They are both included in this dish along with feta cheese for an incredible flavor journey.

Servings: 6

Prep Time: 15 minutes

Cook time: 35 minutes

Energy Value Per Serving: 611 kj

Calories: 146 calories

Protein: 9 g

Total Fat: 5 g

Carbohydrate: 10 g

Ingredients

- 1 large tomato, sliced
- 10 ounces crumbled non-fat feta cheese
- 2 tablespoons extra-virgin olive oil
- 1 medium eggplant, peeled and cut into ½-inch cubes
- 2 cloves fresh garlic, minced
- ¼ teaspoon fresh thyme
- 4 cups canned low-sodium, fat-free chicken broth
- ½ cup dry sherry
- ½ medium onion, thinly sliced and separated into rings
- ½ teaspoon oregano
- salt and freshly ground pepper to taste

Instructions

- Place a skillet over medium heat and olive oil. Add in onion and garlic and saute them until they turn light golden.
- Add eggplant, oregano, and thyme. Continue cooking while stirring constantly until you see the eggplant turn slightly brown.
- Lower the heat to low and add the broth into the skillet. Allow the dish to simmer for about 5 minutes.
- Pour the sherry into the dish, cover it, and allow it to simmer for another 3 minutes. Add salt and pepper for taste, if you prefer. Otherwise, remove the dish from the heat and let it cool a little.
- Preheat the broiler. Take a large bowl safe for oven use and pour the soup into it. Top the soup with feta cheese and tomato slices.
- Place the soup under the broiler until the cheese melts. Take out the soup and serve hot.

MEDITERRANEAN MAINS

We have finally arrived at the "mains" event, pun intended.

Mediterranean mains are packed with so much flavor, it's like the dishes dance on your taste buds. and we are going to explore these majestic flavors in this section.

1. Mediterranean Bowl

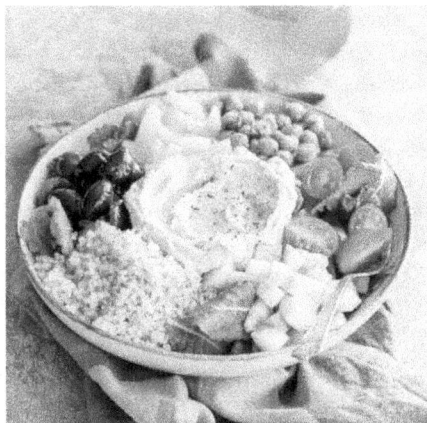

Who is up for some fried rice? You sure can enjoy a lot of it with this healthy and delicious recipe.

Servings: 5

Prep Time: 10 minutes

Cook time: 50 minutes

Energy Value Per Serving: 2,791 kj

Calories: 667 calories

Protein: 75 g

Total Fat: 23 g

Carbohydrate: 34 g

Ingredients for Chicken

- 5 chicken thighs, skin on, bone in
- 1/2 teaspoon salt
- 1 tablespoon dried oregano
- 1 to 2 lemons, you should use the zest and squeeze 4 tablespoon lemon juice
- 4 garlic cloves, minced

Ingredients for Rice

- 2 teaspoon black pepper
- One 1/2 tablespoon olive oil, separated
- 1 small onion, finely diced
- 1 cup long grain rice
- One 1/2 cups chicken broth
- 3/4 cup water
- 1 tablespoon dried oregano
- 3/4 teaspoon salt

Instructions

- Start by placing the chicken in a Ziplock back along with lemon juice, lemon zest, oregano, cloves, and salt. Seal the bag and keep it aside. You can either set it aside for about 20 minutes or keep it refrigerated overnight.

- When you are ready to cook the chicken, then preheat the oven to 350° F.
- Remove the chicken from the ziplock bag but don't throw away the chicken marinade in the bag.
- Place a skillet over medium heat and pour ½ tablespoon of olive oil. Allo the oil to heat a little and then place the chicken with the skin side down. Cook the chicken until it turns golden brown and then flip it over. Cook until the other side turns golden brown as well. Take the chicken off the skillet and keep it aside.
- Remove the oil and fat from the skillet. Clean the skillet using a paper towel to remove any bits that might remain. Place it back over medium heat again.
- Add the remaining olive oil into the skillet and increase the heat to medium high. Add onion and saute until it becomes translucent. Add all the ingredients for rice and the marinade as well into the skillet.
- Reduce the heat to low and allow the ingredients to simmer for about 30 seconds. Add the chicken on top and cover the skillet.
- Transfer the skillet into the oven and bake for about 35 minutes. Remove the lid and continue baking for about 10 minutes more, or until the rice is tender and the liquid has been absorbed.
- Remove from the oven and allow the dish to cool for about 5 to 10 minutes. Serve hot.

2. Turkish Style Meatball Gyro with Tzatziki

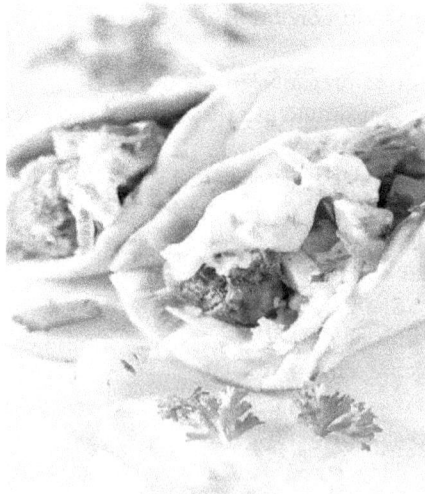

From the land of the famed Hagia Sophia comes a gorgeous dish that reflects the country's flavors and brings in a unique twist.

Servings: 4

Prep Time: 10 minutes

Cook time: 30 minutes

Energy Value Per Serving: 1,795 kj

Calories: 429 calories

Protein: 14 g

Total Fat: 13 g

Carbohydrate: 21 g

Ingredients for Meatball

- 1 pound ground turkey
- 1 teaspoon oregano
- 2 tablespoons olive oil
- 2 garlic cloves, minced
- 1 cup chopped fresh spinach
- 1/4 cup finely diced red onion
- salt and pepper to season

Ingredients for Tzatziki Sauce

- 1/2 cup plain greek yogurt
- 1 cup diced cucumber
- 4 whole wheat flatbreads
- 1/2 teaspoon garlic powder
- 2 tablespoons lemon juice
- 1/2 teaspoon dry dill
- 1/2 cup thinly sliced red onion
- 1 cup diced tomato
- 1/4 cup grated cucumber
- salt to taste

Instructions

- Take a large bowl and add oregano, fresh spinach, minced garlic, ground turkey, diced red onion, salt, and pepper. Use your hands to mix all the ingredients until they stick together. The meat itself will begin to form a ball-like shape.
- Continue using your hands and form meatballs from the mixture. The balls should be around 1 inch in diameter. You should get around 12 meatballs, but don't worry if you managed to get more or got a lot less.
- Place a skillet over medium high heat. Pour olive oil into the pan and allow the oil to heat. Place the meatballs in the skillet and cook for about 3 to 4 minutes until the meatball turns brown. Turn it over to place another side of the meatball on the skillet. Continue cooking this way until the entire meatball is a shade of brown all around. Take the pan off the heat and let it rest.
- Take a small bowl and add garlic powder, grated cucumber, dill, lemon juice, greek yogurt, and salt to taste. Mix all the ingredients together well.

- Time to create the gyros. Take a flatbread (you can even warm them up if you like). Add 3 meatballs, tomato, sliced red onion, and cucumber. Top off the meatballs with your Tzatziki sauce.

3. Artichoke and Spinach Matzo Mina

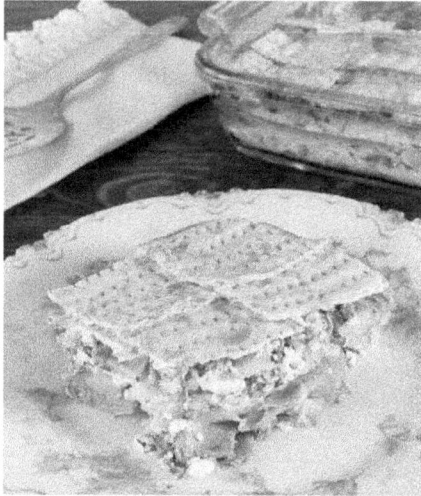

A green dinner that is filled with the incredible duo of artichoke and spinach. Surprisingly, some people have this as an entree. However, the choice on how you are going to have this dish is up to you.

Servings: 2

Prep Time: 10 minutes

Cook time: 30 minutes

Energy Value Per Serving: 1,121 kj

Calories: 268 calories

Protein: 14 g

Total Fat: 13 g

Carbohydrate: 21 g

Ingredients

- 6 sheets matzo more or less
- 3 large eggs divided
- 2 cups frozen artichoke hearts plain
- 2 scallions chopped
- 1/4 cup fresh dill chopped
- 1 tablespoon olive oil
- 1 teaspoon lemon zest
- 1/2 teaspoon crushed red pepper flakes
- 2 cups low-fat cottage cheese
- 8 ounces crumbled feta cheese

- 5 ounces fresh spinach roughly chopped
- salt to taste

Instructions

- Begin by preheating the oven to 350° F. Take out a baking dish and grease it lightly with cooking spray.
- Halve the artichokes if they aren't already halved.
- Place a skillet over medium high heat and pour olive oil into it. Heat the oil and saute the artichokes until they turn brown. Remove the skillet from the heat and allow the ingredients to cool.
- Take a large bowl and add lemon zest, scallions, dill, cottage cheese, spinach,and crushed red pepper. Slowly add the feta into the bowl by crumbling it.
- Take two eggs in a small bowl and beat them well. Pour the eggs into the bowl with scallions. Mix all the ingredients well.
- Place your matzo into a dish filled with water. This softens the matzo, but make sure it does not become too mushy. Dry them by placing them on a towel for about 5 minutes.
- Time to prepare the baking dish. Place a matzo at the bottom. If you notice any gaps in the bottom, then fill them up with pieces of matzo.
- Add the spinach and cheese filling on top, followed by the artichokes. Add another layer of matzo. Then add spinach and cheese later with artichokes again. The final layer will be matzo again.
- Take a brush and apply the eggs on the top layer gently. Don't allow the eggs to collect too much in any area.
- Put the dish into the oven and bake for about 45 minutes.

4. Greek Quesadillas

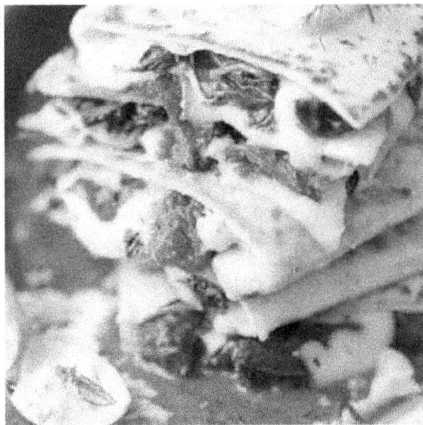

Wait! Aren't quesadillas South American? Not when they receive a major overhaul with some Greek flavors.

Servings: 8
Prep Time: 20 minutes
Cook time: 10 minutes
Energy Value Per Serving: 1,607 kj
Calories: 384 calories
Protein: 14 g
Total Fat: 18 g
Carbohydrate: 32 g

Ingredients

- 8 8-inch flour tortillas
- 1/2 cup julienned sun dried tomatoes in olive oil, drained
- 1 cup crumbled feta cheese
- One 10-ounce package frozen chopped spinach, thawed and drained
- 1 tablespoon fresh dill
- 1/2 cup chopped pitted kalamata olives
- 1 cup shredded mozzarella cheese

Instructions

- The Tzatziki sauce is going to make a return in this recipe. You can find the recipe for the Tzatziki sauce in the *Turkish Style Meatball Gyro with Tzatziki* section.
- Begin by preheating the oven to 400° F. Take out a baking tray and line it with parchment paper.
- Take out a tortilla and add olives, sun dried tomatoes, and cheeses. Add another tortilla on top.
- Repeat the above step until you have 4 quesadillas.
- Transfer the quesadillas into the baking sheet. Place the tray into the oven and bake for about 10 minutes, or until the cheese has melted.
- Serve with tzatziki sauce. Top the quesadillas with dill.

5. Cinnamon and Cayenne Chicken

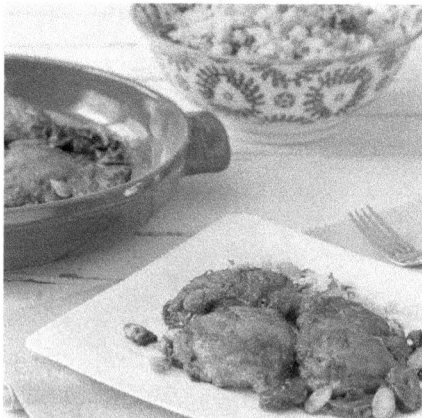

A little bit of cinnamon and a little bit of cayenne gives a whole lot of kick to this delicious dish.

Servings:6

Prep Time: 5 hours (including refrigeration time)

Cook time: 1 hour

Energy Value Per Serving: 2,096 kj

Calories: 501 calories

Protein: 34 g

Total Fat: 37 g

Carbohydrate: 5 g

Ingredients

- 1 whole chicken (3.5 pounds)
- ¼ cup olive oil
- 1 tablespoon kosher salt
- 1 tablespoon ground coriander
- ¼ teaspoon ground cinnamon
- ⅛ teaspoon cayenne
- 2 tablespoons roughly chopped green olives
- 1 tablespoon chopped mint, plus more for garnish
- 8 dried figs, roughly chopped
- 2 tablespoons fresh lemon juice
- 1 cup chicken broth
- 2 tablespoons roughly chopped pitted Kalamata olives

Instructions

- We are going to start by removing the backbone of the chicken. To do so, place it breast down on the chopping board. Remove the backbone using kitchen shears. Use your hands to flatten it into a butterfly shape.
- Take a small bow and add coriander, salt, cinnamon, cayenne, and 2 tablespoons olive oil. Apply the mixture to both sides of the chicken. Place the chicken in an airtight container and refrigerate it for about 5 hours. You can even keep it refrigerated for about 24 hours if you are planning to have it for dinner the next day.
- Preheat the oven to 400° F.
- Take a pan and place it over medium high heat. Pour olive oil and allow it to become hot.
- Gently lower the chicken into the pan with the skin side down and cook until it turns golden brown.
- Place the pan into the oven and then bake for about 30 minutes. Take the pan out, turn over the chicken, and add mint, figs, olives, lemon juice, and chicken broth into the pan. Place the pan back into the oven and cook for another 30 minutes, or until the internal temperature reads 165° F. You can use a thermometer to check the temperature of the chicken.
- Take the chicken out, transfer to a plate, top with mint, and serve with the fig mixture.

6. Roasted Herb Salmon

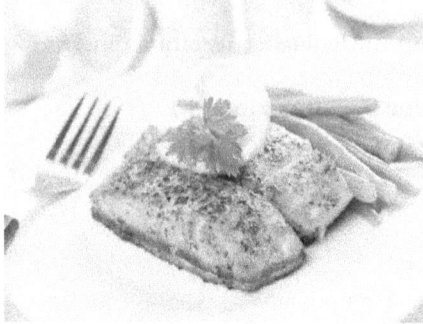

With three different kinds of herbs, you can make this dish into an aromatic treat. So much so that you might not want to eat it, but hang it in a pot!

Servings: 4
Prep Time: 20 minutes
Cook time: 15 minutes

Energy Value Per Serving: 1,347 kj
Calories: 322 calories
Protein: 30 g
Total Fat: 20 g
Carbohydrate: 6 g

Ingredients
- 2 tablespoons Dijon mustard
- 1 small yellow onion, thinly-sliced
- 4 ounces salmon fillets, about One 1/2 inches thick
- 2 tomatoes, thinly-sliced
- 1 tablespoon minced fresh thyme
- 1 tablespoon minced fresh rosemary
- 1 teaspoon dried oregano
- 2 tablespoons fresh lemon juice
- ½ teaspoon salt
- ½ teaspoon ground black pepper

Instructions
- Take your fillet and make four slits on the top, preferably about 2 inches long and ¼ inches deep. It would be better if the slits were evenly spaced.
- Use a large bowl and add in rosemary, lemon juice, mustard, thyme, oregano, salt, and pepper. Mix all the ingredients well.
- Place the salmon into the bowl and coat both sides with the mixture. Use a plastic wrap to cover the bowl and refrigerate for about 20 minutes. Remove the fish from the marinade, but do not dispose of the marinade.

- Preheat the oven to 450° F. Use the cooking spray to coat the baking tray. Place the tomato and onion slices at the bottom and the salmon goes on top of them. Use the marinade you had set aside on top of the salmon.
- Place it in the oven and roast for about 15 minutes, or until the fish is tender. You can check this by poking the fish with a fork.
- Serve hot.

7. Basil Pasta

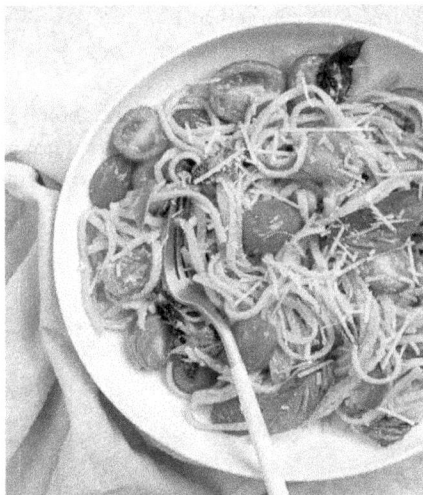

This dish uses a basil tapenade as the pasta sauce. The result is something creamy, but with an herb-like flavor. The best part is that you can use the tapenade as a dip for other recipes.

Servings: 6

Prep Time: 10 minutes

Cook time: 10 minutes

Energy Value Per Serving: 1,569 kj

Calories: 375 calories

Protein: 11 g

Total Fat: 10 g

Carbohydrate: 59 g

Ingredients

- 2 medium cloves of garlic
- 1 tablespoon fresh lemon juice
- 1 cup fresh basil leaves (packed)
- 1 cup flat leaf parsley (packed)
- 1 cup pitted Kalamata olives
- 1 pound linguine
- 3 tablespoons extra virgin olive oil

- parmesan cheese, freshly grated
- salt, to taste

Instructions

- Take a large pot and fill it with water. Add salt and place it over medium high heat. Bring the water to a boil.
- Take the parsley and basil leaves. Clean and dry them before transferring them to a blender. Add lemon juice, garlic, and olives. Pulse the ingredients until they are smooth.
- Transfer the puree into a large bowl.
- Place the paste in the boiling water. Cook as per instructions on the package or until al dente.
- Drain the pasta and transfer it to the puree bowl. Drizzle with olive oil and mix the ingredients well. Sprinkle a generous amount of cheese. Mix all the ingredients together well. Make sure that you are bringing the sauce from the bottom to the top.

8. Vegetarian Flatbread Pizza

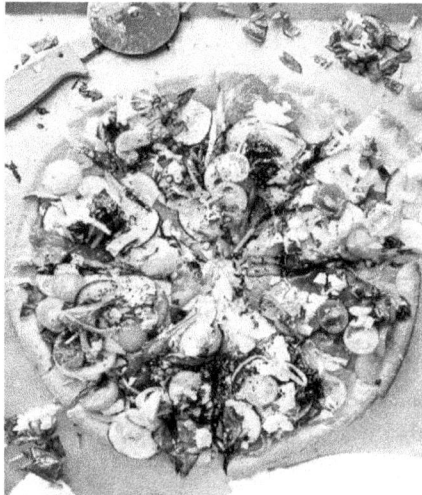

Did someone order a pizza? Well, with this recipe, you won't be ordering from the pizza joint ever again. In fact, your friends and family might start placing orders for your pizza.

Servings: 6

Prep Time: 20 minutes

Cook time: 30 minutes

Energy Value Per Serving: 1,883 kj

Calories: 450 calories

Protein: 17 g

Total Fat: 19 g

Carbohydrate: 57 g

Ingredients

- 3 pieces of pita bread
- 2 ounces crumbled feta cheese with Mediterranean herbs
- 1/8 teaspoon pepper
- 1/2 cup cherry tomatoes
- 1/2 cup marinated artichoke hearts
- 1/4 cup natural almonds
- 1/4 cup fresh basil leaves, torn
- 2 tablespoons water
- 1/4 teaspoon fine sea salt, plus more for sprinkling
- 2/3 cup cannellini beans, drained and rinsed
- 2 cups packed baby spinach
- 1 tablespoon extra-virgin olive oil
- 1/2 medium avocado
- 1/4 small red onion

Instructions

- Preheat the oven to 350° F.
- Take out a baking tray and place the pita bread on it.
- Next, we shall make the pesto. Take baby spinach, white beans, sea salt, almonds, olive oil, basil, water, and pepper in a blender. Pulse the ingredients until they are smooth.
- Transfer the pesto evenly to each bread.
- Chop the artichoke hearts, halve the tomatoes, and slice the red onion and avocado into thin slices. Arrange the ingredients on top of the bread evenly.
- Generously sprinkle some feta cheese on each bread. Add a little sea salt to taste, if you prefer.
- Put the tray into the oven and bake for about 10 minutes, or until the bread becomes mildly crispy. Take the bread out and allow it to cool a little. Serve warm.

9. Stuffed Peppers

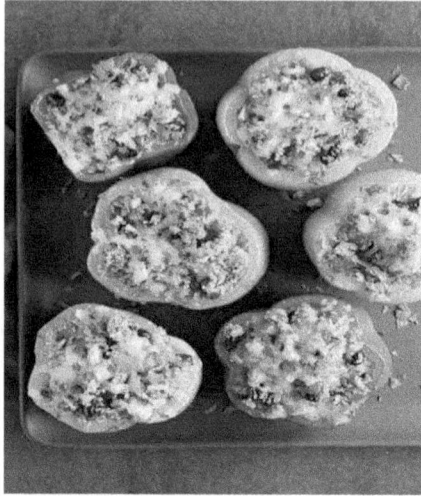

This dish is packed with a lot of protein, since the ingredient used to stuff the peppers is quinoa.

Servings: 4

Prep Time: 15 minutes

Cook time: 1 hour

Energy Value Per Serving: 1,013 kj

Calories: 242 calories

Protein: 10 g

Total Fat: 9 g

Carbohydrate: 33 g

Ingredients

- 1 cup cooked quinoa
- 1 teaspoon olive oil, extra-virgin
- 1 cup water
- 4 medium sweet peppers
- 1 teaspoon table salt
- 1 small uncooked onions, yellow, diced
- ½ teaspoon kosher salt
- 1 teaspoon minced garlic
- 14 ½ ounces canned diced tomatoes, undrained
- 10 medium olives, chopped
- 1 cup canned chickpeas (undrained), rinsed and drained
- 1 ½ tablespoons store-bought-pesto sauce
- ⅓ cup crumbled feta cheese

Instructions

- Preheat the oven to 375° F.
- Take out a baking tray and lightly spray it with cooking spray.

- Place a medium sized pan on medium heat and pour olive oil into it. When the oil is hot enough, add kosher salt and onion. Cook until the onion softens. Toss in the garlic and cook for another 30 seconds. Add quinoa, tomatoes along with their liquid, table salt, and water. Mix all the ingredients well.
- Increase the heat to medium high and bring the mixture to a boil. Then lower the heat to low and cover the pan. Allow the ingredients to simmer for 15 minutes, or until the quinoa becomes tender.
- Remove the tops of the peppers. Take out the seeds, ribs, and core. Check to see if the peppers are sitting flat. If they are not, you simply have to make a thin slice at the bottom.
- Place the peppers on the baking tray.
- Back to the quinoa. Once it has finished cooking, add pesto, chickpeas, and olives. Stir the ingredients well.
- Spoon equal measures of the quinoa into each of the peppers. If some quinoa still remains, then set it aside. Don't try to overstuff the peppers.
- Put the baking tray in the oven and bake for about 25 minutes. Remove the tray from the oven and add crumbled feta on top of the pepper. Put the tray back into the oven for another 5 minutes.

10. Cabbage Steaks with Feta and Basil Pesto

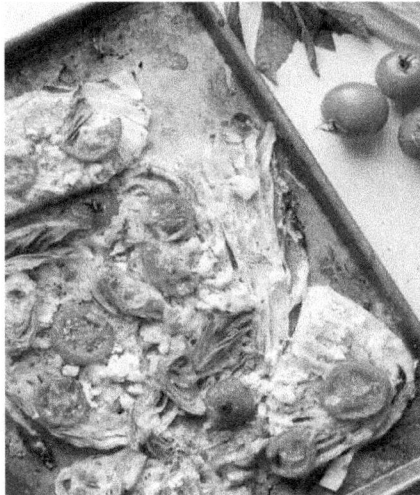

It almost tastes like pizza, but it is not pizza. Yet this dish makes you eat an entire head of cabbage. and you will have no regrets.

Servings: 5
Prep Time: 5 minutes
Cook time: 20 minutes
Energy Value Per Serving: 1,016 kj
Calories: 243 calories

Protein: 12 g

Total Fat: 16 g

Carbohydrate: 16 g

Ingredients

- 2 ounces feta cheese, crumbled
- 4 ounces basil pesto
- 1 tablespoon Mediterranean Seasoning
- 1 small cabbage head, sliced into "steaks"
- 1 cup shredded parmesan cheese
- 2 small tomatoes, sliced
- 6 artichoke halves
- fresh basil, to garnish

Instructions

- Preheat the oven to 400° F. Take out a baking tray and layer it lightly with some cooking spray.
- Place the cabbage as a single layer on the tray. Try to cover the tray as much as possible. Add the artichoke halves on top of the cabbage.
- Add the pesto on the artichokes. Be generous with it since the cabbage will absorb much of the pesto.
- Add tomato and cheese as toppings. Place the tray into the oven and bake for about 20 minutes, or until the cheese is bubbly and cabbage has crispy edges.

11. Stuffed Eggplants with Tahini

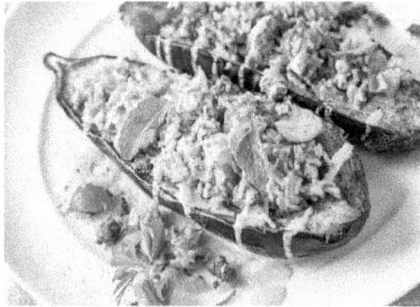

Eggplants have a wonderful sweetness to them. The tahini has a nutty and mildly bitter flavor. Together, they create a unique flavor profile.

Servings: 2

Prep Time: 5 minutes

Cook time: 30 minutes

Energy Value Per Serving: 1,443 kj

Calories: 345 calories

Protein: 9 g

Total Fat: 19 g

Carbohydrate: 38 g

Ingredients

- 1 eggplant
- 1 tablespoon tomato juice
- 2 tablespoons olive oil divided
- 1 tablespoon tahini
- 1 teaspoon lemon juice
- 1/2 teaspoon garlic powder
- 1 medium shallot diced
- 1/2 cup cooked quinoa
- 1/2 teaspoon ground cumin
- 1 cup chopped button mushrooms
- 6 plum tomatoes, chopped
- 2 garlic cloves minced
- 1 tablespoon chopped fresh parsley and more to garnish
- salt and pepper to taste

Instructions

- Preheat the oven to 425° F. Take the eggplant and cut it lengthwise in half. Use a spoon to remove some of the flesh.
- Take out a baking tray and place the eggplant on it. Lightly add 1 tablespoon of the olive oil on top. Sprinkle salt on top.
- Place the tray in the oven and bake for 20 minutes.
- While the eggplant is cooking, take out a large skillet and place it over medium high heat. Pour the remaining oil into it. Add the mushrooms and shallots. Saute the ingredients for about 5 minutes, or until the mushrooms have softened.
- Add the spices, quinoa, and tomato. Cook until the liquid in the skillet has evaporated.
- After the 20 minute bake time, remove the tray and reduce the oven temperature to 350° F. Stuff each half of the eggplant with the tomato mixture. Place the tray back into the oven and bake for about 10 minutes.
- Take a small bowl and add garlic, lemon, tahini, salt, pepper, and water. Mix all the ingredients well. Add the tahini mixture over the eggplants. Top it with a little parsley.

12. Pasta with Escarole and Sausage

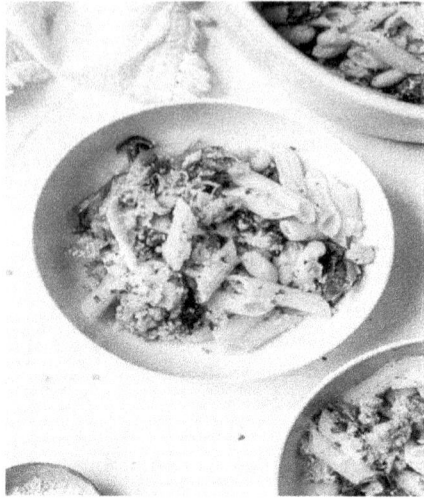

This dinner can be prepared quickly, but the result is a wholesome meal. You can adjust the pepper flakes to increase or decrease the heat level.

Servings: 6

Prep Time: 15 minutes

Cook time: 12 minutes

Energy Value Per Serving: 929 kj

Calories: 222 calories

Protein: 15 g

Total Fat: 5 g

Carbohydrate: 28 g

Ingredients

- 6 ounces uncooked bowtie pasta
- 1 teaspoon olive oil
- ¾ cup canned chicken broth
- 14.5 ounces canned fire-roasted diced tomatoes
- 1 teaspoon crushed red pepper flakes, or to taste
- ¼ cup grated parmesan cheese
- ¼ teaspoon table salt
- 8 ounces uncooked turkey sausage
- 1 small onion, chopped
- 4 medium garlic cloves, sliced
- 8 cups escarole, roughly chopped in bite-size pieces

Instructions

- Place a pot over medium to high heat. Pour water into it and bring it to a boil. Add the pasta into the water and cook as per instructions or until al dente. Drain the pasta but place it back into the pot.
- Take a skillet and place it over medium high heat. Add onion and

sausage. Cook for about 5 minutes, or until the sausage has a brown shade to it. Break apart the sausage into small pieces.

- Add broth, escarole, and garlic to the skillet. Continue cooking for another 5 minutes, or until the escarole is tender. Add the red pepper flakes and tomatoes. Cook for another 1 minute.

- Use a spoon to spread the sauce over the pasta. Add cheese as topping.

13. Penne Pasta with Roasted Leeks, Asparagus, and Tomatoes

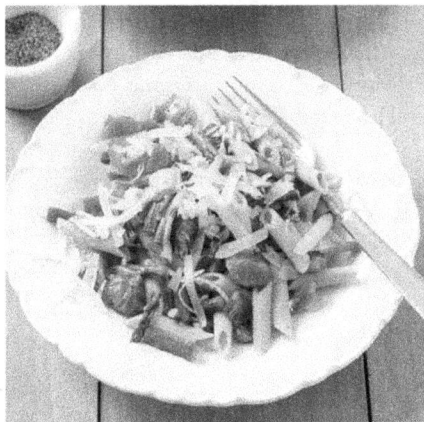

This dish is an example of how you can combine simple ingredients to produce a wholesome meal. It is light and super easy to prepare.

Servings: 6

Prep Time: 15 minutes

Cook time: 40 minutes

Energy Value Per Serving: 1,155 kj

Calories: 276 calories

Protein: 13 g

Total Fat: 7 g

Carbohydrate: 45 g

Ingredients

- 2 pounds uncooked asparagus
- ½ cup chopped basil
- 1 cup shredded Parmigiano Reggiano cheese
- 2 medium uncooked leeks
- ¼ teaspoon black pepper
- 6 cups cherry fresh ingredients
- 2 tablespoons extra virgin olive oil
- 1 teaspoon minced garlic
- 1 teaspoon lemon zest
- 8 ounces uncooked whole wheat pasta, penne

- 1 teaspoon kosher salt to taste

Instructions

- Preheat the oven to 375° F.
- Take out the baking tray and lightly spray it with cooking spray.
- Cut the leeks and soak them in water. Rinse the leeks well and cut the green and white parts separately. Wash the asparagus, rinse it, and trim it into small pieces.
- Add tomatoes, leeks, and asparagus on the baking tray. Top with salt and pepper, and olive oil. Roast for about 35 minutes.
- While the ingredients are roasting, add water to a pot and place it over medium high heat. Add penne to the water and cook it as per the instructions on the package or until al dente. Take out ¼ pasta water and set it aside. Drain the pasta.
- Take a large bowl and add the roasted vegetables, lemon zest, garlic, basil, and the pasta. Pour the pasta water into the bowl. Mix all the ingredients well. Top with parmesan cheese.

14. Chicken Bruschetta Sandwiches

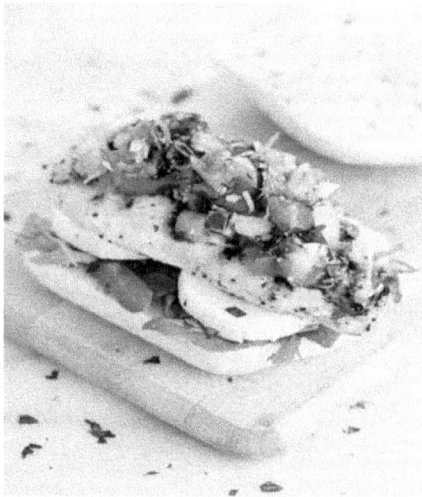

This sandwich features just one whole-grain slice of bread. This allows you to keep the carbs in check while filling your sandwich cravings.

Servings: 4

Prep Time: 10 minutes

Cook time: 15 minutes

Energy Value Per Serving: 1,556 kj

Calories: 372 calories

Protein: 35 g

Total Fat: 17 g

Carbohydrate: 20 g

Ingredients

- 4 slices whole grain bread, sliced
- 1 pound skinless, boneless chicken breast cutlets
- 1 tablespoon canola oil
- 2 teaspoons Italian seasoning
- 3 roma tomatoes, chopped
- ¼ cup fresh basil, chopped
- 2 teaspoons olive oil
- 4 thin slices mozzarella cheese
- ⅓ red onion, chopped
- 1 clove garlic, chopped
- 2 teaspoons olive oil
- 1 teaspoon balsamic vinegar
- salt and pepper to taste

Instructions

- Preheat the oven to 425° F. Take out the baking tray and drizzle it with cooking spray. Place the bread on top and return the tray to the oven. Cook for about 5 minutes, or until the bread turns crispy.
- Take the chicken and cover it with seasonings and oil. Take a skillet and place it over medium high heat. Put the chicken into the skillet and cook for about 4 minutes per side, or until you notice the chicken cooked properly.
- While the bread and chicken are getting ready, take a bowl and add garlic, onion, tomato, balsamic vinegar, oil, and basil. Mix all the ingredients well.
- Take out the bread and at about 2 chicken cutlets. Layer a cheese on top of the chicken. Serve the bread with the bruschetta mix.

15. Baked Feta with Cherry and Grape Tomatoes

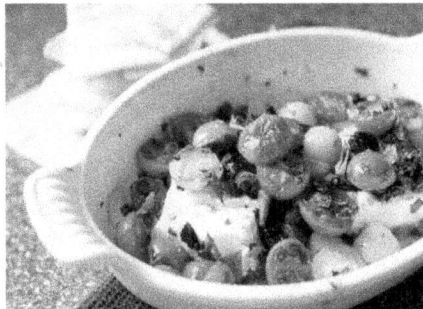

You can combine this dish with polenta and spaghetti, or you can also have it by itself. The grapes add a layer of sweetness that compliments the tomatoes.

Servings: 4

Prep Time: 10 minutes

Cook time: 15 minutes
Energy Value Per Serving: 736 kj
Calories: 176 calories
Protein: 6 g
Total Fat: 13 g
Carbohydrate: 10 g
Ingredients
- 2 tablespoons extra-virgin olive oil, divided
- 1 garlic clove, minced
- 1 4-ounce block feta, cut into thin slabs
- 2 pints multicolored grape and cherry tomatoes
- 1 tablespoon balsamic vinegar
- ½ cup sunflower or other sprouts
- 1 tablespoon sliced fresh basil leaves
- ¼ teaspoon kosher salt
- coarsely ground black pepper

Instructions
- Preheat the oven to 400° F. Take out a baking dish and lightly brush it with 1 tablespoon olive oil.
- Place the feta leaves at the bottom in a single layer. Place the tray aside.
- Take out a large skillet and place it over medium heat. Add the remaining olive oil to it. Introduce the tomatoes to the skillet and cook for about 15 minutes, or until the tomatoes look like they are going to burst open. Add salt, garlic, and balsamic vinegar, and mix the ingredients well. Cook all the ingredients for about 5 minutes, or until the liquid thickens.
- All the tomatoes to cook as you focus on the feta. Bake the feta for about 10 to 12 minutes, or until the feta feels a little springy when you touch it.
- Place equal portions of the feta on plates. Add the tomatoes as topping. Finish it with black pepper, basil, and sprouts as toppings.

MEDITERRANEAN SAUCES

Sauces can be used to complete a dish or simply act as a dip. Whatever your preference, it is always good to have a sauce recipe. A few sauce recipes have been added to certain recipes in the book. The ones mentioned below are not highlighted anywhere else in the book.

1. Ginger and Orange Sauce

Sweet, tangy, and with a little ginger kick, this sauce goes well with salads or as a dip for sandwiches.

Servings: 4
Prep Time: 5 minutes
Cook time: 5 minutes

Energy Value Per Serving: 251 kj

Calories: 60 calories

Protein: 0 g

Total Fat: 0 g

Carbohydrate: 5 g

Ingredients

- juice from 3 fresh oranges
- ¼ cup light mayonnaise
- ¼ teaspoon honey
- ¼ teaspoon ground ginger
- 1 tablespoon extra-virgin olive oil
- 2 tablespoons prepared fresh horseradish
- salt and freshly ground pepper to taste

Instructions

- Place a saucepan over medium heat and add ginger, orange juice, olive oil, mayonnaise, horseradish, honey, and salt and pepper. Mix them properly until the sauce begins to simmer. Cook for an additional 2 minutes.

2. Sweet and Spicy Glaze

This sauce is so simple to prepare that you might just decide to make it every time you sit down to eat something.

Servings: 1

Prep Time: 2 minutes

Cook time: None

Energy Value Per Serving: 423 kj

Calories: 101 calories

Protein: 0 g

Total Fat: 0 g

Carbohydrate: 25 g

Ingredients

- 2 tablespoons spicy chili sauce
- ⅓ cup honey

Instructions

- Take a small bowl and blend the ingredients.
- That's it. No seriously, that's all there is to it. This is probably the shortest recipe in this book.

3. Red Pesto Sauce

Cheesy and complemented by the texture of sundried tomatoes, this pesto sauce is wholesome and flavorful.

Servings: 4

Prep Time: 5 minutes

Cook time: None

Energy Value Per Serving: 983 kj

Calories: 235 calories

Protein: 5 g

Total Fat: 21 g

Carbohydrate: 9 g

Ingredients

- 2 ounces sundried tomatoes
- 1 cup loosely packed fresh basil leaves
- 3 tablespoons pine nuts, lightly toasted
- 4 tablespoons extra-virgin olive oil
- 4 tablespoons freshly grated parmesan cheese
- 2 cloves fresh garlic, minced
- salt and freshly ground pepper to taste
- balsamic vinegar to taste

Instructions

- Put all the ingredients except parmesan into a blender and pulse them until they are smooth.
- Add the parmesan along with a little more salt and pepper. Pulse again until the parmesan has mixed well with the sauce.

4. Olive Sauce

The best part of this sauce is that it can make about ½ cups, which is more than enough to last you for a while, and then some.

Servings: ½ cup

Prep Time: 5 minutes

Cook time: None

Energy Value Per Serving: 4816 kj

Calories: 1,151 calories

Protein: 7 g

Total Fat: 124 g

Carbohydrate: 9 g

Ingredients

- 5 anchovy fillets
- 1 teaspoon dried rosemary
- ½ teaspoon freshly ground pepper
- 5 cloves fresh garlic, chopped
- ½ cup extra-virgin olive oil

Instructions

- Put all the ingredients into a blender and pulse them until they are smooth.

5. Lime Sauce with Almonds

The toasted almonds bring a crunchiness to this sauce while the lime gives it the acidic kick.

Servings: 4

Prep Time: 5 minutes

Cook time: 10 minutes

Energy Value Per Serving: 326 kj

Calories: 78 calories

Protein: 2 g

Total Fat: 6 g

Carbohydrate: 3 g

Ingredients

- 2 tablespoons olive oil
- 1 medium white onion, coarsely chopped
- ½ cup dry red wine
- 4 large cloves fresh garlic, finely chopped
- ½ large green bell pepper, coarsely chopped
- 1 teaspoon dried basil
- 1 teaspoon dried oregano
- 1 large eggplant, peeled and cubed
- 1 28-ounce can peeled Italian tomatoes, drained and broken in pieces by hand
- salt and freshly ground pepper to taste

Instructions

- Take a large skillet and place it over medium heat. Add oil into it and then throw in the garlic and onion. Saute them until the onion is fragrant and soft. Add eggplant, green bell pepper, oregano, tomatoes, wine, basil, and salt and pepper.
- Place the cover on the skillet and let the ingredients simmer for about 30 minutes, or until the peppers and eggplants have become tender. Mix all the ingredients. Serve hot with your favorite pasta dish.

MEDITERRANEAN SNACKS AND DRINKS

When you are in need of something to munch on, then leave it to the Mediterranean diet to provide something delicious and nutritious.

1. Roasted Garlic

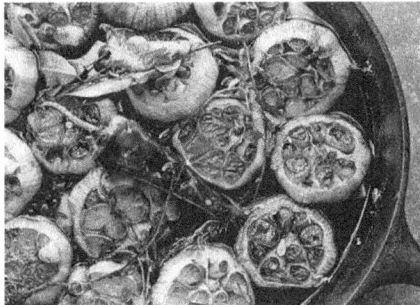

Garlic is an important ingredient in Mediterranean food, so why not dedicate an entire recipe just for it?

Servings: 4

Prep Time: 5 minutes
Cook time: 20 minutes
Energy Value Per Serving: 326 kj
Calories: 59 calories
Protein: 3 g
Total Fat: 0 g
Carbohydrate: 13 g
Ingredients
- 1 jumbo fresh elephant garlic head
- extra-virgin olive oil to drizzle

Instructions
- Preheat the oven to 400° F.
- Remove the top leaf points of each garlic. Place the garlic into a bowl that is over safe. Drizzle a small amount of olive oil on it. Place trimmed garlic head in a tight-fitting oven-safe. Place the garlic in the oven for about 20 minutes, or until it is soft.

2. Garlic and Tomato Bruschetta

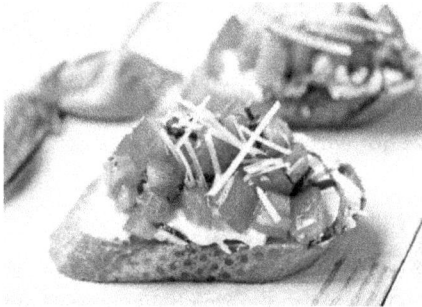

The flavor of garlic and the acidity of balsamic vinegar makes this snack one that you are going to have again and again.

Servings: 8
Prep Time: 5 minutes
Cook time: 5 minutes
Energy Value Per Serving: 238 kj
Calories: 57 calories
Protein: 2 g
Total Fat: 1 g
Carbohydrate: 11 g
Ingredients
- 8 slices ½-inch thick of a French baguette
- 1½ teaspoons minced fresh garlic
- 1¼ cups chopped plum tomatoes
- 1 teaspoon extra-virgin olive oil

- 1 teaspoon balsamic vinegar
- ½ teaspoon dried basil
- ¼ teaspoon of non-caloric sweetener
- ¼ teaspoon freshly ground pepper

Instructions

- Preheat the oven to 500° F.
- Take out a baking tray. Add olive oil to all sides of the baguette. Bake it for about 4 minutes.
- Combine the remaining ingredients in a small bowl. Mix well.
- Add the mixture on the baguette.

3. Crostini

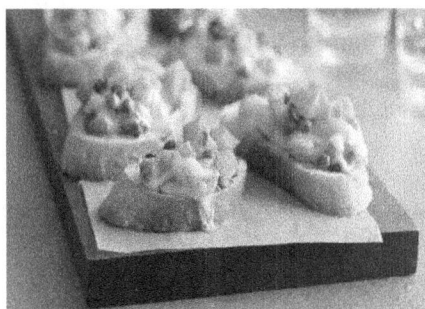

Another snack featuring French baguette. This time, with the addition of herbs.

Servings: 25

Prep Time: 5 minutes

Cook time: None

Energy Value Per Serving: 172 kj

Calories: 41 calories

Protein: 1 g

Total Fat: 1 g

Carbohydrate: 10 g

Ingredients

- 1 French baguette, roughly cut into ½-inch thick slices
- extra-virgin olive oil
- 2½ teaspoons fresh garlic paste
- minced fresh basil
- salt and freshly ground pepper to taste

Instructions

- Preheat the oven to 375° F.
- Take out a baking tray. Add olive oil to all sides of the baguette. Add garlic paste and pepper to taste, if you prefer. Bake it for about 4 minutes.
- Top the baguette with basil and enjoy!

4. Baby Shrimps

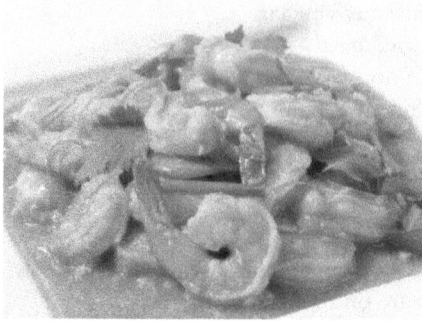

This snack is served on toasted rye along with Dijon mustard, which enhances the flavor profile of the dish.

Servings: 12

Prep Time: 5 minutes

Cook time: 15 minutes

Energy Value Per Serving: 197 kj

Calories: 47 calories

Protein: 2 g

Total Fat: 2 g

Carbohydrate: 4 g

Ingredients

- ½ cup reduced-fat mayonnaise
- 1 tablespoon finely chopped fresh parsley
- 1 teaspoon Dijon mustard
- ½ teaspoon chopped capers
- 2 tablespoons finely minced shallot
- 1 bag cooked salad shrimp, thawed
- ¼ cup freshly squeezed lemon juice
- 16 paper-thin slices lemon
- 16 slices cocktail-sized, thin rye bread
- 2 tablespoons olive oil

Instructions

- Preheat the oven to 300° F.
- In a small bowl, add parsley, mustard, mayonnaise, shallot, and capers. Mix them well and place it in the refrigerator for about an hour. Cover and refrigerate for no less than 1 hour to blend flavors.
- Take a baking tray and place the rye slices. Coat them in olive oil and bake until they become crispy.
- Add 1 teaspoon of mayonnaise on each rye toast. Top with 5 shrimps and sprinkle lemon juice on top. Top it with a slice of lemon.

5. Spicy tomato to baked potatoes

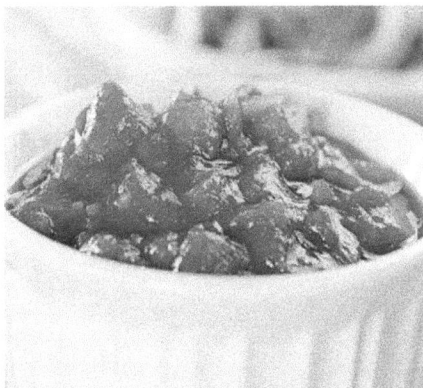

Serve with charcoal-baked or oven-baked potatoes.

Servings: 4

Prep Time: 5 minutes

Cook time: 25 minutes

Energy Value Per Serving:

Calories: 59 calories

Protein: 2 g

Total Fat: 2.5 g

Carbohydrate: 7.6 g

Ingredients

- ½ tbsp Extra virgin olive oil
- 6 cloves Garlic
- 420g Canned tomatoes sliced
- ½ tsp Paprika
- ½ tsp Red Pepper flakes
- ¼ tsp Salt

Instructions

- Heat olive oil in a saucepan. Add chopped garlic and sauté for 1 minute.
- Then add the tomatoes, paprika, red pepper flakes, and salt. Stir and cook for about 15–20 minutes, until the sauce is thickened to a ketchup state

6. Green beans with warm dressing and bacon

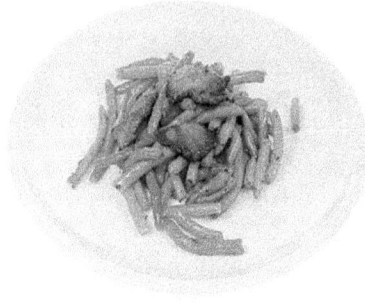

Servings: 2
Prep Time: 5 minutes
Cook time: 25 minutes
Energy Value Per Serving:
Calories: 140 calories
Protein: 7.3 g
Total Fat: 9,2g
Carbohydrate: 7.3 g
Ingredients
- 2 pieces Bacon
- 1 Shallot
- 230g Green String Beans
- 2 tsp White wine vinegar

Instructions

- Please, cook the beans, chopped into small pieces, in boiling salted water until soft, about 8 minutes. Drain and transfer to a bowl.
- Meanwhile, sauté the chopped bacon in a well-heated skillet over medium heat until crisp. Put on a paper towel.
- Put the finely chopped shallots into the pan and sauté for 30 seconds. Remove from heat and cool slightly. Add vinegar, salt, and pepper.
- Pour beans with warm dressing and lay on top slices of bacon.

7. Rolls with lettuce

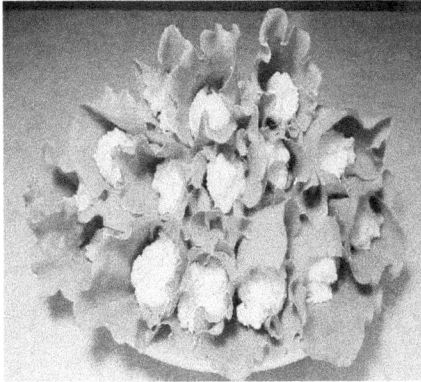

Servings: 2
Prep Time: 5 minutes
Cook time: 15 minutes
Energy Value Per Serving:
Calories: 267 calories
Protein: 25.2 g
Total Fat: 17.2g
Carbohydrate: 1.4 g
Ingredients
* Green salad to taste
* 2 Egg
* 200g Hard cheese
* 200g Peeled shrimp
* Low-calorie Mayonnaise to taste

Instructions

* Prepare the filling for rolls. Boil eggs and finely crush or grate. Grate the cheese. Finely chop the shrimp. Add some mayonnaise.
* Put the cooked mass on lettuce leaves.
* Gently wrap lettuce in rolls.

8. Baked tomatoes with Provencal herbs

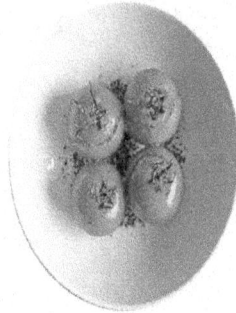

Servings: 2
Prep Time: 5 minutes
Cook time: 15 minutes
Energy Value Per Serving:
Calories: 221 calories
Protein: 1.5 g
Total Fat: 20.5g
Carbohydrate: 8.9 g
Ingredients
• 4 Tomatoes
• 2 tbsp Olive oil
• Salt to taste
• Ground black pepper to taste
• 1 tsp Mixed Herbs
Instructions

- Put the tomatoes in the oven for 15-20 minutes at 180 degrees.
  Plants are ideal when a little cracked, but not turn into puree. In
  the end, you can turn on the oven for 3 minutes.
- Please, drizzle the tomatoes with oil, sprinkle with salt, pepper, and
  herbs.

9. Hummus with roasted peppers

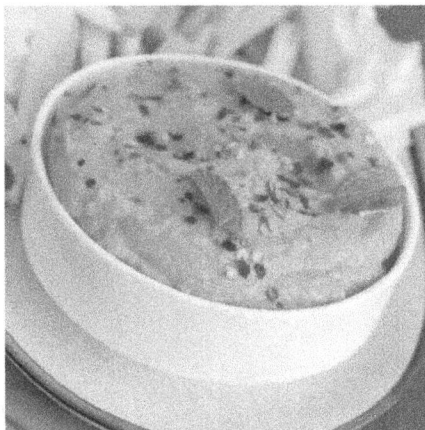

This hummus turns softer taste and less like traditional hummus. It also requires less olive oil because of the liquid which is contained in pepper.

Servings: 4

Prep Time: 5 minutes

Cook time: 15 minutes

Energy Value Per Serving:

Calories: 221 calories

Protein: 6.2 g

Total Fat: 16.2g

Carbohydrate: 12.3g

Ingredients

- 1 Canned jar chickpeas
- 1 Fresh red bell peppers
- 2 tbsp Tahini
- Lemon pieces
- 30ml Olive oil

Instructions

- Preheat the oven to 200 degrees.
- Bake the red pepper for about 20 minutes, then flip and bake for another 20 minutes.
- Remove from the oven and place it in a plastic container with a sealed lid immediately and store it in the refrigerator for 2 hours.
- Please, drain the liquid from the chickpeas.
- Remove the skin from the pepper and coarsely chop.
- Mix in a food processor the chickpeas, red pepper, tahini , and lemon juice.
- Gradually add olive oil to achieve the desired degree of density.
- Please, serve with pitas or pita bread.

10. Octopus Carpaccio

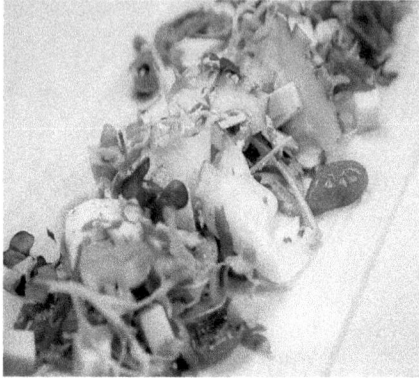

Servings: 1
Prep Time: 5 minutes
Cook time: 15 minutes
Energy Value Per Serving:
Calories: 279 calories
Protein: 18.4 g
Total Fat: 16 g
Carbohydrate: 14.7 g
Ingredients
- 80g Tentacle of the octopus
- 15g Rocket
- 15g Sun-dried tomatoes in oil
- 10g Black olives
- 20g Avocado
- 2g Green onion
- 10ml Olive oil
- 2ml Balsamic vinegar
- 2ml Lemon juice
- 0.2g Pink pepper
- 10g Ciabatta
- 2g Garlic
Instructions

- Boil the octopus (to lower the tentacles into the boiling water at the end to salt).
- Boiled octopus slice and put it on the plate.
- Season with olive oil, lemon juice, and balsamic vinegar.
- Put the arugula, dressed with olive oil, salt, pepper.
- Diced avocado, green onions, and black olives ring.

- Place them on a dish, add the sun-dried tomatoes, sprinkle top with crushed crackers ciabatta.
- Please, decorate with lettuce leaves.

11. The Babaganoush with Roasted Peppers

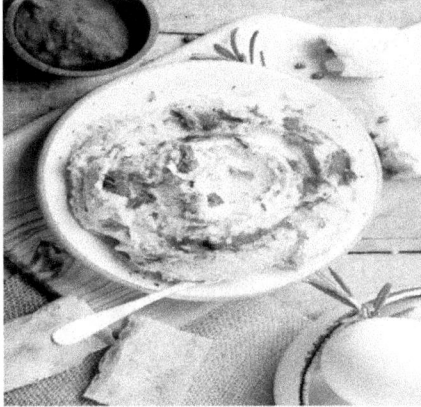

For babaganoush vegetables, it is better to bake in advance the night before. You can also add chopped cilantro, green onions, or mint.

Servings: 2
Prep Time: 10 minutes
Cook time: 20 minutes
Energy Value Per Serving:
Calories: 176 calories
Protein: 6.5 g
Total Fat: 11.2 g
Carbohydrate: 12.1 g
Ingredients
- 2 Eggplants
- 2 Fresh red chilli
- 3 tbsp Tahini
- 1 Lemon
- 1 tbsp Paprika
Instructions

- Preheat the oven to 180 degrees.
- Eggplant fry in a hot pan grill to black markings and bake in the oven for 40 minutes, pre-pinhole with a fork.
- After 20 minutes, add red pepper. Remove from the oven and place in a plastic container and store in the refrigerator.
- The flesh of the eggplant, remove with a spoon from the peel and

finely chop.

- Pepper peel and white films and also cut into small pieces and mix with eggplant. Add fresh tahini and lemon juice to pasta (do not be afraid that it will be too sour, as the eggplant will absorb it) and mix well. Sprinkle with paprika powder.
- Serve as a snack, on a side dish to grilled meat or with pitas.

12. Olives with Orange Zest, Cumin, and Caraway Seeds

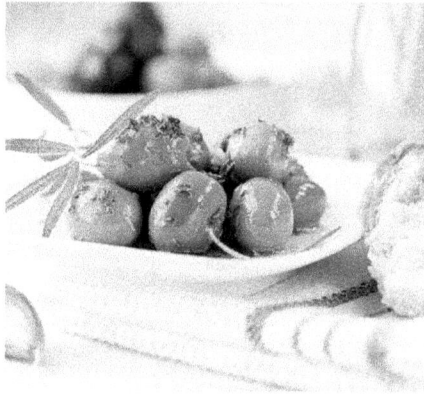

Servings: 4
Prep Time: 10 minutes
Cook time: 20 minutes
Energy Value Per Serving:
Calories: 181 calories
Protein: 1.5 g
Total Fat: 17.1 g
Carbohydrate: 8.4 g
Ingredients
- 2 tsp Cumin seeds
- 1 tsp Cumin seeds
- Red pepper
- 3 Oranges, zested
- 2 tbsp Extra virgin Olive oil
- 2 cups Olive oil
Instructions

- In a small bowl, lightly grind cumin seeds, then add cumin, red pepper flakes, and olive oil.
- Add the olives and mix well. Leave it for a while.

13. Cheese Baskets with Mussels

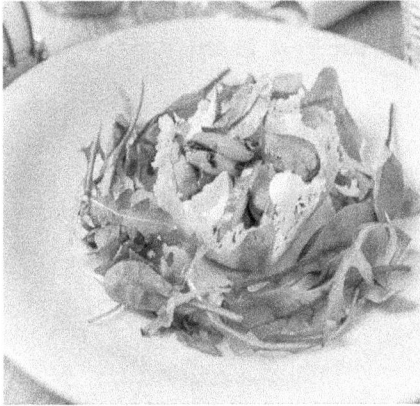

Servings: 8
Prep Time: 10 minutes
Cook time: 30 minutes
Energy Value Per Serving:
Calories: 111 calories
Protein: 9.1 g
Total Fat: 7.5 g
Carbohydrate: 0.6 g

Ingredients
- 350g Frozen mussels
- 100g Grated Parmesan cheese
- 2 cucumber
- 1 tbsp Vegetable oil
- 8 Quail egg
- 20g salat Arugula
- 1tbsp Lemon juice

Instructions

- Prepare the pastry: the Cup bottom diameter 5-6 cm, cut the A4 sheet of paper a circle with diameter 2 times more glass, grate cheese on a fine grater. Over medium heat preheat the pan, remove from heat, add cheese, allow to melt and cool slightly, then place on the bottom of the glass to form the shape. Baskets ready!
- Prepare the mussels: wipe the pan, add 1 tbsp oil, to evaporate the liquid from the molds, pour lemon juice. The mussels are ready, allow them to cool.
- Eggs boiled and cut into 2-4 pieces. Cucumbers cut into strips.

- To complete cooking before serving. Toppings: onion, cucumber, mayonnaise, mix, and put in baskets. Decorate eggs and greens!

14. Scallops under the Pear Pesto

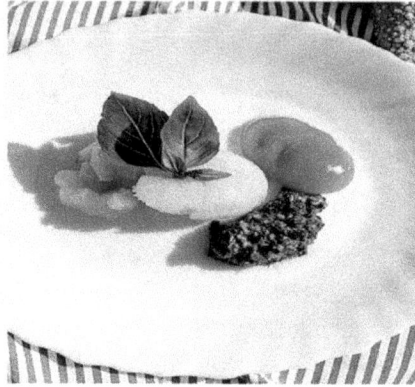

Servings: 2
Prep Time: 10 minutes
Cook time: 20 minutes
Energy Value Per Serving:
Calories: 165 calories
Protein: 10.5 g
Total Fat: 8.5 g
Carbohydrate: 12.7 g
Ingredient
- 3 Scallops
- 1 Pear
- 3 Cherry tomatoes
- Basil leaves
- 1 tbsp Pine nuts
- 10 ml Olive oil
- 1 clove garlic, finely chopped
- Salt to taste

Instructions

- Please, pear wash, dry, cut small cubes.
- Please, the pan heat, pour a little olive oil, put the bag. Add a little water and simmer for 10-15 minutes.
- The scallops are rinsed, dried with a paper towel, season with salt, put in a pan with the peas, sauté 4-6 minutes.
- Basil washed, dried, placed in a container, add the pine nuts,

chopped garlic, olive oil, and carefully beat with a blender until a homogeneous mass.

- Prepared scallops on a platter, garnish of stewed pears obtained with pesto, thinly sliced tomatoes, and sprig of Basil.

15. Zucchini in Greek

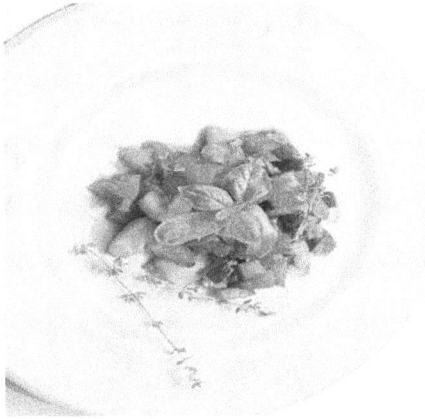

Servings: 2
Prep Time: 10 minutes
Cook time: 30 minutes
Energy Value Per Serving:
Calories: 136 calories
Protein: 1.5 g
Total Fat: 10.3 g
Carbohydrate: 10 g
Ingredients
- 120g Zucchini
- 5g Wheat flour
- 1 Onion
- 20g Spinach
- 20ml Vegetable oil
- 10g Green salad
- 20g Sweet pepper
- Parsley
- 1 Tomatoes
- Salt to taste
Instructions

- Clean young zucchini peeled, cut into neat slices thickness of about

1 cm. Put on the table a little flour and roll it, slice zucchini. Saute on a low heat until golden brown.
- Chop the green onion, fry it in vegetable oil. Then add the onions chopped spinach, lettuce, bell pepper, parsley, tomatoes , and cook vegetable mixture for 10-15 minutes.
- Season the boiled vegetables with salt and pepper, and then pour this mixture into the courgettes and cook all together in the oven for 15-20 minutes.
- Cool the zucchini and serve sprinkled with chopped dill.

16. Blueberry and Whey Smoothie

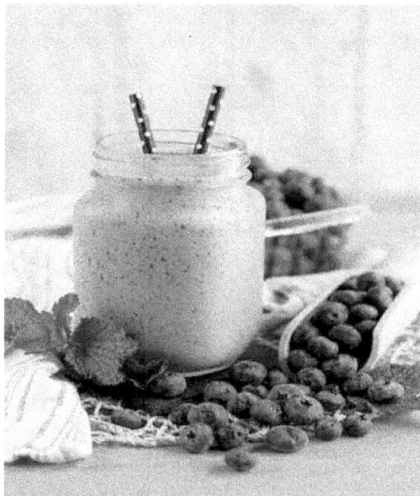

Not only does this drink have no sweeteners at all, it also includes non-fat yogurt to give it a creamy texture.

Servings: 1
Prep Time: 10 minutes
Cook time: None
Energy Value Per Serving: 519 kj
Calories: 22 calories
Protein: 1 g
Total Fat: 10 g
Carbohydrate: 4 g
Ingredients
- ¼ cup fresh or unsweetened frozen blueberries
- ¼ cup plain non-fat yogurt
- 1 scoop natural-flavored whey protein powder
- ½ cup cold water

- 8 ice cubes
- sprinkle of crushed almonds for garnish

Instructions
- Put all the ingredients in a blender and pulse until they are smooth.
- Serve with almonds as toppings.

17. Mediterranean Lemonade

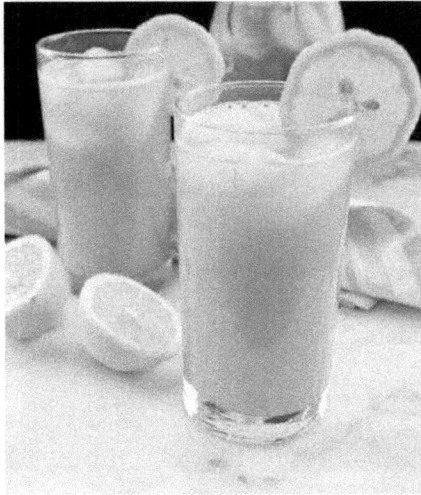

Who can say no to a classic lemonade?

Servings: 4
Prep Time: 10 minutes
Cook time: None

Energy Value Per Serving: 172 kj
Calories: 41 calories
Protein: 2 g
Total Fat: 4 g
Carbohydrate: 3 g

Ingredients
- 2 cups crushed ice
- 4 cups water
- juice of 1 large lemon
- 1 bunch fresh mint leaves, stems removed, more for later
- 2 large lemons, washed, cut into small pieces, and seeds removed

Instructions
- Put all the ingredients in a blender and pulse until they are smooth.
- Serve with more ice, if required.

18. Raspberry Mojito

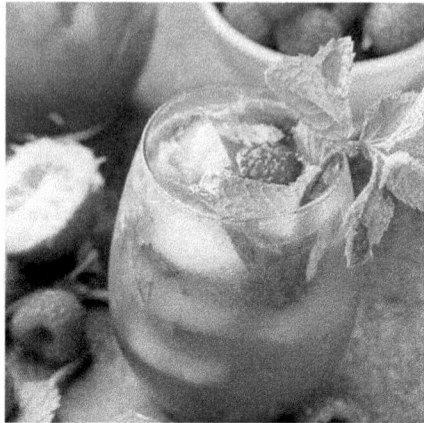

Fresh raspberry mojito without the alcohol. Perfect for when kids are around.
Servings: 4
Prep Time: 10 minutes
Cook time: None
Energy Value Per Serving: 565 kj
Calories: 135 calories
Protein: 1 g
Total Fat: 1 g
Carbohydrate: 23 g
Ingredients
- 4 fresh raspberries plus more for garnish
- 6 mint leaves
- 2 tablespoon fresh lime juice
- 1/2 cup sparkling mineral water
- 1/4 cup raspberry juice
Instructions
- Put all the ingredients except the sparkling water in a blender and pulse until they are smooth.
- Transfer the ingredients to a glass and pour in sparkling water.
19. Apple Pie Smoothie

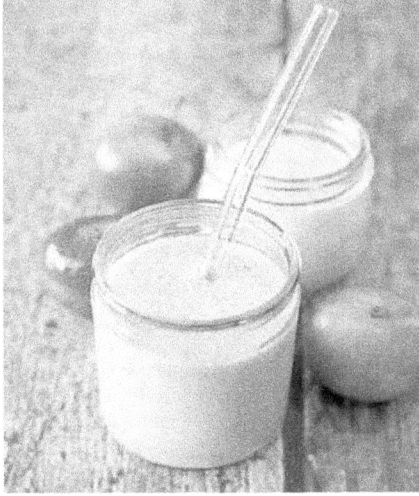

Enjoy apple pie in a smoothie form with a wonderful cinnamon twist.

Servings: 1

Prep Time: 10 minutes

Cook time: None

Energy Value Per Serving: 2,092 kj

Calories: 500 calories

Protein: 4 g

Total Fat: 29 g

Carbohydrate: 59 g

Ingredients

- 1 frozen banana
- 1 gala apple
- 1/2 cup unsweetened almond milk
- 1/4 teaspoon cinnamon
- 1 pinch nutmeg
- 1/2 cup plain low-fat Greek yogurt

Instructions

- Put all the ingredients in a blender and pulse until they are smooth.

20. Chocolate Mousse Smoothie

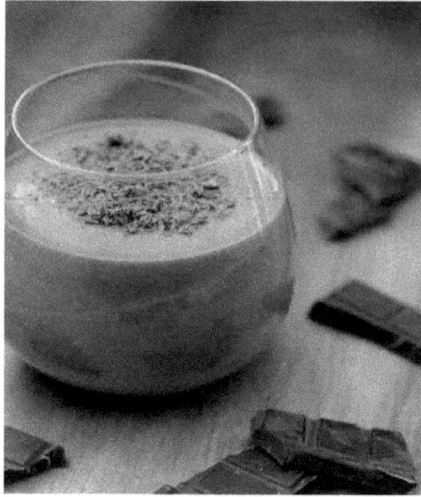

When your chocolate cravings reach a fever pitch, then you might need to try this smoothie.

Servings: 1

Prep Time: 10 minutes

Cook time: None

Energy Value Per Serving: 607 kj

Calories: 145 calories

Protein: 24 g

Total Fat: 1 g

Carbohydrate: 11 g

Ingredients

- ½ cup cold water
- 1 scoop natural-flavored whey protein powder
- 1 tablespoon fat-free, sugar-free chocolate syrup
- 1 teaspoon almond extract
- 8 ice cubes
- ½ cup plain fat-free yogurt
- fat-free whipped cream
- fat-free, sugar-free chocolate syrup to drizzle

Instructions

- Put all the ingredients, except the whipped cream and chocolate syrup, in a blender and pulse until they are smooth.

Serve in a glass and top it off with the whipped cream and drizzle.

21. Smoothie pineapple raspberry

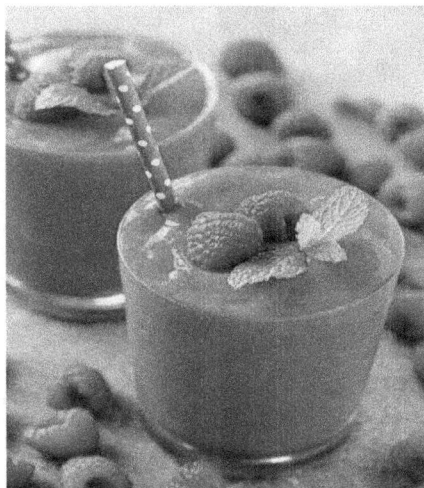

Buckwheat flakes can be replaced by oat or any other, to taste.
Servings: 4
Prep Time: 20 minutes
Cook time: None
Energy Value Per Serving:
Calories: 178 calories
Protein: 2.9 g
Total Fat: 1.4 g
Carbohydrate: 37.3 g
Ingredients
- 700g Pineapple
- 300g Frozen raspberries
- 300ml Vanilla rice milk
- 3 tbsp Buckwheat flakes
- Mint to taste

Instructions

- Please cut the pineapple into slices, clean and remove the core. Cut into medium pieces.
- Put the raspberries can be frozen can be defrosted during the night on the top shelf of the refrigerator.
- Take 200 ml of rice milk (in the absence of it, of course, you can substitute no fat milk), buckwheat flakes, slices of Mandarin , and pineapple and punch at high speed in a blender.
- Let stand for about 10-15 minutes — during this time, the oat flakes will swell.
- Add another 100 ml of rice drink and a punch in the blender again.

If the smoothie is still thick, bring the water or rice drink to need concentration. Garnish with leaves of fresh mint.

22. Beet-pineapple smoothie with fennel

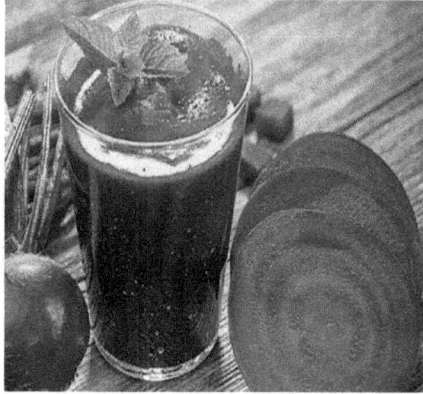

Servings: 2
Prep Time: 10 minutes
Cook time: None
Energy Value Per Serving:
Calories: 136 calories
Protein: 3.1 g
Total Fat: 10.5 g
Carbohydrate: 29.5 g
Ingredients
* 300g Beets
* 1/3 Pineapple
* 1 Fennel
* 1 Lime

Instructions

* Clean ⅓ of the pineapple and remove the core.
* Clean the beets and squeeze the juice of fennel. Squeeze the juice of a lime.
* Put all the ingredients in a blender and run at maximum speed until smooth.

23. Grape smoothie with green tea

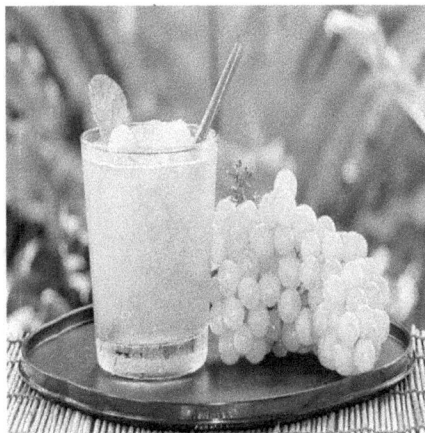

Servings: 2
Prep Time: 25 minutes
Cook time: None
Energy Value Per Serving:
Calories: 109 calories
Protein: 1 g
Total Fat: 0.4 g
Carbohydrate: 27.2 g
Ingredients
• 125ml Water
• 250g Green seedless grapes
• 125g Pineapple
• 6 Ice cubes
• 1 tsp Green tea
Instructions

• Pour green tea with hot (but not boiling) water. Cover and let it brew for 5 minutes. Please, strain and cool completely.
• Place all the ingredients in the blender bowl: grapes, pineapple slices, tea, and ice cubes. Beat until smooth.
• Pour into a glass and serve immediately.

24. Black cream smoothie

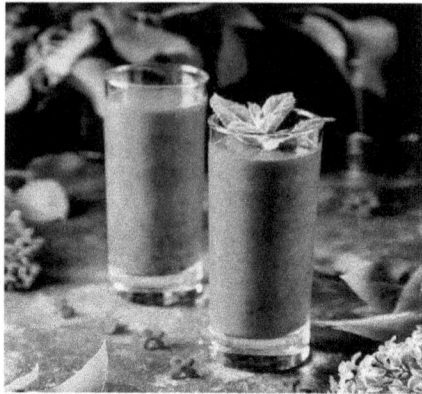

Servings: 1
Prep Time: 5 minutes
Cook time: None
Energy Value Per Serving:
Calories: 208 calories
Protein: 3.9 g
Total Fat: 0.9 g
Carbohydrate: 49.5 g
Ingredients
- Frozen blueberries to taste
- 1 Bananas
- 2 Strawberry
- 2.5ml Cream
- 5g Oatmeal

Instructions

- Place fruits and cereals in a blender.
- Please, pulsate.
- Put in a glass.
- Add cream.

25. Berry cranberry and blackberry smoothie

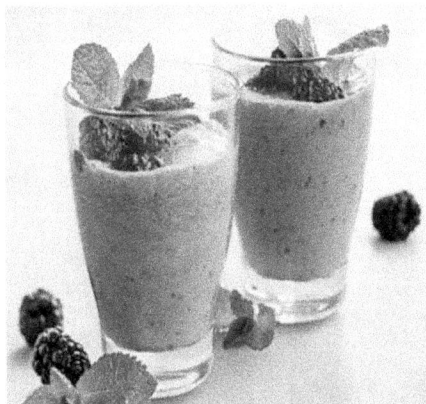

Servings: 2
Prep Time: 5 minutes
Cook time: None
Energy Value Per Serving:
Calories: 201 calories
Protein: 7.3 g
Total Fat: 3.5 g
Carbohydrate: 36.8 g
Ingredients
- ½ cup Cranberry fruit drink
- 160g Cranberries
- 190g Blackberry
- 250g Raspberry yogurt

Instructions

- Beat in a blender until smooth all the ingredients, adding a little ice.
- Pour into glasses and serve.

26. Blueberry Shake with Honey

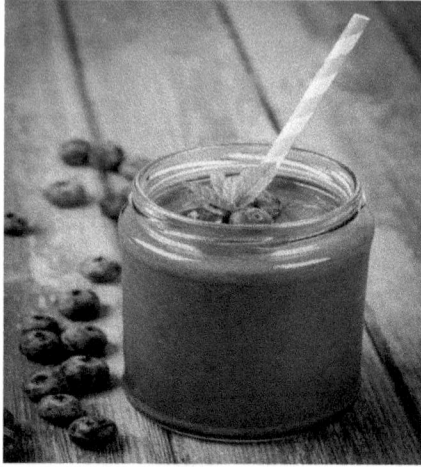

Servings: 4
Prep Time: 25 minutes
Cook time: None
Energy Value Per Serving:
Calories: 72 calories
Protein: 2.8 g
Total Fat: 2.2 g
Carbohydrate: 9.6 g
Ingredients

- 2 tbsp Honey 2 tablespoons
- 100g Blueberries 100 g
- 125ml Milk 125 ml
- 125g Natural yogurt 125 g
- 5 Ice cubes5 pieces

Instructions

- All ingredients are put in a blender bowl (do not defrost frozen berries beforehand) and grind.

27. Raspberry cooler with lemon

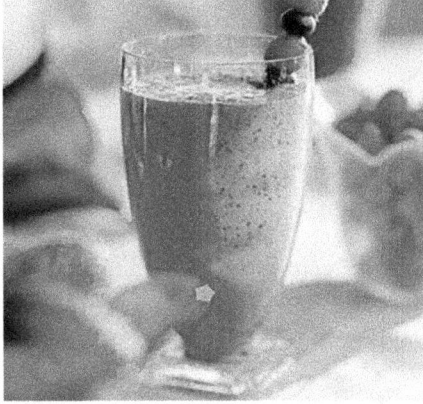

Servings: 4
Prep Time: 30 minutes
Cook time: None
Energy Value Per Serving:
Calories: 139 calories
Protein: 1.7 g
Total Fat: 0.8 g
Carbohydrate: 28.4 g
Ingredients
- 1 Lemon
- 720g Raspberry
- 1 Vanilla pod
- ¼ cups Sugar
- 3 cups Sparkling water

Instructions

- In a bowl, mix the berries, sliced into thin slices of lemon, vanilla pod, from which remove the seeds and put the same in the beans and sugar. Put in a water bath and cook, stirring, for about 12 minutes, until the berries give away the juice.
- Wipe the mass through a sieve, squeezing all the juice. Chill.
- Pour the syrup into 3 ice-filled glasses and fill it with sparkling water. Serve immediately, garnishing with lemon slices.

Mediterranean Instant Pot Cookbook

100 + New Recipes to Your Life

WHAT IS THE MEDITERRANEAN DIET

Almost anywhere you go, you will find people have something to boast about in regards to their food. And for good reason, with so much great food out there, you want yours to be considered the best, or at least in the running for the top spot. Consisting of a large landmass that surrounds the Mediterranean Sea, it is a vast region depicting numerous different types of people, and a mixed bag of cultures. As such this provides a wide array of meal choices. This diet has slowly spread out across the globe and has become popular in just about every corner of the world. Although many people have gone to a Mediterranean or Greek restaurant at some point, they do not understand exactly what the diet consists of or the many benefits it provides. For this reason is why we are here, creating this text to spread the word.

What Does It Entail?

Based on the traditional cuisine of the region surrounding the Mediterranean Sea, this diet boasts many heart-healthy, low fat, healthy fat, and delicious meal options for almost every palette. While there is no exact definition of the Mediterranean diet, the main components consist of:

- Fruits and vegetables - Most fruits and vegetables are acceptable as long as they are fresh, and it is recommended to have several servings throughout the day.
- Whole grains - These are different from refined grains because they retain all of their nutritional values.
- Beans, nuts, and seeds - These can include almonds, cashews, pistachios, garbanzo beans, chickpeas, chia seeds, and so much more.
- Fatty fishes and poultry - Fatty fishes include mackerel, herring, tuna, and salmon.
- Olive oil - This is considered a healthy fat and a great alternative to butter and other unhealthy saturated fats.

Consuming the Mediterranean diet will consist of eating these various food groups regularly, in addition to different herbs and spices, like garlic, ginger, black pepper, parsley, oregano, and coriander. Including these herbs and spices adds flavor to the food, which will eliminate the need for excess salt. While red meat can certainly be indulged, it is not commonly included due to the heavy fat and cholesterol content. The Mediterranean diet promotes more plant-based proteins than meat-based but if you are to consume red meat, lean meats are what is recommended.

HEALTH BENEFITS

Not only is Mediterranean cuisine some of the most delicious food in the world, but it is also some of the healthiest, maybe some of the healthiest you can find. But only, and this part is important, if you use the correct ingredients and are eating it fresh. Try substituting these meals in place of your regular diet for a few days, and see the difference in how it makes you feel as a whole. You will notice that you have more energy and your mood is improved drastically. Overall, you will just feel like a more healthy person.

The Mediterranean diet has not only been instrumental in helping people prevent disease, but also reversing some of the processes of advanced illness. The food groups and ingredients involved have many beneficial outcomes which will positively affect your heart, brain, kidneys, blood, digestive tract and your entire body system. The health benefits are immense and you will feel the changes almost instantly when making the switch.

Instant Pot

An instant pot is a convenient cookware that essentially does the job of seven different appliances to make life easier. It works as a pressure cooker, slow cooker, rice cooker, browning pan, steamer, yogurt maker, and warming pot. It is quickly becoming one of the most popular appliances among cooking pros and enthusiasts. Whatever recipes we include in this book that requires cooking can be done in your instant pot. But before jumping right in it's good to get better acquainted with this tool and, take time to learn about your instant pot. You can do a quick internet search or scroll on You tube for a number of helpful resources.

MEDITERRANEAN STYLE BREAKFAST

I. Fall Instant Pot Shakshuka
Servings: 4
Prep Time: 15 minutes
Cook time: 30 minutes

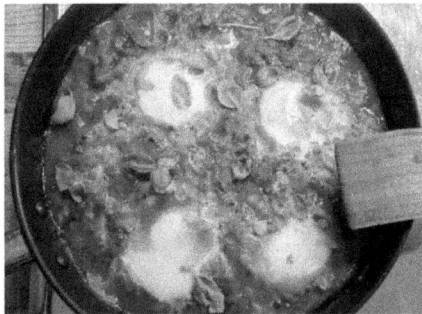

Energy Value Per Serving:
Calories: 217
Protein: 13 grams
Total Fat: 11 grams
Carbohydrate: 18 grams
Ingredients:

- 1 tablespoon olive oil
- ½ large yellow onion, diced
- 1 green bell pepper, diced
- ¼ teaspoon salt
- ¼ teaspoon black pepper
- 1 garlic clove, minced
- 2 cups butternut squash, diced
- 28-ounce can whole plum tomatoes with juice
- 1 teaspoon chili powder
- ½ teaspoon smoked paprika
- ½ teaspoon dried oregano
- ¼ teaspoon red pepper flakes
- 2 tablespoons fresh parsley, minced
- 4 free-range eggs
- ¼ cup crumbled feta
- 1 tablespoon shelled pumpkin seeds

Instructions:

- Set instant pot to saute, to heat the olive oil. Add onions, bell pepper, salt, and pepper. Cook and stir for 4-5 minutes or until onions are translucent. Add garlic and cook for another minute while stirring, or until the garlic is fragrant.
- Add squash, tomatoes, chili powder, smoked paprika, oregano, and red pepper flakes. Stir.
- Cover the pressure cooker, making sure to set the valve to "seal." Cook on high pressure for 8 minutes, then quick release the pressure and remove the lid.
- Stir in the parsley and then add free-range eggs. Replace the cover and set the valve to "seal." Cook on high pressure for less than a minute, then quick release the valve and remove the lid again.
- You can top with parsley for extra garnish, feta, and pumpkin seeds. The shakshuka is now ready to serve and enjoy.

2. Pesto Instant Pot Eggs
Servings: 2
Total Time: 35 Minutes

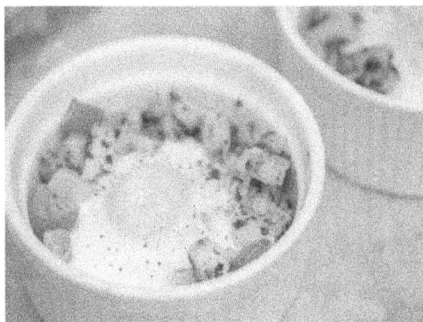

Energy Value Per Serving:
Calories: 440
Protein: 19.9 grams
Total Fat: 34.2 grams
Carbohydrates: 15.2 grams

Ingredients:

- 2 eggs
- 1 cup of greens filled with basil, kale, and spinach
- ¼ cup olive oil
- 1 clove garlic
- 1 cup chopped vegetables like potatoes, bell peppers, and onions

Instructions:

- Break the eggs and add a cup of greens and mix in a bowl.
- Turn the instant pot on saute, add olive oil to the bottom and allow to heat for 1-2 minutes.
- Add garlic and vegetables, allow it to heat for 2-3 minutes.
- Take out of the instant pot and serve.

3. Instant Pot Mediterranean Spinach-Feta Pie
Servings: 6
Total Time: 55 minutes

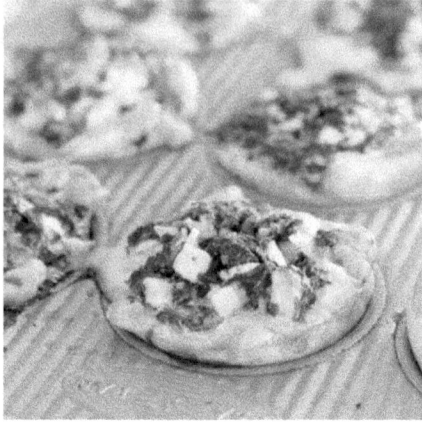

Energy Value Per Serving:
Calories: 50
Protein: 1.2 grams
Total Fat: 3.3 grams
Carbohydrates: 4 grams

Ingredients:
- 2 tablespoons ghee, plus a little extra for greasing the dish
- 1 small onion, diced
- 4 cloves garlic, minced
- 1-½ pounds of spinach washed, dried and chopped
- 3 organic eggs
- ½ cup heavy cream
- 1 teaspoon of sea salt
- 1 lemon zest
- ¼ cup fresh Italian parsley, chopped
- 2 tablespoons fresh dill, chopped
- ¼ teaspoon ground nutmeg, freshly grated
- ½ cup of Parmesan cheese, shredded
- 1-½ cups feta cheese
- 1 cup of water

Instructions:

- Add the ghee to your instant pot and turn the setting to saute. Allow it to melt and add the onion and garlic. Saute for 7 minutes, until lightly caramelized.
- Add the spinach and saute for 3 minutes, or until the spinach is wilted. Press the keep warm button on the pot.
- With the ghee, grease a 1-½ quart casserole dish that fits inside the instant pot. Set this aside.

- In a large mixing bowl, whisk together eggs and cream until the eggs are fully incorporated.
- Add the sea salt, lemon zest, parsley, dill, and nutmeg, then gently stir to combine.
- Add the Parmesan cheese and the onion-garlic-spinach mixture, stir to combine. Pour mixture into the greased casserole dish from before.
- Evenly add crumbles of feta into the filling.
- Place the glass lid on top of the casserole dish. Place the instant pot trivet inside of the instant pot. Pour 1 cup of water into the instant pot, then carefully transfer the covered casserole dish to the instant pot on top of the trivet.
- Place the lid on the instant pot, and make sure the steam release valve closed. Press manual and change the time to 20 minutes.
- When the instant pot beeps, press keep warm. Allow the pressure to release naturally for 10 minutes, and then quick release.
- When the venting of steam stops, carefully open the lid.
- Remove the casserole dish.
- Allow to cool and serve.

4. Instant Pot Mediterranean Chicken And Quinoa Stew

Servings: 6
Total time: 30 minutes

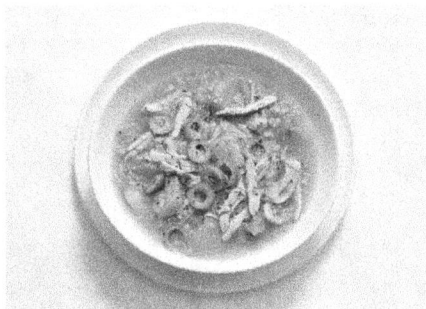

Energy Value Per Serving:
Calories: 234
Protein: 25 grams
Total Fat: 6 grams
Carbohydrates: 24 grams

Ingredients:
- 1-¼ pound of chicken thighs, boneless and skinless
- 4 cups butternut squash, chopped and peeled
- 4 cups unsalted chicken stock

- 1 cup chopped yellow onion
- 2 garlic cloves
- 1 bay leaf
- 1-¼ teaspoon kosher salt
- 1 teaspoon dried oregano
- 1 teaspoon ground fennel seeds
- ½ teaspoon of black pepper
- ½ cup uncooked quinoa
- 1 ounce olives, pitted

Instructions:

- Combine the chicken, squash, stock, onion, garlic, bay leaf, salt, oregano, fennel seeds, and pepper in the instant pot. Cover with lid and turn to manual.
- Turn lid valve to seal and set pressure to high for 8 minutes.
- Carefully release the valve until the steam stops. Uncover and transfer the chicken to a cutting board.
- Add the quinoa. Turn to saute and cook, occasionally stirring, until quinoa is tender.
- Shred the chicken and stir into the stew. Discard bay leaf and divide soup evenly into 6 bowls. Sprinkle the olives over the stew.

5. Instant Pot Breakfast Egg Casserole
Servings: 8
Total Time: 27 Minutes

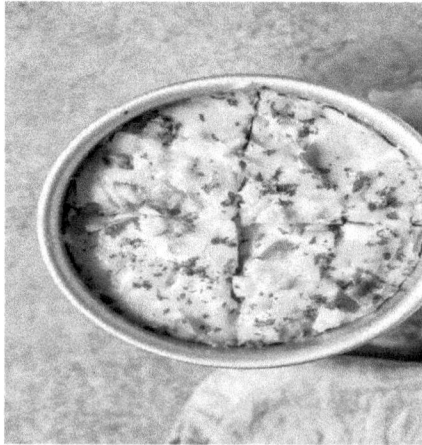

Energy Value Per Serving:
Calories: 223.6
Protein: 13.2 grams

Total Fat: 15.4 grams
Carbohydrates: 7.6 grams

Ingredients:

- 3 slices bacon, chopped
- 1 pound turkey breakfast sausage
- ¼ teaspoon salt
- ¼ cup of onions, chopped
- 10 large eggs
- 2/3 cup of milk
- ¼ teaspoon salt
- 2 cloves of garlic, minced
- ½ teaspoon dried basil
- ½ teaspoon dried oregano
- 1-½ cup shredded Italian blend cheese
- 1 cup of water
- 2 ounces crumbled feta

Instructions:

- Set the instant pot to saute. Add the chopped bacon and cook until browned. Remove bacon and set aside.
- Add the sausage to the pan. Crumble and cook until no longer pink.
- Add the onions and cook until they have softened. Remove meat mixture and set aside.
- Add all but 1 tablespoon of chopped bacon to the sausage mixture.
- Spray an 8-inch cake pan with non-stick spray.
- In a bowl, whisk together eggs, milk, salt, garlic, basil, and oregano.
- Spread the cheese on the bottom of the pan, followed by the meat mixture. Pour egg mixture over the meat.
- Place the trivet inside of the instant pot. Add 1 cup of water. Place the baking pan on the trivet. Place the lid on the pressure cooker and set it on high for 12 minutes.
- Carefully quick release after this, remove the lid carefully, and allow the casserole to stand for 10 minutes.
- Top with feta cheese and remaining bacon.

6. Instant Pot Barley

Servings: 4
Total Time: 28 Minutes

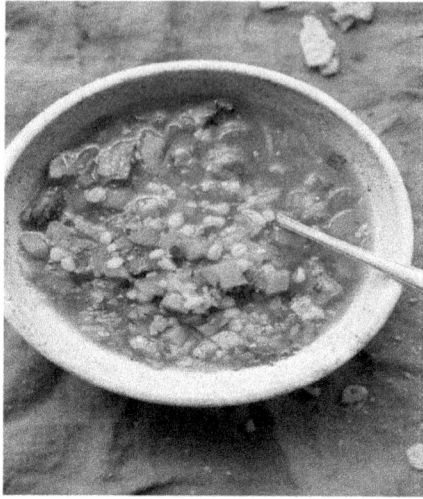

Energy Value Per Servings:
Calories: 217
Protein: 14 grams
Total Fat: 10 grams
Carbohydrates: 15 grams
Ingredients:
- 1 tablespoon olive oil
- 1 cup pearl barley
- ¼ cup red onion, finely chopped
- 4 cups of liquid, water and broth
- 1 teaspoon sea salt
- 4 ounces turkey ham, diced small
- 4 ounces baby kale
- 4 eggs, cooked to your preference

Instructions:

- Add olive oil to instant pot and set it to manual for 18 minutes.
- Add barley and onion. Saute until it smells a bit toasty.
- Add liquid and stir.
- Lock lid in place.
- Dice ham while the barley cooks.
- When the pressure cooker completes cooking, quick release the pressure. Drain most of the liquid. Return the pot to saute and add diced ham. Saute while stirring occasionally.
- Prepare eggs and when they are ready, add the arugula to the pot and stir to combine. You just want to wilt the greens a little.
- Scoop the barley mixture into bowls and top with egg.

7. Instant Pot Frittata

Servings: 4
Total Time: 30 minutes

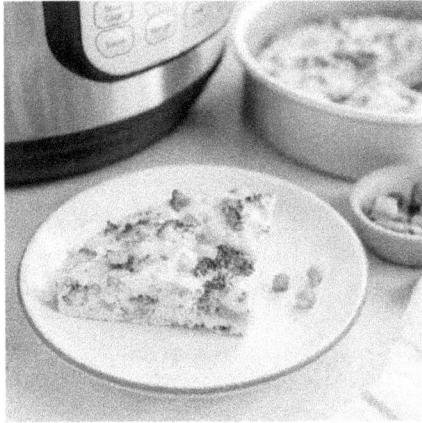

Energy Value Per Serving:
Calories: 195
Protein: 14 grams
Total Fat: 12 grams
Carbohydrates: 5 grams

Ingredients:
- 6 eggs
- ½ teaspoon fine sea salt
- black pepper
- 8 ounces broccoli florets
- 3 green onions, chopped
- ½ cup of cheddar cheese, shredded
- 1 cup of water

Instructions:

- In a large bowl, beat the eggs, salt, and several grinds of black pepper. Add in the chopped broccoli, green onions, and cheddar
- Grease a 7-inch pan, then pour in the egg mixture. Pour 1 cup of water into the bottom of your instant pot and place a trivet over the water.
- Place the pan on top of the trivet and close the lid. Move the valve to sealing. Use the manual to cook on high pressure for 10 minutes.
- When cooking is completed, let the pressure release for 10 minutes. You can then do a quick release to remove the remainder of the pressure.

- Open the lid carefully and remove the frittata pan. Any excess liquid will evaporate.
- Slice frittata into 4 slices and serve warm.

8. Instant Pot Sous Vide Egg Bites
Servings: 7
Total Time: 15 Minutes

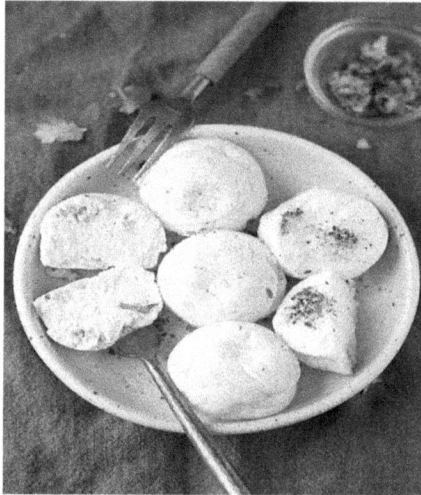

Energy Value Per Serving:
Calories: 310
Protein: 19 grams
Total Fat: 14 grams
Carbohydrates: 9 grams
Ingredients:
- 4 eggs
- 1 cup of smoked gouda, shredded
- ½ cup cottage cheese
- ¼ cup of 2% milk
- ½ teaspoon salt
- ¼ cup of basil, finely chopped
- 4 tablespoons of ham, chopped
- 1 cup of water

Instructions:

- Add 1 cup of water to the bottom of the instant pot, and place the trivet inside.
- Add eggs, cheese, cottage cheese, milk and salt to your blender and

blend until smooth. Stir in the basil.

- Equally divide ham among the individual cups in a silicone baby food maker mold. Pour the egg mixture equally over the ham. Cover with foil and place on top of the trivet in the pot.
- Cover the instant pot, select steam, and set a timer for 8 minutes. Allow the instant pot to slowly release for 10 minutes, then quick release pressure.
- Remove silicone mold from the instant pot and allow it to cool completely. Take the egg bites out of the mold and serve on a plate.

9. Instant Pot Oatmeal

Servings: 2
Total Time: 25 Minutes

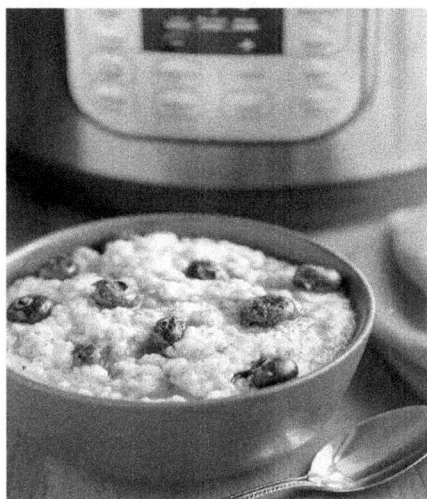

Energy Value Per Serving:
Calories: 506
Protein: 20 grams
Total Fat: 11 grams
Carbohydrates: 84 grams
Ingredients:
- 2 cups water
- 1 cup vanilla almond milk
- 1 cup steel cut oats
- 1 cinnamon stick
- kosher salt
Instructions:

- Add the oatmeal and the liquid ratio that matches your instant pot. Add kosher salt and cinnamon stick.
- Press the manual setting and set the cooking time on high for 3 minutes.
- Once the cooking time ends, allow the oatmeal to sit in the pot and the natural pressure release for 20 minutes. Quick release after this period.
- Open the lid, remove oatmeal, and add toppings of your choice, like honey or fresh berries.

10. Instant Pot Mini Frittatas
Servings: 7
Total Time: 1 hour 15 minutes

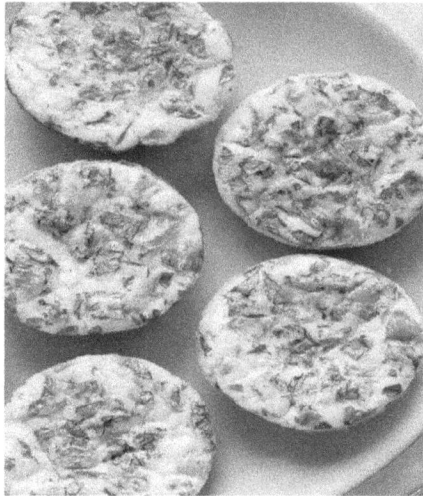

Energy Value Per Serving:
Calories: 342.5
Protein: 25 grams
Total Fat: 23.7 grams
Carbohydrates: 8.2 grams
Ingredients:
- 2 slices of bacon, cut into pieces
- 1 cup of button mushrooms
- ½ teaspoon fresh thyme leaves
- kosher salt
- freshly ground black pepper
- ⅓ cup baby spinach, chopped
- ¼ cup of sharp cheddar cheese, grated

- 5 large eggs
- ⅓ cup heavy cream
- pinch of nutmeg
- 1 cup of water

Instructions:

- Add the bacon to the instant pot and turn on the saute mode. Cook bacon for 10 minutes, until golden brown.
- Add mushrooms to the pot, along with the thyme and a pinch of salt.
- Stir occasionally until the mushrooms have reduced and are golden brown.
- Remove mushrooms from pot, divide them among silicone egg bite molds as well as the spinach, cheese, and bacon.
- Whisk eggs with the cream, nutmeg, and ½ teaspoon of salt with a few grinds of pepper in a medium bowl.
- Pour egg custard over mushroom fillings in each cup.
- Add water to the pot, place egg cups on the rack, and cover tightly with foil. Lower rack into the pot and lock the lid. Set the pressure cook on low for 6 minutes.
- After the pressure cycle is complete, allow the natural release of pressure for 10 minutes, then quick release.
- Remove the tray and let the mini frittatas stand for 5 minutes.

11. Instant Pot Keto Crustless Quiche

Servings: 6
Total Time: 40 Minutes

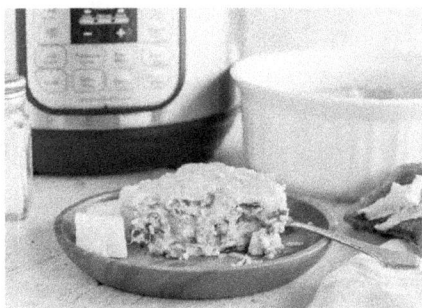

Energy Values Per Serving:

Calories: 293
Protein: 14 grams
Total Fat: 24 grams
Carbohydrates: 4 grams

Ingredients:
- 6 large eggs
- ¾ cup of heavy cream
- ⅓ cup of fresh spinach, chopped
- ¼ cup of sun-dried tomatoes, chopped
- ¾ cup of fontina cheese, shredded
- 1 teaspoon fresh rosemary, chopped
- ¼ teaspoon crushed red pepper
- salt and pepper
- 1 ½ cups of water

Instructions:

- Butter a 7-8 cup souffle dish. Place the rack inside the instant pot. Add water and place the dish on top of the rack.
- Crack the eggs into a mixing bowl and whisk. Whisk in the cream, salt, and black pepper.
- Stir in all remaining ingredients. Pour mixture into the souffle dish.
- Lock the instant pot lid into place, set on manual pressure cook high for 30 minutes. Once the timer goes off, press quick release and turn off.
- Allow the quiche to sit in the pot for 10 minutes. Unlock the lid and carefully lift and take out the souffle.
- Cut and serve.

12. Instant Pot Hard Boiled Eggs
Servings: 6
Total Time: 20 Minutes

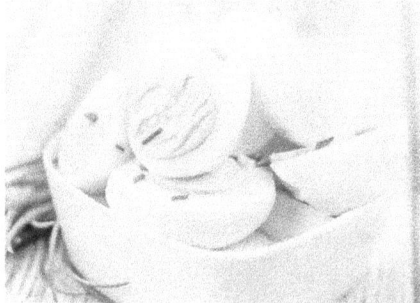

Energy Value Per Serving:
Calories: 78
Protein: 6 grams
Total Fat: 5 grams
Carbohydrates: 0.6 grams

Ingredients:
- 1 cup of water
- 1 teaspoon of oregano
- 6 large eggs
- salt and freshly ground black pepper

Instructions:

- Add water to your instant pot. Place the metal trivet into the pot. Gently add the eggs on top of the trivet.
- Select manual setting, adjust to high pressure for 3-7 minutes. Quick release the pressure.
- Cool eggs in a bowl of water, drain well, and peel.
- Cut eggs in half, sprinkle evenly the oregano, salt, and pepper.

13. Instant Pot Cream Cheese Scallion Omelet
Servings: 3
Total Time: 20 Minutes

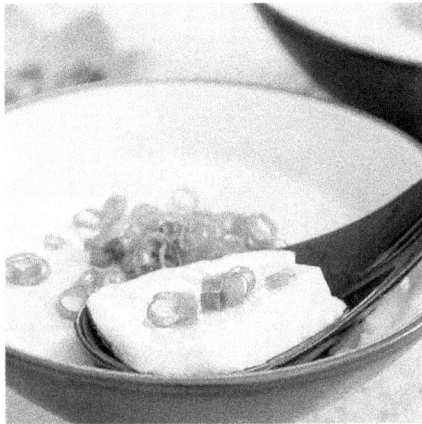

Energy Value Per Serving:
Calories: 295
Protein: 12 grams
Total Fat: 27 grams
Carbohydrates: 1 gram

Ingredients:
- 3 large eggs
- ½ cup of water
- 1 teaspoon of garlic powder
- 3 scallions, chopped
- 1 teaspoon of sesame seeds

- ½ tablespoon of olive oil
- 3 tablespoons of cream cheese
- salt and freshly ground black pepper to taste

Instructions:

- Arrange the trivet at the bottom of the instant pot, and add 1 cup of water.
- In a heatproof bowl, add eggs, water, garlic powder, salt and black pepper and beat until well-combined.
- Stir in the scallions and sesame seeds.
- Place bowl on top of trivet.
- Secure the lid and lock it. Cook under Manual high pressure for 5 minutes. Turn instant pot off and do a quick release.
- Take out of pot and serve immediately.

14. Instant Pot Egg Bites
Servings: 14 bites
Total Time: 15 Minutes

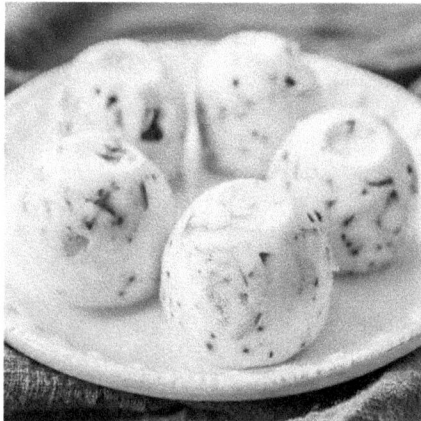

Energy Value Per Serving:
Calories: 72
Protein: 6 grams
Total Fat: 5 grams
Carbohydrates: 1 grams

Ingredients:
- 8 large eggs
- ¼ cup of milk
- ¼ teaspoon salt
- ⅛ teaspoon of freshly ground black pepper

- ½ cup of diced ham
- ⅓ cup of cheddar cheese, shredded

Instructions:

- Spray two silicone baby food tray with nonstick cooking spray. Whisk together eggs, milk, salt, and pepper in a large bowl until combined. Evenly divide the meat among the silicone cups. Pour the egg mixture over the ham until the cups are ⅔ full. Sprinkle the cheddar cheese evenly.
- Pour 1/2 cup of water into the instant pot and place a trivet at the bottom. Place the silicone tray on top of the trivet and them lock the instant pot lid. Select high pressure cooking for 11 minutes.
- Turn off the pressure cooker and let the pressure release naturally for 5 minutes, then press quick release. Remove the silicone tray using mitts, place on a wire rack to allow to cool. After 5 minutes. Squeeze out the bites and they are ready to serve.

15. Instant Pot Quinoa Breakfast Porridge

Servings: 4
Total Time: 5 Minutes

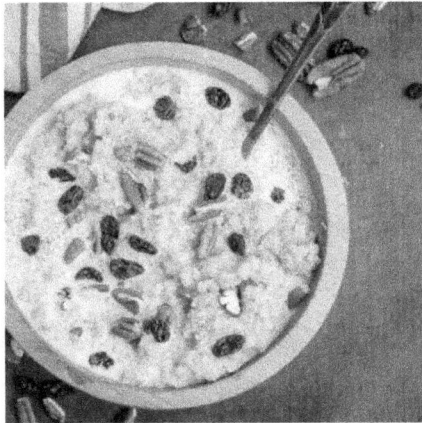

Energy Value Per Serving:
Calories: 400
Protein: 5.5 grams
Total Fat: 23.1 grams
Carbohydrates: 43.9 grams

Ingredients:

- 2 Cups Quinoa
- 2 Tablespoons apple cider vinegar

- 1.5 cups of filtered water
- 2 Cup of regular coconut milk
- ⅓ Cup Maple syrup
- 1 Teaspoon salt

Instructions:

- Place Quinoa and apple cider vinegar in a glass bowl and cover in water to let soak for about 8 hours.
- Drain the quinoa and rinse until the water is clear. Then add the quinoa to instant pot with 1.5 cups of water.
- Pour in the coconut milk. Place the lid on the instant pot, seal the vent and push manual button. Adjust time to 3 minutes for high pressure.
- When complete, so a natural pressure release for 10 minutes.
- Open the instant pot, stir the contents and then serve. May serve with topping of maple syrup and salt if desired.

MEDITERRANEAN SALADS

1. Instant Pot Green Beans With Lemon

Servings: 4
Total Time: 11 Minutes

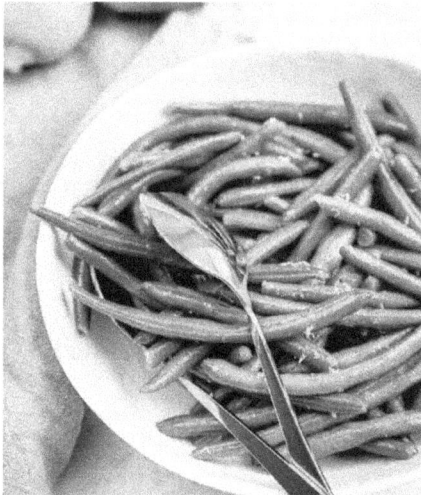

Energy Value Per Serving:
Calories: 67
Protein: 2.1 grams
Total Fat: 3.8

Carbohydrates: 8.5 grams
Ingredients:
- 1 pound of green beans
- 1 tablespoon olive oil
- 1 tablespoon lemon juice
- ½ teaspoon kosher salt
- fresh ground black pepper
- ½ cup of water

Instructions:

- Trim green beans, add them to instant pot with water. Lock lid. Place vent to sealing.
- Select high-pressure setting for cooking.
- After cooking and instant pot beeps, press quick release to remove pressure.
- Open lid, carefully remove beans to a bowl, drain all water. Toss with a pinch of kosher salt and black pepper.

2. Quinoa Instant Pot Greek Bowl Salad
Servings: 8
Total Time: 12 Minutes

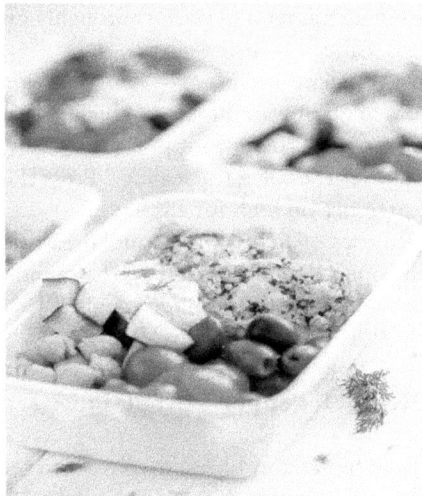

Energy Value Per Serving:
Calories: 136
Protein: 7 grams
Total Fat: 3 grams
Carbohydrates: 22 grams

Ingredients:
- 1 cup of quinoa
- 15 ounce low-sodium chickpeas
- 1 cup of water
- salt and pepper
- 5 black olives
- 3 sliced pepperoncini
- ¼ cup of sliced red onion
- ½ cup cherry tomatoes, cut in half
- 4 handfuls of baby spinach leaves
- 2 tablespoons cut feta cheese
- ½ cup of sliced radish
- 1 cucumber
- 1 tablespoon fresh parsley, chopped

Spicy Roasted Red Bell Pepper Sauce Ingredients:
- ¼ cup of roasted red bell peppers
- 3 garlic bulbs
- 2 tablespoons lemon juice
- 1 teaspoon hot sauce
- salt to taste

Instructions:

- Put the quinoa in a strainer and wash thoroughly until the water is clear. Set quinoa aside.
- Strain the can of chickpeas, rinse.
- Add the quinoa, 1 cup of water, 1 can of chickpeas, and some salt and pepper to taste into the instant pot.
- Close the lid and set the valve to "sealing." Press the manual cook mode and set pressure on high for 2 minutes.
- When the timer goes off, allow the natural pressure release to occur. Carefully open the lid and fluff up the quinoa using a fork. Allow the quinoa to come to room temperature.
- Prepare the olives and pepperoncini.

Spicy Roasted Red Bell Pepper Instructions:

- Take a high-speed blender. Add ¼ cup of roasted red bell peppers and garlic bulbs after peeling. Also, add the lemon juice, hot sauce, and salt to taste. Blend all ingredients until they are smooth.
- Once the quinoa and chickpea mix has cooled off, add toppings and cover with spicy roasted red pepper sauce.

3. Instant Pot Mediterranean Potato Salad
Servings: 8

Total Time: 13 minutes

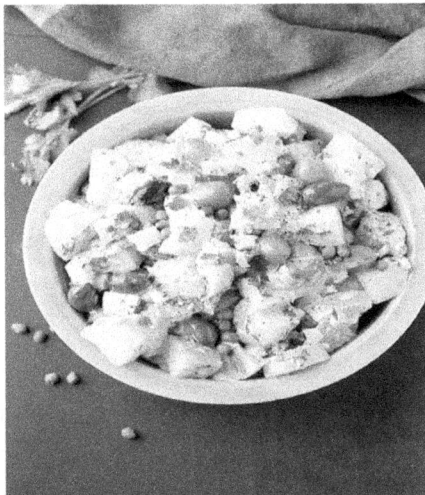

Energy Value Per Serving:
Calories: 120
Protein: 1 gram
Total Fat: 7 grams
Carbohydrates: 13 grams

Ingredients:
- 5 cups of yellow potatoes, cubed
- 1 cup of onions, chopped
- 3 cups of water
- 1 cup mixed olives, halved
- 1 cup feta cheese
- 2 tablespoons capers
- ½ teaspoon oregano
- ⅓ cup of light mayo
- 1 tablespoon olive oil
- 1 pinch salt and pepper to taste
- ¼ teaspoon red pepper flakes
- 1 handful fresh parsley

Instructions:

- Wash the potatoes thoroughly. Leave the skin on and cut into bite-sized pieces. Add them to the instant pot. Then add the chopped onions and 3 cups of water. Cover and seal the valve and cook on high pressure for three minutes.
- When done, press the quick-release carefully to remove the

pressure. Remove the potatoes and allow to cool.

- While the potatoes are cooling, grab a small glass bowl and mix in the light mayo and halved olive oil.
- When the potatoes are cooled off, add the olives, capers, and feta cheese, then season with oregano, red pepper flakes, sea salt, and pepper.
- Add the mayo mixture and mix gently. Top with fresh parsley and it is now ready to serve.

4. Instant Pot Mediterranean Couscous Salad
Servings: 4
Total Time: Total Time

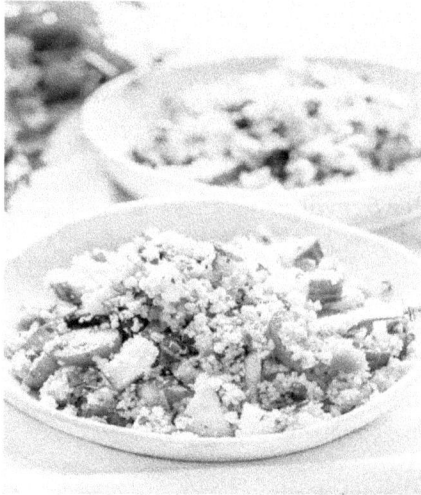

Energy Value Per Serving:
Calories: 533
Protein: 20 grams
Total Fat: 8.5 grams
Carbohydrates: 95.9 grams
Ingredients:
- 2 tablespoons olive oil
- 2 cups couscous
- ½ cup dry mung beans
- 4 cups vegetable broth
- 2 teaspoons salt, divided
- 1 cucumber, diced
- 2 tomatoes, diced
- 1 juiced lemon

- 1 tablespoon cilantro, chopped
- ½ teaspoon ground black pepper

Instructions:

- Turn on the instant pot and select saute. Add olive oil and when heated add the couscous and mung beans. Cook and stir for 2 minutes and then add vegetable broth and 1 teaspoon of salt. Close the lid and lock. Put on high pressure and set timer for 20 minutes.
- Release the pressure for 10 minutes and then quick release for remaining pressure. Carefully unlock and remove the lid and fluff up the couscous with a fork. Let it cool for about 10 minutes.
- Combine the couscous, mung beans, cucumber, tomatoes, lemon juice, and cilantro in a bowl and mix.
- Sprinkle with salt and pepper and serve.

5. Instant Pot Chickpea Greek Salad
Servings: 6
Total Time: 16 Minutes

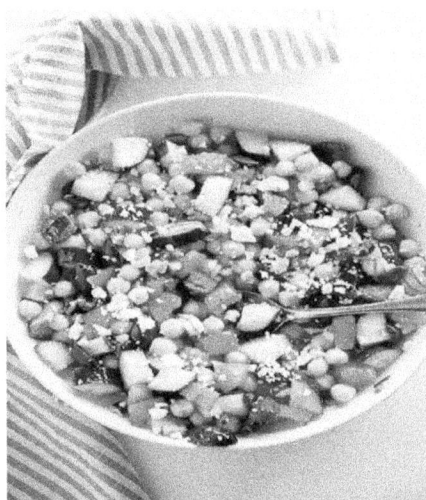

Energy Value Per Serving:
Calories: 125
Protein: 4 grams
Total Fat: 7 grams
Carbohydrates: 13 grams

Ingredients:
- 1 cup dried chickpeas
- 3 cups water

- 2 tablespoons extra virgin olive oil
- 1 tablespoon red wine vinegar
- 1 teaspoon kosher salt
- ½ teaspoon freshly ground black pepper
- ½ cup onions, finely chopped
- 10 cherry tomatoes, cut in half
- 10 pitted black olive, cut in half
- 1 cucumber cut into small dices
- ¼ cup of fresh green bell pepper, chopped
- 2 tablespoons of fresh cilantro, chopped
- 1 ounce of vegan feta cheese, crumbled

Instructions:

- Submerge the chickpeas in cold water for 6-8 hours, drain and rinse.
- Pour water into instant pot and add the soaked chickpeas. Lock the lid and select the high pressure. Adjust the timer to 15 minutes.
- After completing, naturally release the pressure. Carefully unlock and remove the lid. Drain the beans and allow them to cool for 5 minutes.
- While preparing the chickpeas, you can also prepare the dressing. In a small bowl, combine the olive oil, vinegar, salt, and black pepper. Whisk thoroughly.
- In a large bowl, combine the chickpeas, onions, tomatoes, olives, bell pepper, and cilantro. Add dressing and then top with feta. Ready to serve cold.

6. Mediterranean Farro Salad

Servings: 2
Total Time: 25 Minutes

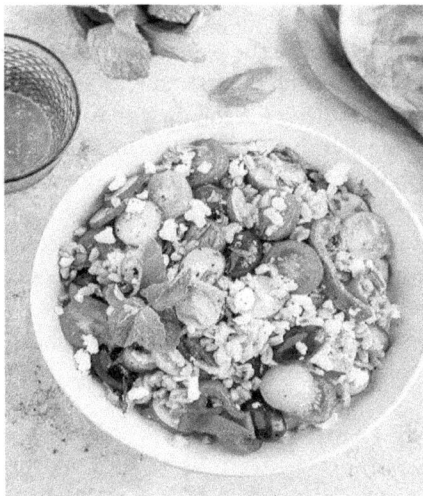

Energy Value Per Serving:

Calories: 637

Protein: 36 grams

Total Fat: 40 grams

Carbohydrates: 32 grams

Ingredients:

- 1 cup cooked farro
- 2 chicken thighs
- ½ tablespoon butter
- ½ tablespoon olive oil
- 1 tablespoon poultry seasoning
- ½ english cucumber
- ½ cup grape tomatoes
- ¼ red onion
- ½ cup fresh parsley, chopped
- 1 cup parmesan cheese, freshly grated
- pinch sea salt
- pepper
- ½ lemon
- honey
- ½ cup green olives

Instructions:

- Rinse 1 cup of farro and transfer to the instant pot. Add 1 cup of water and sea salt. Lock the lid and turn the valve to sealing position. set on high pressure for 22 minutes, then let the pressure release naturally.

- Preheat skillet over medium heat for 6-7 minutes.
- Add butter and olive oil to the pan, wait until melted and coats the pan. Then add the chicken thighs and season with poultry seasoning. Fry for another 6-8 minutes on each side. Reduce heat to the lowest setting and then cover the pan. Cook another 5 minutes.
- Wash and chop the cucumbers, grape tomatoes, and parsley. Peel and chop the red onion.
- Add the vegetables, herbs, the cooked farro, green olives, parmesan cheese to a large bowl, and then season with sea salt, pepper, olive oil, lemon juice, and honey. Mix together well.
- Top the farro salad with pan-fried chicken thigh, and it is ready to serve.

7. Mediterranean Lentil Salad
Servings: 4
Total Time: 50 minutes

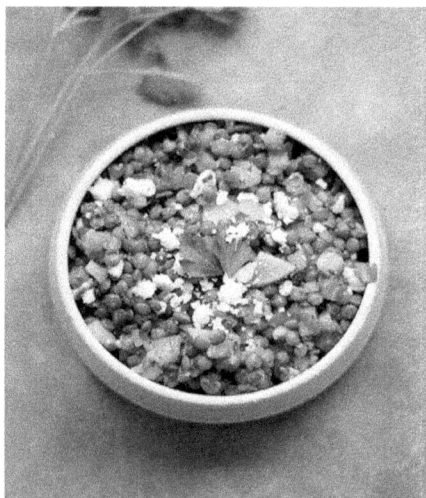

Energy Value Per Serving:
Calories: 240
Protein: 8 grams
Total fat: 17.2 grams
Carbohydrates: 15.5 grams
Ingredients:
- 1 ½ cups chickpeas
- 1 sprig thyme
- 1 teaspoon parsley
- 3 cups of water

- 5 tablespoons olive oil
- 1 cup French green lentils
- 1 teaspoon Herbes de Provence (Dried herbs mixture)
- ½ teaspoon kosher salt
- 1-¾ cups vegetable broth
- 4 tablespoons dry white wine
- 1 clove minced garlic
- ½ cup mint
- ½ ounce cherry tomatoes
- ¼ cup black olives
- ½ cup feta cheese

Instructions:

- Combine the chickpeas, thyme, parsley, water, and 1 tablespoon of oil into your instant pot. Stir well.
- Close the lid, lock it, and turn the valve to sealing. Change the time to 38 minutes for pressure cooking on high.
- When the timer beeps, press cancel and let it stand covered until the float valve drops down. Turn the valve handle to venting and carefully remove the lid.
- The chickpeas should be tender by now, but if not, cover the pot and press saute. Cook and stir for 3-5 minutes.
- Drain and rinse the chickpeas and set aside.
- Combine the chickpeas, lentils, Herbes de Provence, salt, broth, and 1 tablespoon of wine in the inner pot.
- Place the pot inside the instant pot, lock the lid and turn the steam release handle to venting.
- Press slow cook. The indicator will read "Normal." Adjust the heat level to "less." Decrease the time to 3 minutes.
- When it beeps, remove the lid and make sure the lentils are firm-tender.
- In a small bowl, whisk together the garlic, mint, and the remaining wine.
- Gradually whisk in remaining oil. Drizzle over the mixture in the pot. Stir in the tomatoes and olives.
- Transfer the salad to a serving dish and garnish with feta.

8. Instant Pot Greek Chicken Bowls

Servings: 4
Total Time: 50 minutes

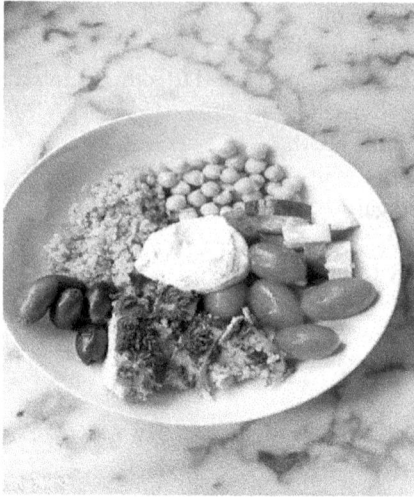

Energy Value Per Serving:

Calories: 481

Protein: 33 grams

Total Fat: 32 grams

Carbohydrates: 17 grams

Ingredients:

- ½ teaspoon of dried oregano
- ½ teaspoon spanish paprika
- A pinch crushed red pepper flakes
- ¼ cup plus two extra tablespoons olive oil
- 3 cloves garlic, grated
- 1.5 pounds chicken breasts, boneless, skinless, sliced 1.2-inch thick
- kosher salt
- fresh ground pepper
- 1 cup couscous
- 1 cup regular Greek yogurt
- juice from 1 lemon
- 1 chopped english cucumber
- 1 cup cherry tomatoes, chopped
- ½ cup pitted kalamata olives, chopped
- ½ cup crumbled feta
- 2 tablespoons fresh dill, chopped
- ½ cup and 1 tablespoon of water

Instructions:

- Whisk together the oregano, paprika, red pepper flakes, ¼ olive oil, 2 cloves garlic, and water in instant pot.

- Then add the chicken, 2 teaspoons salt, black pepper and toss until well coated.
- Lock the lid and cook on high for 3 minutes. After cooking is completed, press the quick release to remove the pressure. Transfer the chicken to a medium-sized bowl and turn off the instant pot.
- Add the couscous, ½ teaspoon of salt and some black pepper to the pot and stir to combine well. Place the glass lid on top and allow the couscous to sit until tender and fluffy.
- Mix together the yogurt, lemon juice, remaining garlic, 1 tablespoon water in a medium bowl. Spread ¼ cup of yogurt sauce on the bottom of the plate. Top with a quarter of the couscous, cucumbers, tomatoes, kalamata olives, and feta. Repeat for 3 more plates. Garnish each plate with the dill and drizzle the remaining 2 tablespoons of olive oil.

9. Roasted Beet Salad With Crispy Kale And Almonds
Servings: 6
Total Time: 1 Hour and 10 Minutes

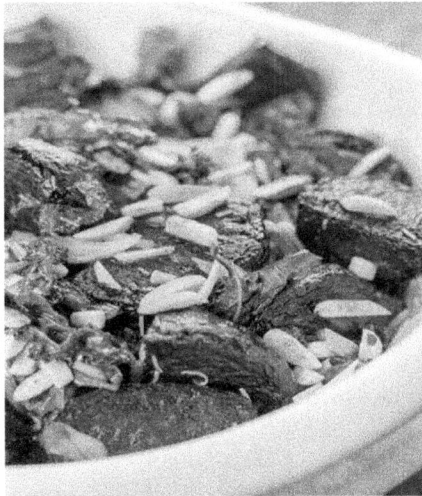

Energy Value Per Serving:
Calories: 192
Protein: 3.8 grams
Total Fat: 11.5 grams
Carbohydrates: 21.7 grams
Ingredients:
- 1 bunch kale, cleaned and ribs removed
- 2 ½ pounds of beets

- salt and pepper to taste
- extra virgin olive oil
- 1 shallot, sliced
- 3 tablespoons almonds, slivered

Ingredients For Lemon-Honey Vinaigrette:

- ¼ cup extra virgin olive oil
- 2 tablespoons lemon juice
- 3 tablespoons of raw honey
- 1 chopped garlic clove
- 1-¼ teaspoon dried organic rosemary
- salt and pepper to taste

Instructions:

- Wash and trim beets. Add basket insert into the instant pot and then 1 cup of water. Place the beets in a single layer over the insert.
- Lock the lid and make sure the valve is pointed at the "sealing" position.
- Cook on high pressure for 15 minutes. When finished, quick release the pressure. When all of the pressure is released, carefully unlock the lid. Remove the beets from the pot.
- Mix all of the vinaigrette ingredients in a small bowl and whisk to combine.
- Toast the slivered almonds in a dry, non-stick skillet. Toss the almonds frequently to get an even toast. They should be golden brown.
- Transfer the beets to a mixing bowl and add shallots.
- Pour vinaigrette dressing on top and give the beets and shallots a nice toss. Add crispy kale and toss again gently.
- Transfer the beets to a bowl or serving platter and then add almonds. Enjoy warm or room temperature.

10. Mediterranean Quinoa Salad With Chicken

Servings: 4
Total Time: 15 Minutes

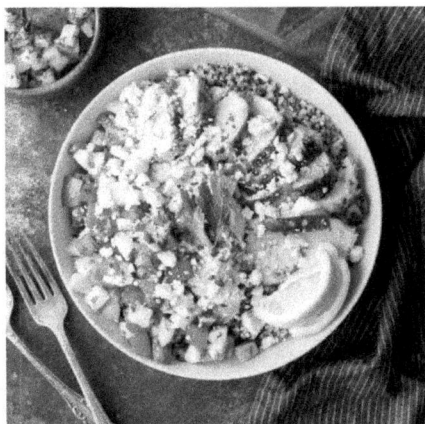

Energy Value Per Serving:
Calories: 361
Protein: 14 grams
Total Fat: 20 grams
Carbohydrates: 31 grams

Ingredients:
- 1 cup uncooked quinoa
- 1.5 cups of water
- 1 chicken breast, boneless and skinless
- 1 tablespoon salt
- ¼ cup red pepper, diced
- ¼ cup black olives, diced
- ¼ cup cucumber cut lengthwise
- 2 tablespoons red onions, diced
- ¼ cup feta cheese
- 2 tablespoons fresh parsley, chopped
- 1 tablespoon Greek seasoning
- ¼ cup of olive oil

Instructions:

- Rinse the quinoa. Add water and quinoa to the instant pot. Lock the lid and seal. Cook on manual high pressure for a minute, then allow natural release for 10 minutes. Flip the valve to venting, carefully open the lid and fluff quinoa with a fork.
- Season the chicken breast with salt on both sides. Pour some olive oil into a pan and allow the chicken breast to cook for 10 minutes on medium heat until the juices run clear and the internal temperature reaches 165 degrees F. Allow chicken to cool, then cut into cubes.

- Cut and dice the red pepper, black olives, cucumber, red onion, and parsley.
- Combine the quinoa, chicken, and vegetables in a bowl. Top with feta cheese, fresh parsley, Greek seasoning, and olive oil and mix everything together.

11. Matbucha (Israeli Hot Salad)
Servings: 4-6
Total Time: 40 Minutes

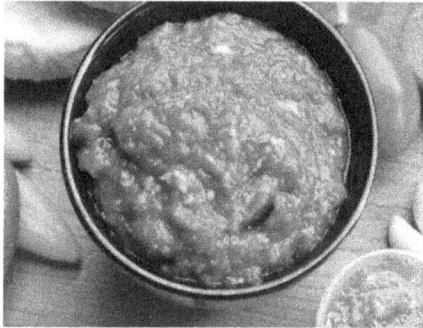

Energy Value Per Serving:
Calories: 183
Protein: 2 grams
Total Fat: 12 grams
Carbohydrates: 18 grams
Ingredients:
- 3 garlic cloves, crushed
- 1 diced onion
- olive oil
- 1 teaspoon paprika
- 1 teaspoon cumin
- 1 teaspoon sea salt
- 1 tablespoon brown sugar
- ½ teaspoon of red pepper flakes
- 7 roma tomatoes, chopped
- 1 green pepper and 1 red pepper
- 1 jalapeno, chopped

Instructions:

- Set the instant pot to saute. Add 1-2 tablespoons of olive oil and then allow it to heat. Add chopped onions, minced garlic, and the rest of the seasonings and stir.

- Leave for 10 minutes to saute and stir every few minutes.
- Meanwhile, chop the tomatoes, peppers, and jalapeno. Add these to the pot and change the setting to beans/chili. Cover and lock the pot, then set steam to sealing.
- Allow to cook until the timer beeps. Quick-release pressure, open the lid and pour off the extra liquid into a quart container.
- Serve warm or at room temperature.

12. Pressure-Cooker Buddha Bowl

Servings: 4
Total Time: 40 Minutes

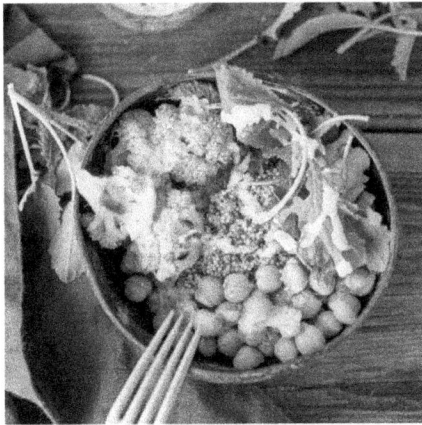

Energy Value Per Serving:
Calories: 514
Protein: 15.1 grams
Total Fat: 22 grams
Carbohydrates: 66.9 grams

Ingredients:

- 4 tablespoons extra virgin olive oil
- 1 large sweet potato, peeled and cut into small pieces
- 1 cup quinoa
- 2 tablespoons harissa
- 1 large minced garlic clove
- ½ teaspoon salt
- 4 cups chopped kale
- 1 tablespoon lime juice
- 15-ounce of chickpeas, no salt added
- ¼ cup scallions, sliced
- ¼ cup chopped, unsalted pistachios

Instructions:

- Turn on the instant pot, add 2 tablespoons of olive oil and heat on the saute mode. Add the sweet potato, quinoa, 1 tablespoon harissa, garlic, and salt. Cook and stir 2 minutes, until the garlic is fragrant.
- Turn off the heat, and then stir in kale and water. Close the lid and lock, then cook on high pressure for 8 minutes.
- Quick-release pressure, remove the lid, and let stand for 5 minutes.
- Meanwhile, combine the remaining two tablespoons of olive oil, the remaining tablespoon of harissa, and lime juice in a small bowl.
- Divide the quinoa mixture among 4 bowls. Top each portion with chickpeas, scallions, and pistachios. Drizzle the sauce over the bowls. Serve and enjoy.

13. Instant Pot Couscous And Vegetables
Servings: 6
Total Time: 13 Minutes

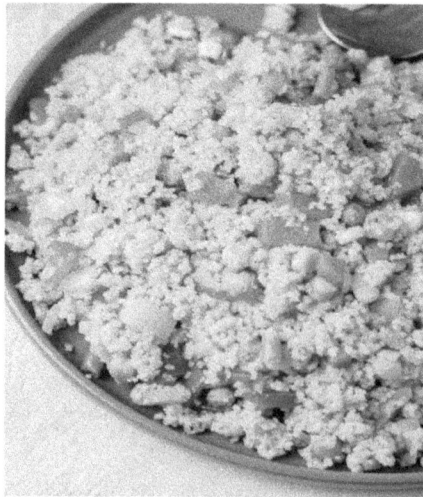

Energy Value Per Serving:
Calories: 460
Protein: 6.5 grams
Total Fat: 4 grams
Carbohydrates: 36 grams
Ingredients:
- 4 cups couscous
- 2 cups water
- 5 grated carrots

- 2 bay leaves
- 2 chopped bell peppers
- 1 chopped onion
- 2 tablespoons olive oil
- 2 tablespoons lemon juice
- 2 teaspoons of turmeric
- salt and black pepper

Instructions:

- Pour olive oil into the instant pot, and add onion and bay leaves.
- Press the saute setting and cook for 2 minutes. The onions should be golden brown.
- Add carrots and bell peppers, then cook for another 2 minutes, until the veggies turn soft.
- Add the couscous, water, turmeric, salt, and pepper to the mix.
- Cook at high pressure for 2 minutes, and then quick release the steam.
- Remove bay leaves, add lemon juice and stir well.

14. Instant Pot Pasta With Mediterranean Vegetables

Servings: 6
Total Time: 14 Minutes

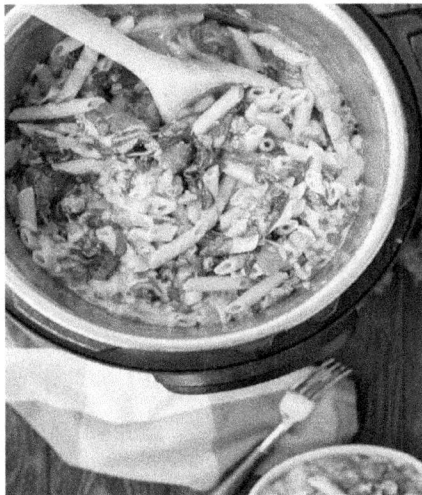

Energy Value Per Serving:
Calories: 399
Protein: 12 grams
Total Fat: 6 grams

Carbohydrates: 73 grams
Ingredients:
- 1 tablespoon olive oil
- 1 red onion, chopped
- 2 garlic cloves, crushed
- 1 aubergine, chopped
- 1 red pepper, chopped
- 2 cups of tomatoes, chopped
- 2 cups of pasta
- vegetable stock to cover the pasta
- ½ cup black olives
- fresh parsley
- Parmesan for serving
- salt and freshly ground black pepper to taste

Instructions:

- Set your instant pot to saute and add olive oil, red onion and garlic cloves. Heat for a couple of minutes until softened. Then add the aubergine and pepper and cook for another 3-5 minutes.
- Add the pasta to the instant pot and pour in the chopped tomatoes and vegetable stock to cover the pasta. Season with salt and pepper to taste.
- Cook on the manual high pressure setting for 4 minutes. Quick release the pressure and then stir in the olives. Transfer to a bowl and serve topped with chopped parsley and parmesan.

15. Instant Pot Mediterranean Quinoa Bowl With Lemon Garlic Chicken

Servings: 6
Total Time: 30 minutes

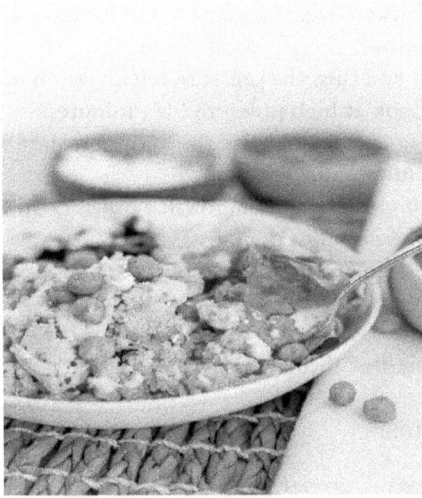

Energy Value Per Serving:
Calories: 247
Protein: 22.7 grams
Total Fat: 6.6 grams
Carbohydrates: 25.4 grams

Ingredients:
- 3 garlic cloves, minced
- 2 tablespoons of dried parsley
- zest of 1 lemon
- 1 teaspoon of kosher salt
- ½ teaspoon black pepper
- 1 tablespoon olive oil
- 1 pound of chicken breast, boneless and skinless, cut into larger bite-size pieces

Ingredients For Quinoa:
- 1 cup uncooked quinoa
- 1.5 cups of low sodium chicken broth
- juice from 1 lemon
- pinch of salt

Instructions:

- In a medium-sized bowl, mix the marinade ingredients and toss in the chicken to coat. Place in the fridge to marinate for 6-10 hours, or cook it right away.
- Place quinoa, chicken broth, lemon juice, and salt into the instant pot, making sure the quinoa is immersed.

- Scatter the chicken over the quinoa, and make sure they are not clumping together.
- Secure the lid and turn the pressure release knob to the sealed position — Cook at high pressure for 1 minute.
- When cooking is complete, use the natural release. Stir and the chicken and fluff quinoa.
- Put a scoop of chicken and quinoa in a bowl. Load with toppings of your choice like hummus or your favorite sauce.

MEDITERRANEAN SOUPS

1. Chickpea Instant Pot Soup

Servings: 6
Total Time: 35 Minutes

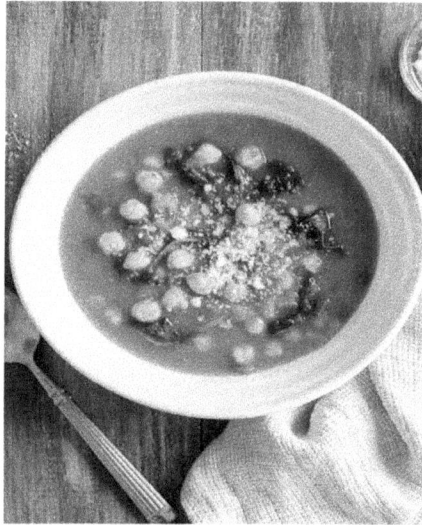

Energy Value Per Serving:
Calories: 367
Protein: 20.1 grams
Total Fat: 9.8 grams
Carbohydrates: 12.1 grams
Ingredients:
- 2 cups of dry chickpeas
- 2 tablespoons extra virgin olive oil
- 1 yellow onion, chopped
- 3 garlic cloves, minced
- salt to taste

- 2 carrots, chopped
- 1 green bell pepper, cored and chopped
- 3-4 red chili peppers
- 1 teaspoon ground coriander
- 1 teaspoon ground cumin
- a teaspoon of Aleppo pepper (A Middle Eastern spice)
- ½ teaspoon of ground turmeric
- ½ teaspoon of ground allspice
- 15 ounces of chopped tomatoes with the juice
- 6 cups of low-sodium vegetable broth
- juice from 1 lemon
- 1-ounce fresh cilantro, chopped

Instructions:

- Place the dry chickpeas in a bowl and submerge them in water. Let them soak overnight and then drain well.
- Preheat your instant pot using the saute setting and adjust the heat to high. Add extra virgin olive oil and heat until simmering. Add the onions, garlic, and a pinch of salt. Cook for 3 minutes, while stirring regularly.
- Add the carrots, bell peppers, and spices. Cook for another 4 minutes, while stirring until the vegetables have softened a bit.
- Add the chickpeas, tomatoes, and the broth. Make sure to add the juice from the tomatoes too. Lock the instant pot lid, and put the pressure cooking setting on high. Set a timer for 15 minutes.
- After cooking, allow natural release of pressure. After 10 minutes, you can press the quick release to remove any extra pressure.
- Carefully unlock and remove the lid. Stir in the lemon juice and fresh cilantro.
- Transfer the contents to serving bowls and drizzle a little extra olive oil.

2. Instant Pot Mediterranean Chicken And Quinoa Stew

Servings: 6
Total Time: 30 Minutes

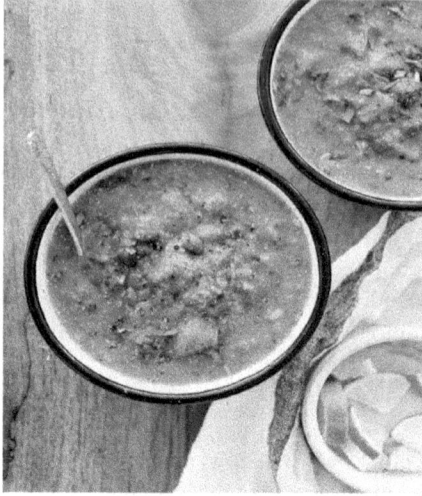

Energy Value Per Serving:
Calories: 243
Protein: 25 grams
Total Fat: 6 grams
Carbohydrates: 24 grams

Ingredients:
- 1-¼ pounds of chicken thighs, boneless and skinless
- 4 cups of butternut squash, peeled and chopped
- 4 cups unsalted chicken stock
- 1 cup yellow onion, chopped
- 2 garlic cloves, chopped
- 1 bay leaf
- 1-¼ teaspoons of kosher salt
- 1 teaspoon of dried oregano
- 1 teaspoon of ground fennel seeds
- ½ cup of uncooked quinoa
- 1-ounce of olives, sliced and pitted

Instructions:

- Combine the chicken, squash, stock, onion, garlic, bay leaf, salt, ground fennel seeds, oregano, and pepper in your instant pot. Cover the lid, turn the valve to seal and cook on high pressure for 8 minutes.
- Release the valve carefully, using mitts or tongs. Quick-release until the steam and pressure go down. Remove chicken, then add quinoa to the instant pot, turn to saute and cook while occasionally stirring until the quinoa is tender.

- Shred the chicken and stir into stew. Discard bay leaf.
- Serve the soup up into separate bowls, and sprinkle sliced olives.

3. Greek Vegetable Soup

Servings: 4
Total Time: 55 minutes

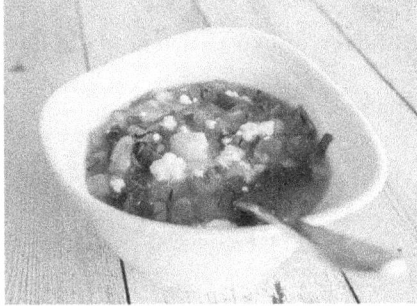

Energy Value Per Serving:

Calories: 412.9
Protein: 6.3 grams
Total Fat: 26.1 grams
Carbohydrates: 43.2 grams

Ingredients:

- 3 tablespoons of olive oil
- 1 onion, chopped
- 1 clove garlic, minced
- 3 cups of cabbage, shredded
- 2 medium carrots, chopped
- 2 celery stocks, chopped
- 2 cups of cooked chickpeas
- 4 cups of vegetable broth
- 15-ounce fire-roasted tomatoes, diced
- salt and pepper to taste

Instructions:

- Add olive oil to the instant pot and set to medium heat saute.
- Add the onions and cook until soft. Add garlic and cabbage and cook for another 5 minutes. When the cabbage softens, add the carrots, celery, and chickpeas. Stir everything to combine and cook for 5 minutes longer
- Add the broth and canned tomatoes, then season with salt and pepper.

- Press cancel to end saute mode and cover the pot with the lid set to sealing mode.
- Set to soup mode and adjust the time to 10 minutes.
- After completion, release the pressure manually and serve immediately.
- You may garnish the soup with parsley, feta, or anything you like on soup.

4. Instant Pot Mediterranean Lentil And Collard Soup
Servings: 6
Total Time: 30 Minutes

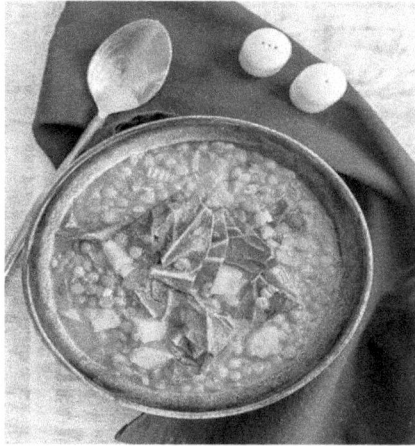

Energy Value Per Serving:
Calories: 127.9
Protein: 7.3 grams
Total Fat: 0.8 grams
Carbohydrates: 25.9 grams
Ingredients:
- 2 tablespoons of extra virgin olive oil
- 1 medium yellow onion, chopped
- 2 medium celery stocks, diced
- 3 garlic cloves, minced
- 2 teaspoons of ground cumin
- 1 teaspoon of ground turmeric
- 4 cups of low-sodium vegetable broth
- 1 ¼ cup of water
- 1 1/2 cups dry brown lentils, rinsed in water
- 2 carrots, peeled and diced
- 1 bay leaf

- 1 teaspoon himalayan salt
- ½ teaspoon of ground black pepper
- 3 collard leaves, cut into strips
- 1 teaspoon of lemon juice

Instructions:

- Set instant pot to saute, then add the olive oil, heat, and add onions and celery. Stir often for 5 minutes. Turn the instant pot off.
- Stir in the garlic, cumin, and turmeric until combined.
- Add broth, water, lentils, carrots, bay leaf, salt, and pepper. Lock the lid and close the valve. Set to manual and cook on high pressure for 13 minutes.
- After completion, quick release the pressure, carefully remove the lid and stir in collards and lemon juice.
- Close the lid and set to manual and cook for 2 more minutes on high. Quick-release the pressure, open the lid, and it's ready to serve.

5. Instant Pot Golden Lentil And Spinach Soup

Servings: 4
Total Time 35 Minutes

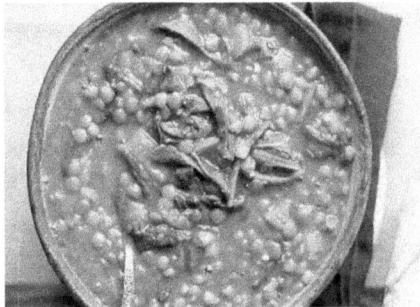

Energy Value Per Serving:
Calories: 134
Protein: 9 grams
Total Fat: 3 grams
Carbohydrates: 17 grams

Ingredients:

- 2 teaspoons of olive oil
- ½ medium yellow onion, diced
- 2 medium carrots
- 1 medium celery stock, diced
- 4 medium garlic cloves, minced

- 2 teaspoons of ground cumin
- 1 teaspoon ground turmeric
- 1 teaspoon of dried thyme
- ½ teaspoon of kosher salt
- ¼ teaspoon of freshly ground black pepper
- 1 cup of dry brown lentils, rinsed well
- 4 cups of vegetable broth
- 8 ounces of baby spinach

Instructions:

- Put the instant pot on the saute setting, and add oil. When heated, add onions, carrots, and celery, stirring occasionally for 5 minutes, then add garlic, cumin, turmeric, thyme, salt and pepper. Cook and stir continuously for 1 minute.
- Add the lentils and pour in the broth, then stir.
- Place the lid on the instant pot and make sure the release valve is on sealing. Select manual setting and set the timer to 12 minutes.
- After 12 minute mark, Quick release to vent the pressure.
- Remove the lid carefully, stir in the spinach. Add additional salt and pepper to taste.
- It is now ready to serve.

6. Instant Pot Italian Beef Stew
Servings: 6
Total Time: 45 Minutes

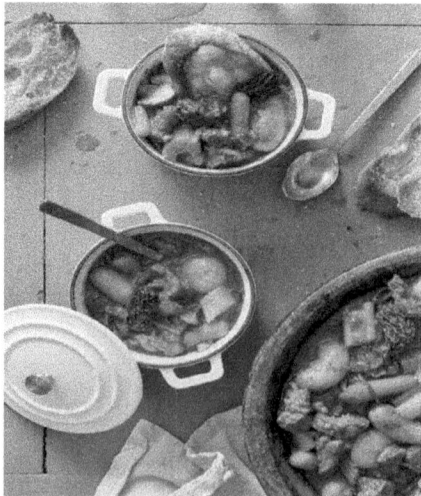

Energy Value Per Serving:

Calories: 385
Protein: 54 grams
Total Fat: 12 grams
Carbohydrates: 12 grams

Ingredients:

- 3 pounds of beef stew
- 1 onion, diced
- 4 carrots, diced
- 8-ounce baby portabella mushrooms, sliced
- 24-ounces of beef broth
- 15 ounce diced tomatoes, canned
- 3 tablespoons of white flour
- 1 teaspoon of dried basil leaves
- 1 teaspoon of dried thyme leaves
- 1 teaspoon of salt
- 1 teaspoon of pepper
- dried parsley

Instructions:

- Place meat in the instant pot.
- Add in carrots, broth, flour, basil, thyme, salt, pepper, and tomatoes to instant pot and stir.
- Place the lid on the pot and then close.
- Cook on high pressure for 35 minutes.
- Quick release the pressure and carefully remove the lid.
- Stir in the mushroom, stir the soup and then serve.

7. Instant Pot Fish Stew

Servings: 4
Total Time: 20 minutes

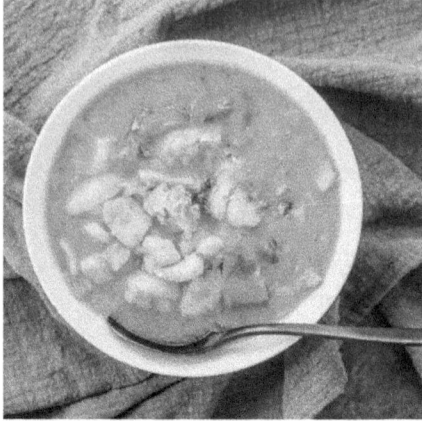

Energy Value Per Serving:
Calories: 471
Protein: 43 grams
Total Fat: 20 grams
Carbohydrates: 24 grams

Ingredients:
- 4 tablespoons of extra-virgin olive oil
- 1 medium red onion, chopped
- 4 garlic cloves, chopped
- ½ cup of dry white wine
- 8-ounce clam juice
- 2 1/2 cups of water
- ½ pound potatoes, diced
- 1 1/2 cups of fresh tomatoes with juices
- kosher salt
- black pepper for taste
- pinch of crushed red pepper for taste
- 2 pounds sea bass cut into 2-inch pieces
- 2 tablespoons lemon juice
- 2 tablespoons of fresh dill, chopped

Instructions:

- Use saute setting on your instant pot and cook onions in 2 tablespoons of olive oil for 3 minutes, until golden brown.
- Add the chopped garlic, saute until fragrant.
- Add the white wine, scrape up any brown bits, until about half of the wine has evaporated.
- Add the clam juice, water, potatoes, tomatoes, salt, pepper, and a pinch of crushed red pepper.

- Turn the saute off, cover and seal your instant pot, and set to manual high pressure for 5 minutes.
- After this, quick release the pressure. Open the instant pot and turn the saute setting back on. Once the soup is simmering, add the pieces of fish, and simmer for about 5 minutes, until the fish flakes apart easily.
- Turn off saute mode, stir in lemon juice and fresh dill and remaining olive oil. Season to taste and serve.

8. Crushed Lentil Soup
Servings: 8
Total Time: 40 Minutes

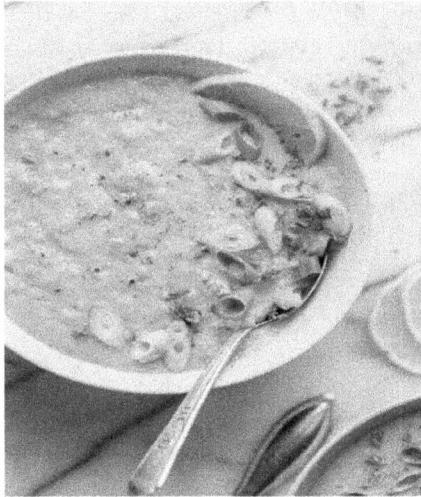

Energy Value Per Serving:
Calories: 191
Protein: 11.8 grams
Total Fat: 1.2
Carbohydrates: 34.4
Ingredients:
- 2 tablespoons vegetable broth
- 1 onion, finely chopped
- 4 garlic cloves, minced
- 4 cups unsalted vegetable broth
- 2 cups of water
- 2 cups red split lentils
- 1 small pinch saffron
- 1 teaspoon coriander

- 1 teaspoon cumin
- ½ teaspoon freshly ground black pepper
- 1 teaspoon sea salt
- ½ teaspoon of red pepper flakes
- 2 bay leaves
- 2 tablespoons fresh lemon juice

Instructions:

- Set the instant pot to saute, add the vegetable broth, 2 tablespoons. Then add the garlic and onions and cook until they are soft, about 4-5 minutes.
- Add remaining ingredients except for bay leaves and lemon juice. Stir and then lock the lid of the instant pot.
- Press cancel and choose the soup function. Set timer for 30 minutes. After the 30 minutes, let it sit for another 20 minutes to release the pressure.
- Open the lid and add bay leaves and lemon juice, then stir for 5 minutes.
- Remove bay leaves and serve.

9. Lemony Lentil Soup
Servings: 4
Total Time: 35 Minutes

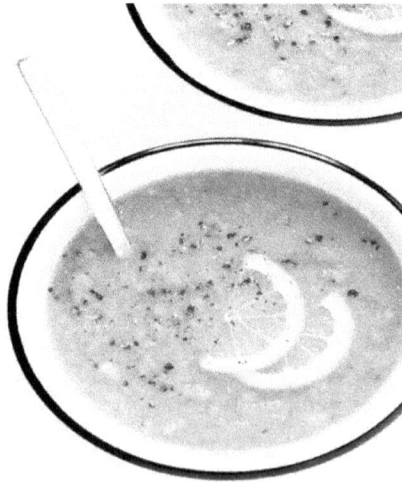

Energy Value Per Serving:
Calories: 260
Protein: 16 grams

Total Fat: 6 grams

Carbohydrates: 40 grams

Ingredients:

- 1 tablespoon of olive oil
- 1 medium onion, peeled and diced
- 2 carrots, diced
- 5 garlic cloves, minced
- 6 cups of vegetable stock
- 1 1/2 cup of red lentils
- ⅔ cup of whole kernel corn
- 2 teaspoons of ground cumin
- 1 teaspoon of curry powder
- zest and juice of 1 lemon
- sea salt and fresh black pepper to taste

Instructions:

- Choose the saute function on your instant pot and add oil. Add the onions and carrots and saute for 5 minutes. Stir occasionally until the onions are soft and translucent. Add garlic and saute for 1 more minute, until fragrant.
- Stir in the vegetable stock, lentils, corn, cumin, and curry powder until combined
- Close the lid and set to "sealing."
- Press and set for manual high pressure, and adjust the timer for 8 minutes. Cook, then carefully turn to venting for quick release. Once vented, remove the lid carefully.
- Using a blender, puree the soup until it reaches your desired consistency.
- Return the puree to the instant pot and stir in lemon zest and juice until combined.
- Season with sea salt and black pepper to taste.
- Serve warm.

10. Instant Pot Vegetable Soup

Servings: 5

Total Time: 30 Minutes

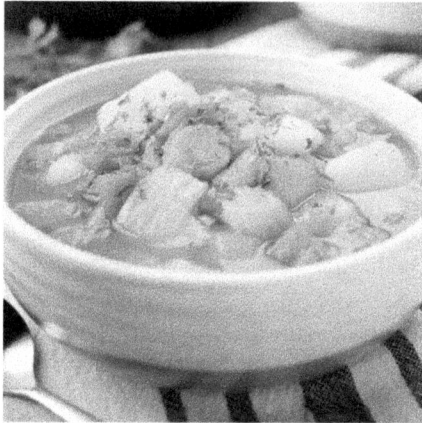

Energy Value Per Serving:
Calories: 192
Protein: 7.3 grams
Total Fat: 6.6 grams
Carbohydrates: 26 grams

Ingredients:
- 2 tablespoons extra virgin olive oil
- ½ onion, chopped
- ½ green bell pepper, chopped
- 2 cloves garlic, minced
- 1 1/2 cups green cabbage, chopped
- 1 1/2 cups small cauliflower florets
- 1 cup chopped carrots
- ½ cup green beans, cut into small pieces
- 4 cups low-sodium vegetable broth
- 14 ounce can diced tomatoes, no salt added
- 1 bay leaf
- ½ teaspoon salt
- 4 cups of chopped spinach
- 15 ounce cannellini beans, rinsed
- ¼ cup chopped basil

Instructions:

- Place olive oil in the instant pot and set to saute. Add onions, bell peppers, and garlic, then cook, stirring often until starting to soften, which will take 2-3 minutes.
- Add cabbage, cauliflower, carrots, and green beans and cook for 4-5 minutes, stirring often.
- Add the broth, tomatoes, bay leaf, and salt. Turn off the heat, lock

the lid, and cook on high for 5 minutes.

- Release the pressure using quick release, open the lid carefully, and remove bay leaf. Stir in the spinach, basil, and beans.
- Ready to serve. May drizzle more olive oil on top if desired.

11. Instant Pot Golden Lentil And Spinach Soup

Servings: 4
Total Time: 35 Minutes

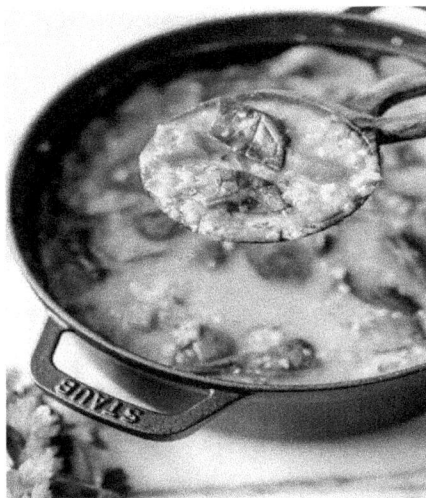

Energy Value Per Serving:
Calories: 134
Protein: 9 grams
Total Fat: 3 grams
Carbohydrates: 17 grams

Ingredients:

- 2 teaspoons of olive oil
- ½ yellow onion, diced
- 2 carrots, peeled and diced
- 1 celery stock, diced
- 4 garlic cloves, minced
- 2 teaspoons ground cumin
- 1 teaspoon ground turmeric
- 1 teaspoon dried thyme
- 1 teaspoon kosher salt
- ¼ teaspoon freshly ground black pepper
- 1 cup dry brown lentils, rinsed well
- 4 cups low-sodium vegetable broth

- 8 ounces baby spinach

Instructions:

- Choose saute function of the instant pot and add oil. When hot, add onions, carrots, and celery. Saute, occasionally stirring, until tender, about 5 minutes.
- Add garlic, cumin, turmeric, thyme, salt, and pepper. Cook and stir for one minute.
- Stir in lentil and broth.
- Place lid on instant pot and put the valve to "sealing." Press manual high pressure and set a timer for 12 minutes.
- After 12 minutes, quick release pressure and then carefully remove the lid when done. Stir in the spinach, and add salt and pepper to taste.

12. Mediterranean Bamyeh Okra Tomato Stew

Servings: 4
Total Time: 12 Minutes

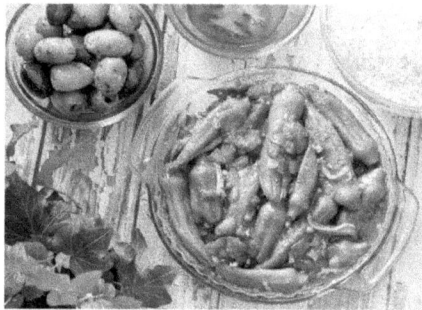

Energy Value Per Serving:
Calories: 85
Protein: 4 grams
Total Fat: 5 grams
Carbohydrates: 19 grams

Ingredients:

- ¼ cup of water
- 2 tablespoons apple cider vinegar
- 1 cup onions, chopped
- 1 tablespoon minced garlic
- 14.5 ounce canned tomatoes
- 1 tablespoon vegetable broth
- 1 teaspoon smoked paprika
- ½ teaspoon ground allspice

- 1 teaspoon salt
- 1 1/2 pounds fresh okra

Instructions:

- Place all ingredients except for the lemon juice and tomato paste into instant pot. Put in okra last.
- Cook on high pressure for 2 minutes, let it rest for 5 minutes.
- Quick release the pressure.
- Open the lid carefully and add tomato paste in water and then the lemon juice. Stir gently and serve.

13. Instant Pot Minestrone Soup

Servings: 6
Total Time: 45 Minutes

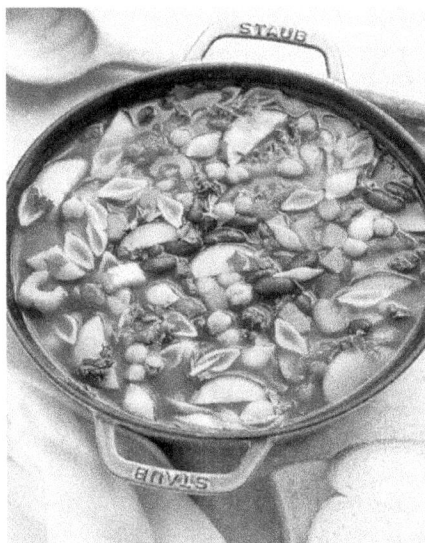

Energy Value Per Serving:

Calories: 227
Protein: 14 grams
Total Fat: 7 grams
Carbohydrates: 26 grams

Ingredients:

- 2 tablespoons olive oil
- 3 cloves garlic, minced
- 1 onion, diced
- 2 carrots, peeled and diced
- 2 celery stalks, diced

- 1 ½ teaspoons fresh basil
- 1 teaspoon dried oregano
- ½ teaspoon fennel seed
- 6 cups low-sodium chicken broth
- 28 ounce can tomatoes, diced
- 16 ounce can kidney beans, drained and rinsed
- 1 zucchini, chopped
- 1 Parmesan rind
- 1 bay leaf
- 1 bunch kale, chopped and stems removed
- 2 teaspoons red wine vinegar
- kosher salt and freshly ground black pepper
- ⅓ cup Parmesan, grated
- 2 tablespoons fresh parsley leaves, chopped

Instructions:

- Set instant pot to saute, add olive oil, garlic, onion, carrots, and celery. Cook, occasionally stirring, until tender. Stir in basil, oregano, and fennel seeds, for a minute, until fragrant.
- Stir in the chicken stock, tomatoes, kidney beans, zucchini, parmesan rind, and bay leaf. Select the manual high pressure setting and set for 5 minutes.
- When completed, press quick release to remove all pressure.
- Stir in the kale for about 2 minutes, then stir in red wine vinegar and season with salt and pepper to taste. Ready to serve.

14. Instant Pot Greek Beef Stew
Servings: 4
Total Time: 55 Minutes

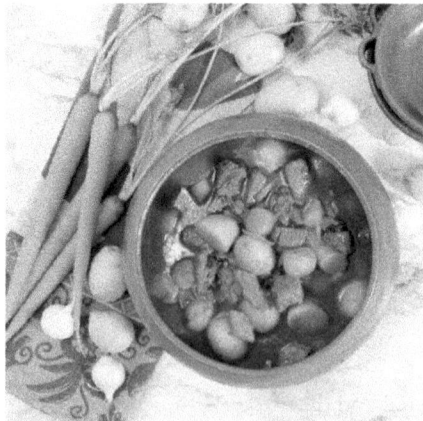

Energy Value Per Serving:
Calories: 479
Protein: 43 grams
Total Fat: 20 grams
Carbohydrates: 31 grams

Ingredients:
- 1 ½ pounds stew beef cut into small cubes
- ¼ cup of butter
- 8 small onions
- 8 small potatoes
- 2-3 carrots, sliced
- ¾ cups tomato paste
- 1 teaspoon cinnamon

Instructions:

- Set instant pot to saute mode and cook beef in the butter until browned. This will take about 5 minutes. Then remove.
- Add onions to the pot and saute about 5 minutes.
- Stop saute mode. Add beef back to the pot and then add carrots, potatoes, tomato paste, and cinnamon. Add 2-3 cups of water.
- Lock the lid and set pressure to high and cook for 35 minutes.
- Allow steam to release naturally for 10 minutes and then quick release remaining pressure.
- Ready to serve.

15. Instant Pot Bean Soup
Servings: 6
Total Time: 1 Hour 45 Minutes

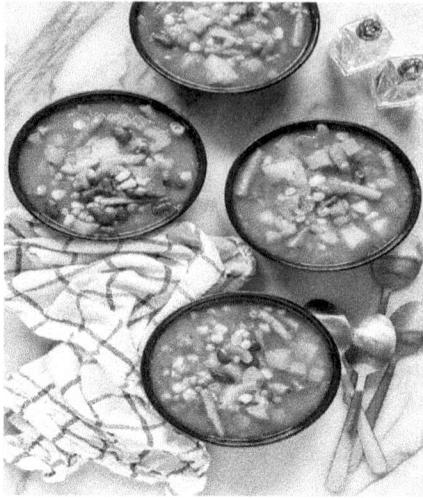

Energy Value Per Serving:
Calories: 86
Protein: 2.8 grams
Total Fat: 5 grams
Carbohydrates: 9.7 grams

Ingredients:
- 1 pound white beans
- 1 ¼ pound of beef shanks with bone
- 1 white onion, chopped
- 1 green bell pepper, chopped
- 2 carrots, chopped
- 4 tablespoons olive oil
- 2 tablespoons fresh parsley, chopped
- ½ teaspoon garlic, minced
- ½ tablespoon salt
- 1 can tomatoes, diced
- 1 liter water
- 3 bay leaves
- ½ teaspoon paprika

Instructions:

- Soak beans in a pot of cold water overnight.
- Place the beef shanks and olive oil in instant pot and turn on saute setting. Brown on both sides
- Remove the beans from water, and rinse. Add beans, diced tomatoes, paprika, bay leaves, and garlic.
- Add water, close the lid, and cook on the manual high setting for 1

hour. Check if the beans are soft, and if not, cook for another 30 minutes. Serve.

MEDITERRANEAN MAINS

1. Instant Pot Low-Carb Chicken Tacos

Servings: 8
Total time: 8 minutes

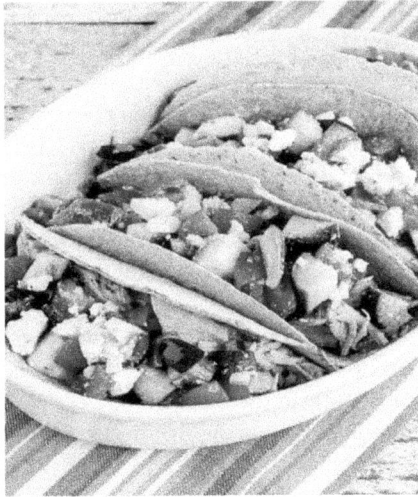

Energy Value Per Serving:
Calories: 240
Protein: 29 grams
Total Fat: 11 grams
Carbohydrates: 11.5 grams

Ingredients:
- 4 large chicken breasts, trimmed and cut
- juice and zest of 2 lemons
- 1 tablespoon Greek seasoning
- 1 tablespoon extra-virgin olive oil
- ¼ cup chicken stock
- ½ teaspoon fresh oregano
- ½ teaspoon fresh ground black pepper
- 8 small low-carb tortillas

Greek Salsa Ingredients:
- 3 medium cucumbers, chopped
- 1 cup cherry tomatoes, chopped
- ¼ cup chopped kalamata olives

- ¼ cup red onions that are finely chopped
- 4 ounce crumbled feta cheese
- ¼ cup low-sugar Italian dressing

Instructions:

- Trim the chicken breast and cut lengthwise into 2 or 3 strips. Put the chicken into the instant pot.
- Grate the lemon zest. Cut the lemons in half and squeeze the juice.
- Whisk the zest and juice together with the Greek seasoning, olive oil, chicken stock, Greek oregano, and black pepper to make the cooking sauce. Pour over the chicken in the instant pot.
- Set the instant pot to high pressure for 8 minutes. Then do a natural release for 10 minutes before you release the rest of the pressure.
- After the pressure has been released, remove chicken and place it on a cutting board. Leave the sauce in the instant pot.
- Shred the chicken and put it back into the instant pot. Stir gently until the chicken is coated. Put the instant pot on the warm setting while preparing other ingredients.
- For the Greek salsa, chop the cucumbers, tomatoes, kalamata olives, and red onions and put these together in a bowl. Stir in the Italian dressing and stir in the feta cheese.
- Heat the tortillas in a dry pan on high heat until they are softened. Then fill in each tortilla with taco meat, and top with salsa.

2. Healthy Instant Pot Mediterranean Chicken
Servings: 4
Total Time: 20 minutes

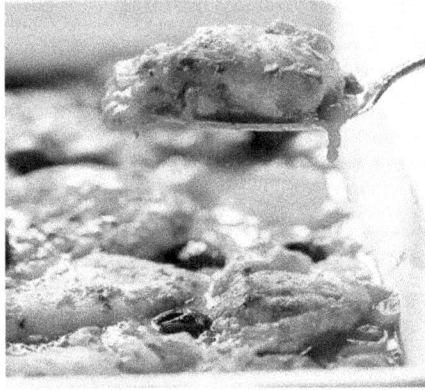

Energy Value Per Serving:

Calories: 228

Protein: 11.1 grams

Total Fat: 10.7 grams

Carbohydrates: 25 grams

Ingredients:

- 4 chicken breasts, skinless and boneless
- 1 can tomatoes with no salt, diced
- ½ onion, diced
- 2 tablespoons garlic, minced
- 25 kalamata or black olives, pitted
- 2 tablespoons extra virgin olive oil
- 2 tablespoons Greek seasoning
- fresh oregano sprigs for garnish

Instructions:

- Cut each chicken breast into 4-5 large pieces.
- Turn instant pot to the saute setting.
- Add the olive oil, onion, and garlic to the pot. Cook for 3-4 minutes.
- Sprinkle Greek seasoning on both sides of chicken pieces.
- Take ½ of chicken breasts and place them in the instant pot. Brown on both sides, which will take about 3 minutes. Remove this first batch of chicken and add in the second. Once this chicken is done, remove from the pot.
- Add the tomatoes, olives and dried oregano.
- Nestle the chicken breasts into olive oil mixture.

- Set the instant pot to Manual high for 15 minutes.
- Allow to self-release for 10 minutes and then pressure release until all of the steam is gone.
- Serve this chicken over your favorite rice.

3. Mediterranean Instant Pot Chicken And Potatoes
Servings: 6
Total Time: 14 Minutes

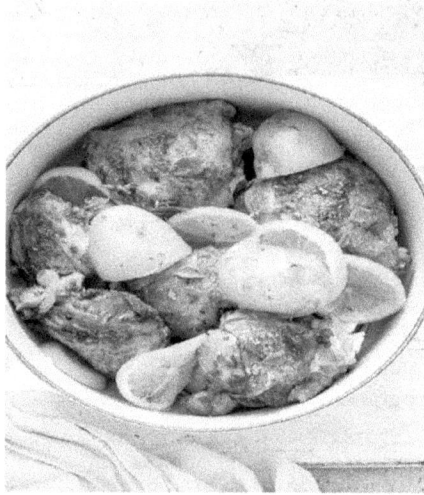

Energy Value Per Serving:
Calories: 273
Protein: 24 grams
Total Fat: 10 grams
Carbohydrates: 21 grams
Ingredients:
- 2 tablespoons of olive oil
- ½ teaspoon of ground pimento
- 1 teaspoon of smoked paprika
- 6 chicken thighs, bone in and skin on
- 1 cup of chicken broth
- 1 teaspoon of garlic puree
- juice from 1 lemon
- 2 tablespoons of honey
- 1 pound of potatoes, cut in half
- 1 teaspoon of fresh oregano
Instructions:

- In a bowl, combine 1 tablespoon of olive oil with salt, smoked paprika and pimento.
- Add in the chicken thighs and coat well with the sauce.
- Take the other tablespoon of olive oil in the instant pot using the saute setting. Add the chicken thighs and brown on both sides, about 6 minutes.
- Turn the instant pot off. Remove any excess oil before going further.
- Pour in chicken broth.
- Add in remaining ingredients, put on the lid and lock. Set the valve to the sealing position.
- Set the instant pot to pressure cook, high pressure for 8 minutes.
- Allow for 5 minutes of natural pressure release, then perform quick pressure release for remaining.

4. Instant Pot Steamed Artichokes With Mediterranean Aioli
Servings: 3
Total Time: 15 minutes

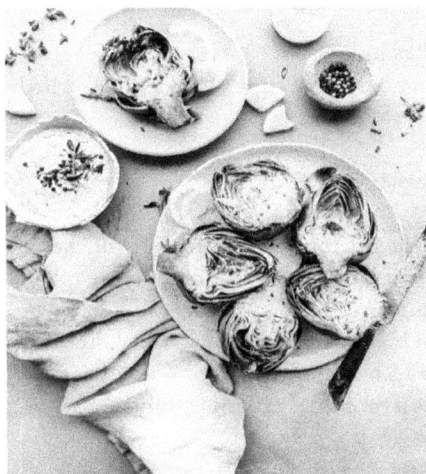

Energy Value Per Serving:
Calories: 135
Protein: 0.7 grams
Total Fat: 12 grams
Carbohydrates: 0.5 grams
Ingredients:
- 3 medium artichokes with the stems cut off
- 1 cup vegetable broth
Aioli Ingredients:

- 2 tablespoons fresh oregano and rosemary, chopped
- 2 teaspoons of garlic
- ½ teaspoon ground coriander
- a pinch of cumin
- 1 teaspoon crushed red pepper flakes
- 2 egg yolks
- 1 tablespoon mustard
- 2 teaspoons lemon juice
- ⅔ cup olive oil
- sea salt and pepper

Instructions:

- Cut stems off artichokes and place upside down on wire trivet in instant pot. Pour vegetable broth over the artichokes and around the instant pot.
- Lock the lid with vent closed. Press the steam mode and set the timer to 10 minutes. Allow for slow release when done. The lid will unlock when done.
- Remove artichokes from instant pot. Save ¼ cup of the broth for later.
- Slice artichokes in half.
- Place the artichokes on a large plate. Drizzle a little bit of broth on both halves.

Aioli Instructions:

- Place all ingredients for the aioli, except for the oil, in the food processor. Blend until creamy. Drizzle in the oil and then blend for 1-2 more minutes.
- Remove from blender and place in a bowl. Let this mixture sit in the fridge for 10 minutes.
- Spread the aioli on top of artichokes and enjoy.

5. Instant Pot Greek Chicken

Servings: 6
Total Time: 30 minutes

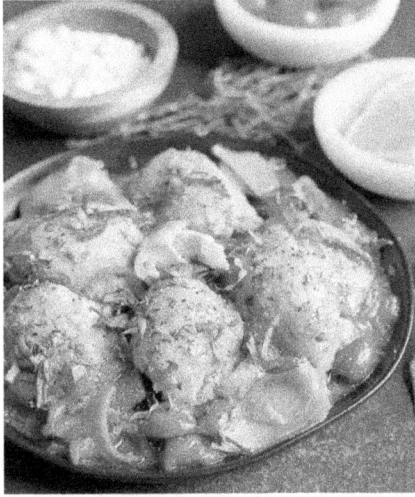

Energy Value Per Serving:

Calories: 433

Protein: 24 grams

Total Fat: 34 grams

Carbohydrates: 6 grams

Ingredients:

- 2 tablespoons olive oil
- 3 garlic cloves
- 2 pounds chicken thighs, boneless and skinless
- ½ teaspoon salt
- ¼ teaspoon black pepper
- 12 ounce jar roasted red peppers, diced and rinsed
- 8 ounce jar marinated artichoke hearts, drained
- 1 cup kalamata olives
- ½ sliced red onion
- ⅔ cup chicken broth
- ¼ cup red wine vinegar
- juice from ½ of a lemon
- 1 teaspoon dried oregano
- 1 teaspoon dried thyme
- 1-2 tablespoon arrowroot starch
- ½ cup crumbled feta

Instructions:

- Choose saute on the instant pot. Sprinkle salt and pepper to each side of chicken thighs. Add oil to the pot, then add garlic. Cook for

1 minute and then add the chicken. Sear chicken on each side for about 2 minutes.

- Arrange the artichoke hearts, peppers, and olives around the chicken, filling in the gaps on the bottom of the instant pot. Top with the sliced red onion.
- Mix the chicken broth, vinegar, lemon, dried oregano, and thyme in a bowl. Pour mixture on top of the chicken and vegetables. Secure lid.
- Select the manual function and cook on high pressure for 7 minutes.
- Use quick release and then open the lid.
- Take out some of the juice from the instant pot and place into a small bowl. Add 2 tablespoons of starch, mix, and then pour back into the instant pot. Allow sauce to thicken.
- Serve over rice. Add fresh herbs, feta, salt and pepper to taste.

6. Instant Pot Moroccan Chicken

Servings: 4
Total Time: 30 minutes

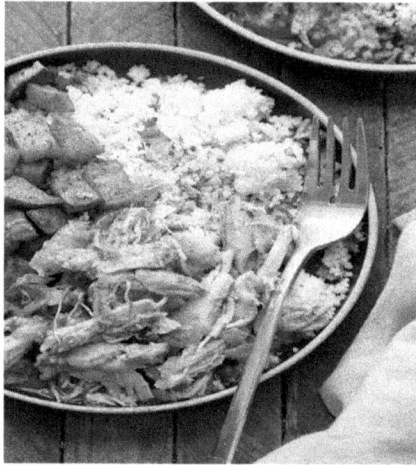

Energy Value Per Serving:

Calories: 194.2
Protein: 28.1 grams
Total Fat: 6.7 grams
Carbohydrates: 5.3 grams

Ingredients:

- 1 teaspoon paprika
- 1 teaspoon turmeric

- 1 teaspoon ground cumin
- ½ teaspoon salt
- ¼ teaspoon black pepper
- 3 tablespoons olive oil
- 1 ½ pounds chicken thighs, boneless and skinless
- 1 ½ cups chicken broth
- 2 garlic cloves, minced
- ½ cup onions, diced
- 1 teaspoon ginger, minced
- ¾ cup quinoa, uncooked
- 1 can chickpeas, drained
- ½ cup dried cherries
- chopped cilantro leaves

Instructions:

- Mix together paprika, turmeric, cumin, salt, and pepper in a small bowl.
- Coat the chicken thighs with spice rub. Set aside.
- Add 2 tablespoons of olive oil to the bottom of the instant pot.
- Select saute mode.
- Add chicken to the instant pot and cook both sides until slightly brown. Remove from the instant pot and set aside on a plate.
- Add another tablespoon of olive oil to the bottom of the pot.
- Add garlic, onions, and ginger, then saute for 2 minutes while stirring slowly.
- Add quinoa, dried cherries, chickpeas, chicken broth, and the browned chicken.
- Close the lid and seal.
- Press poultry and set for 10 minutes.
- At the end of the 10 minutes, use tongs to carefully turn the knob for quick release of pressure.
- Once the pressure is released, carefully open the lid.
- Check the chicken and make sure it is 165 degrees F before serving.
- Serve on a plate with cilantro garnish.

7. Mediterranean Instant Pot Shredded Beef
Servings: 8
Total Time: 25 minutes

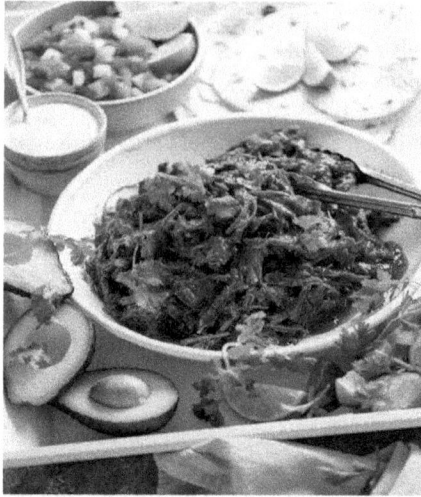

Energy Value Per Serving:
Calories: 190.2
Protein: 23.5 grams
Total Fat: 6.3 grams
Carbohydrates: 8.9 grams

Ingredients:
- 2 pounds Chuck beef roast
- 1 teaspoon salt
- 1 cup white onion, chopped
- ¾ cup carrots, chopped
- ¾ cup yellow bell pepper, chopped
- 14.5 ounce can of fire-roasted tomatoes
- 2 tablespoons red wine vinegar
- 1 tablespoon garlic, minced
- 1 tablespoon Italian seasoning blend
- 1/2 tablespoon dried red pepper flakes

Instructions:

- Cut the beef roast into small chunks, and trim away any excess fat. Season with salt.
- Place the small beef cubes into the instant pot and then top with onions, carrots, and yellow bell peppers.
- Open the can of fire-roasted tomatoes and stir in the vinegar, garlic, Italian dressing, and red pepper flakes. Pour mixture over the beef in the instant pot.
- Secure the lid and set the vent to sealed. Set for 20 minutes on the high-pressure setting.

- When the timer goes off, quick release to remove pressure, remove lid carefully, and let stand for 5-10 minutes.
- Use a large fork to shred beef into bite-sized pieces and then serve.

8. Mediterranean Greek Shredded Chicken And Brown Rice Bowl
Servings: 4
Total Time: 57 Minutes

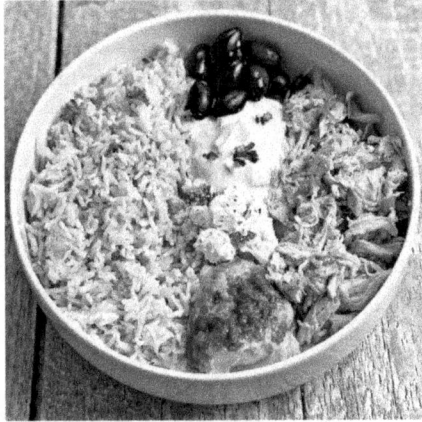

Energy Value Per Serving:
Calories: 426
Protein: 29 grams
Total Fat: 17 grams
Carbohydrates: 42 grams
Ingredients:
- 2 chicken breasts, skinless
- 1 cup low-sodium chicken broth
- 2 cups basmati or brown rice
- 2 ½ cups of water
- ½ teaspoon turmeric
- ½ teaspoon thyme
- ½ teaspoon cumin
- ½ teaspoon paprika
- ½ teaspoon red pepper
- salt and pepper to taste
- 4 tablespoons plain hummus
- 4 tablespoon tzatziki sauce
- ½ cup kalamata olives
- 4 tablespoons feta cheese
Instructions:

- Season chicken breast with thyme, cumin, turmeric, paprika, red pepper, salt and pepper.
- Add the chicken and broth to the instant pot.
- Cook for 10 minutes on manual high pressure setting.
- When the instant pot beeps, allow the natural release of steam for 10 minutes.
- Remove chicken and shred.
- Rinse the rice with water in a large bowl and drain.
- Add the rice to the instant pot and pour in water.
- Cook for 22 minutes on manual high pressure.
- Allow the steam to release naturally for 10 minutes. Do not use the quick release at this time.
- Remove rice from the pot.
- Create your bowls with the desired amount of the chicken, rice, olives, feta cheese, hummus, and tzatziki sauce.

9. Instant Pot Mediterranean Spiced Chicken
Servings: 4
Total Time: 45 minutes

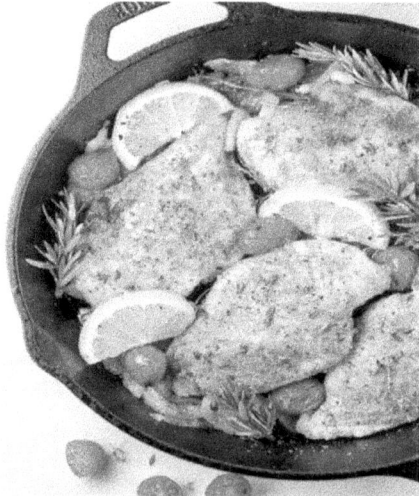

Energy Value Per Serving:
Calories: 244
Protein: 23.2 grams
Total Fat: 16.1 grams
Carbohydrates: 0.6 grams
Ingredients:
- 1 tablespoon olive oil

- 2 pounds chicken thighs, boneless and cut into large pieces
- 2 red peppers, cut into chunks
- 1 large onion, diced
- 4 garlic cloves, diced
- 2 roma tomatoes, cut into chunks
- 1 can chickpeas
- 1 teaspoon salt
- ½ teaspoon black pepper
- 1 teaspoon cumin
- ½ teaspoon coriander
- 1 teaspoon dried parsley
- ½ teaspoon of red pepper flakes
- 1 cup tomato sauce

Instructions:

- Set instant pot to saute.
- Pour oil into pot and allow to heat. Add onion and garlic. Saute for 5 minutes.
- Add the pieces of chicken and brown them on all sides, 3-5 minutes.
- Add remaining ingredients, mix, and cook on manual. Set timer for 10 minutes.
- Quick release the steam and serve. Served over pita bread or any favorite base.

10. Instant Pot Mediterranean Tomato, Chicken, And Rice Dinner

Servings: 4
Total Time: 30 Minutes

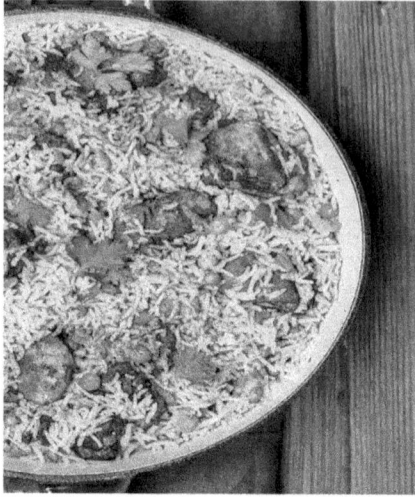

Energy Value Per Serving:
Calories: 259
Protein: 18 grams
Total Fat: 11 grams
Carbohydrates: 17 grams
Ingredients:
- 2 tablespoons extra virgin olive oil
- 1 small onion
- 1 tablespoon garlic and ginger, chopped
- ½ teaspoon cumin
- ¼ teaspoon chili flakes
- ½ teaspoon coriander powder
- ¼ teaspoon black pepper
- salt to taste
- 1 tablespoon tomato paste
- 2 cups basmati rice, rinsed
- 2 ½ cups chicken broth (plus extra ¼ cup)
- 1 chicken breast, cut into small cubes

Instructions:

- Turn instant pot to saute on medium.
- After heating, add oil and onions and allow them to turn golden brown. Add the fresh ginger and garlic and let it cook for a minute. Add the extra ¼ cup of stock that you have.
- Add the spices you have and allow the mixture to simmer for a minute. Add the tomato paste and mix it all together. Add chicken to the mixture once it has thickened a bit and allow it to coat

thoroughly.
- Immediately add the rice and stock, then give it a good stir.
- Lock the lid.
- Turn the pot on and select manual and adjust to 7 minutes.
- Once it is done cooking, wait 5 minutes and then quick release the pressure. After the pressure is released, open the lid and fluff the rice. Serve.

11. Instant Pot Orzo With Shrimp, Tomatoes, And Feta
Servings: 4
Total Time: 30 Minutes

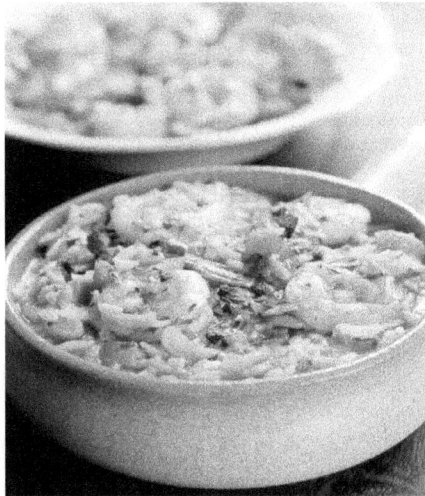

Energy Value Per Serving:
Calories: 395
Protein: 38 grams
Total Fat: 11 grams
Carbohydrates: 33 grams
Ingredients:
- 1 tablespoon olive oil
- 1 medium onion, diced
- 2 cloves garlic, minced
- two, 14-ounce cans diced tomatoes
- 2 tablespoons fresh parsley
- 2 tablespoons fresh dill
- 1-¼ pounds medium shrimp, peeled and deveined
- ¼ teaspoon salt
- ¼ teaspoon freshly ground black pepper

- ⅔ cup of feta cheese, crumbled
- 1-¼ cups chicken stock
- ¾ cup orzo

Instructions:

- Set your instant pot to saute. Then add the olive oil, onion, and garlic. Cook, stirring until softened and translucent, which takes about 3 minutes. Deglaze with a splash of water to prevent sticking.
- Next, add the tomatoes and chicken stock and bring to a boil, and stir.
- Add the orzo, dill, and parsley and mix well.
- Add shrimp and season with salt and pepper and add feta cheese.
- Set instant pot on manual high pressure for 3 minutes.
- After 3 minutes, press the quick release to avoid overcooking the shrimp and orzo. Serve.

12. Instant Pot Mediterranean Chicken Wings

Servings: 2
Total Time: 13 minutes

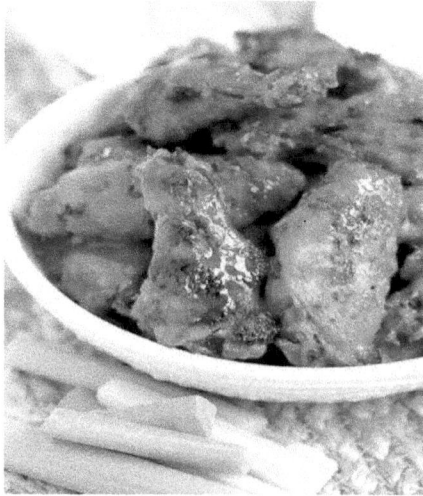

Energy Value Per Serving:

Calories: 545
Protein: 26 grams
Total Fat: 42 grams
Carbohydrates: 8 grams

Ingredients:

- 1 pound of chicken wings

- 1 tablespoon garlic puree
- 3 tablespoons coconut oil
- 6 tablespoons white wine
- 1 tablespoon chicken seasoning
- 3 tablespoons tarragon
- 1 tablespoon oregano
- 1 tablespoon basil
- salt and pepper to taste
- 1 cup of water

Instructions:

- Split the marinade ingredients between two foil sheets.
- Split the chicken wings between the two parcels and rub well into the mixture. Seal each package up and shake so everything has a good coating.
- Add one cup of water to your instant pot and place the steaming shelf on top.
- Place chicken wing packets on top of the steaming shelf.
- Place the lid on your instant pot and set the valve to sealing, then press manual button for 10 minutes.
- Ready to serve in foil packets.

13. Instant Pot Salmon

Servings: 4
Marination Time: 1 hour
Total Time: 1 hour and 20 minutes

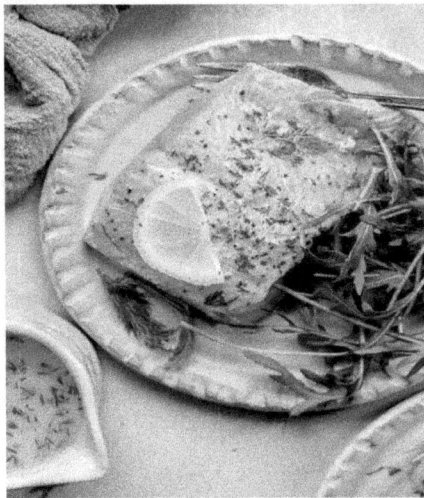

Energy Value Per Serving:
Calories: 161
Protein: 22 grams
Total Fat: 7 grams
Carbohydrates: 1.8 grams

Ingredients:
- 1 pound wild-caught Alaskan salmon
- salt and pepper
- 1 cup of water

Instructions:

- Cut salmon into 4 fillets.
- Pour water into the instant pot and place the metal trivet on top.
- Place the salmon fillets on top of the trivet in a single layer and sprinkle light salt and pepper to taste.
- Secure the lid and turn pressure to sealing. Use the manual setting to cook on high pressure for 3 minutes.
- When this is complete quick release the pressure.
- Serve warm.

14. Paella With Cauliflower Rice
Servings: 6
Total Time: 40 minutes

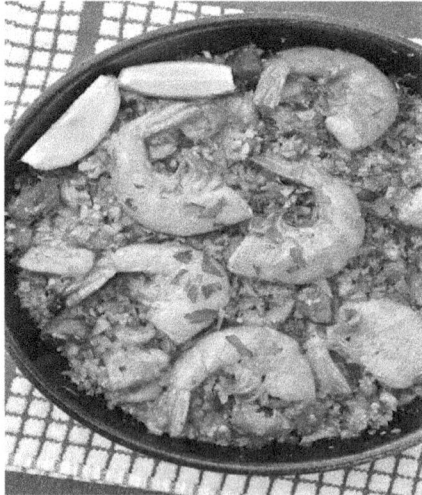

Energy Value Per Serving:
Calories: 218
Protein: 24 grams

Total Fat: 10 grams

Carbohydrates: 6 grams

Ingredients:

- ¾ pound chicken breast, boneless and skinless cut into small chunks
- 3 tablespoons olive oil
- 2 teaspoons smoked paprika
- 1 teaspoon dried oregano
- 1 large head cauliflower, grated
- 1 tablespoon turmeric
- 2 teaspoons sea salt
- 2 sausage links, cut into small slices
- 12 ounces large shrimp, peeled and deveined
- ½ cup yellow onions, diced
- 1 tablespoon garlic, minced
- 1 cup chicken stock
- 6 sprigs of thyme
- 2 tablespoons fresh parsley, chopped

Instructions:

- Combine the chicken, 1 tablespoon of olive oil, paprika, and oregano into a small bowl and marinate for 1 hour.
- Grate the cauliflower into rice sized pieces.
- Turn instant pot on the saute setting. Once hot, add 2 tablespoons of oil. Add the sausage and brown on both sides. Then set aside for later.
- Add chicken and marinade to the pot and cook for about 7-8 minutes. Remove and set aside.
- Add onions to the instant pot and saute until translucent. This will take about 3 minutes. Add garlic and continue cooking for another 30 seconds.
- Add the grated cauliflower, turmeric and salt to instant pot, and mix well. Then add the stock, chicken, sausage and mix thoroughly again.
- Add thyme sprigs and shrimp on top in an even layer.
- Lock the lid and cook for 1 minute at high pressure.
- Once the cooking time is completed, quick release the pressure and carefully remove the lid. Turn off the instant pot.
- Remove the shrimp and set aside. Discard the thyme.
- Pour all of the contents of the instant pot into a strainer to remove liquid and then return the pot and mix in parsley.
- Remove from the pot and place in a bowl. Serve.

15. Instant Pot Lemon Pepper Salmon

Servings: 4

Total Time: 15 minutes

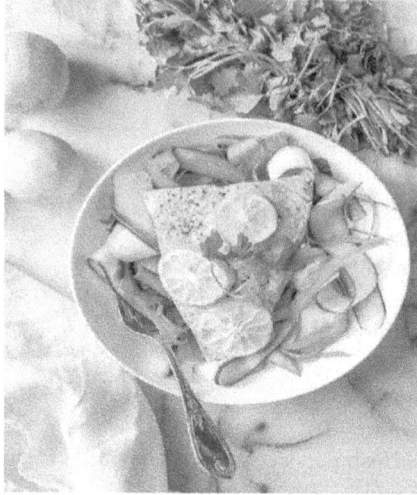

Energy Value Per Serving:
Calories: 296
Protein: 31 grams
Total Fat: 15 grams
Carbohydrates: 8 grams

Ingredients:

- ¾ cup of water
- a few sprigs parsley, tarragon, and basil
- 1 pound salmon filet, skin on
- 3 teaspoons ghee butter
- ¼ teaspoon salt, or to taste
- ½ teaspoon pepper, or to taste
- ½ lemon, thinly sliced
- 1 zucchini
- 1 red bell pepper
- 1 carrot

Instructions:

- Put the water and herbs in the instant pot and then the steamer.
- Place the salmon with the skin side down on the rack.
- Drizzle on some ghee, season with salt and pepper for desired taste, and cover with lemon slices.
- Close the instant pot and make sure the vent is turned to "sealing." Press the steam button and set for 3 minutes.

- While the salmon is cooking, cut all the veggies into small, thin strips.
- When the instant pot is done, quick release the pressure carefully. After pressure is released, press keep warm.
- Open the lid using mitts and carefully remove the rack with the salmon on it and set on a plate.
- Discard the herbs. Add the veggies and put the lid back on, then press the saute setting. Let the veggies cook for 1-2 minutes.
- Serve veggies with salmon and add remaining teaspoon of ghee to the pot.

MEDITERRANEAN RECIPES FOR SAUCES AND MARINADES

1. Instant Pot Hummus

Servings: 6-8
Total Time: 1 Hour

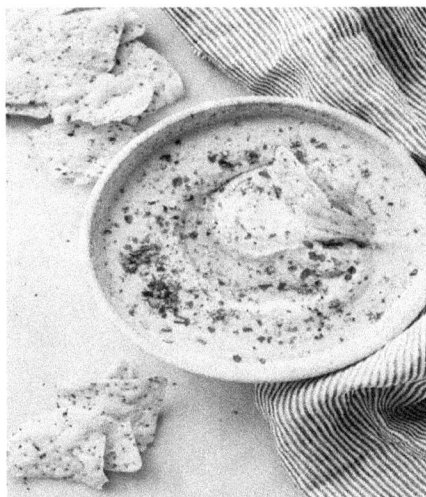

Energy Value Per Serving:
Calories: 293
Protein: 11 grams
Total Fat: 18 grams
Carbohydrates: 27 grams
Ingredients:
- 1 cup dried chickpeas
- 1 head of garlic, crushed
- 2 bay leaves
- 1 onion, cut in half

- 1 ½ teaspoon fine salt
- 4 cups of cold water
- 1 teaspoon ground cumin
- 6 garlic cloves, crushed
- 1 cup tahini
- ¼ cup lemon juice

Instructions:

- Rinse chickpeas thoroughly under cold water.
- Add chickpeas, bay leaves, garlic head, and onion half into the instant pot. Add salt. Pour in water, and mix. Place knob to venting position, close the lid, and turn the knob to sealing position. Cook on high pressure for 60 minutes, and then natural release for 20 minutes. Open the lid carefully.
- Soak 6 cloves of garlic in freshly squeezed lemon juice in a blender for 20-30 minutes before blending. Discard the onions and bay leaves. Drain the chickpeas and garlic cloves well and then set aside chickpeas and liquid. Blend the garlic and lemon juice in blender.
- Add chickpeas, cooked garlic clove, ground cumin, and ¾ cup chickpea liquid to the garlic lemon juice in the blender. Blend the chickpeas at the lowest speed, then increase slowly to high speed. Blend until smooth
- Season with salt to taste.

2. Instant Pot Tomato Sauce

Servings: 3 cups
Total Time: 50 minutes

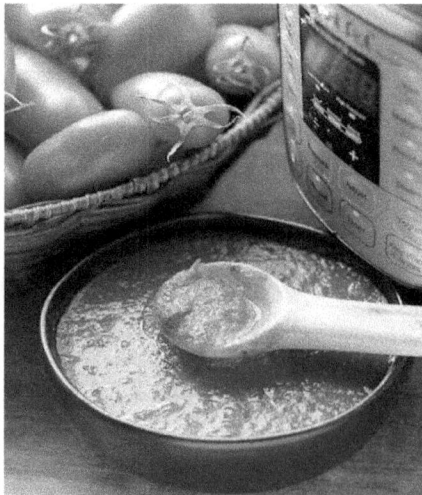

Energy Value For Serving:
Calories: 121
Protein: 1 gram
Total Fat: 12 grams
Carbohydrates: 4 grams
Ingredients:
- 4 medium ripe tomatoes, chopped
- 1 small onion, peeled, trimmed at root and cut in half
- 6 tablespoons butter
- 4 sprigs basil
- 1 teaspoon sea salt

Instructions:

- Place all of the ingredients in the instant pot, place the valve to sealing, and then push manual high pressure to adjust time to 8 minutes.
- Push "Keep Warm/Cancel" to turn off warming mode. Quick release the pressure. When finished, remove the lid.
- Puree the sauce in a blender until you reach your desired consistency. Leave the onion in while blending, or remove.

3. Instant Pot Homemade Spaghetti Sauce
Servings: 6 cups
Total Time: 25 Minutes

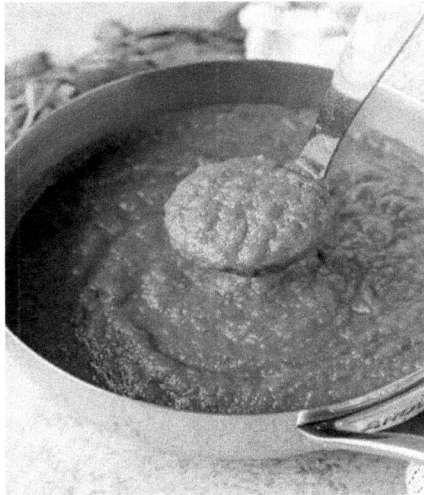

Energy Value Per Serving:
Calories: 145

Protein: 7 grams
Total Fat: 9 grams
Carbohydrates: 8 grams

Ingredients:

- 1 pound ground Italian sausage
- 1 yellow onion, diced
- 1 cup beef broth
- 28 ounce can crushed tomatoes
- 14 ½ ounce can diced tomatoes
- 2 tablespoons tomato paste
- 1 bay leaf
- 2 teaspoons dried basil
- 1 teaspoon garlic powder
- ½ teaspoon dried oregano
- 1 teaspoon brown sugar
- salt and pepper

Instructions:

- Turn your instant pot to saute mode and then add the sausage when heated. Use a wooden spoon to move sausage around and brown on all sides. Add in onions and let them soften for 3 minutes.
- Deglaze the pot with beef broth, then add all of the tomatoes, tomato paste, bay leaf, basil, garlic powder, oregano, and brown sugar.
- Cover the pot and secure the lid. Make sure the valve setting is sealing. Set manual to high pressure and cook for 10 minutes. Let the pressure release naturally for 10 minutes, and then quick release.
- Remove the lid carefully and stir the sauce. Discard bay leaf and add salt and pepper to taste. The sauce is now ready.

4. Instant Pot Sicilian Meat Sauce

Servings: 12
Total Time: 70 Minutes

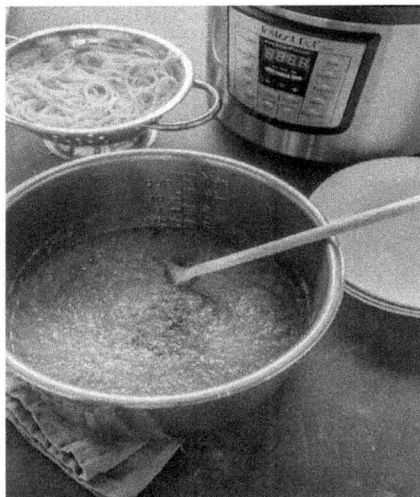

Energy Value Per Serving:
Calories: 214
Protein: 16 grams
Total Fat: 11 grams
Carbohydrates: 13 grams

Ingredients:
- 3 tablespoons olive oil
- 2 pounds boneless pork ribs, trimmed
- 1 onion, chopped
- 5 garlic cloves, minced
- 2, 28 ounce cans diced tomatoes
- 1 can Italian tomato paste
- 3 bay leaves
- 2 tablespoons fresh parsley, chopped
- 2 tablespoons capers, chopped
- ½ teaspoon dried basil
- ½ teaspoon crushed dried rosemary
- ½ teaspoon dried thyme
- ½ teaspoon crushed red pepper flakes
- ½ teaspoon salt
- ½ teaspoon sugar
- 1 cup beef broth
- ½ cup dry red wine

Instructions:

- Select the saute option on instant pot and add 2 tablespoons of olive oil. Brown the pork on both sides in the pot. Then remove and set aside.

- Add remaining oil, saute onion for 2 minutes, then add garlic and cook for another minute.
- Add the remainder of the ingredients and then transfer the meat back to the instant pot. Pour in the broth and red wine, and bring to a boil. Lock the lid and adjust to manual high pressure for 35 minutes.
- When finished cooking, allow pressure to release naturally for 10 minutes and then quick release the rest of the pressure.
- Remove meat from the pressure cooker, shred, discard bone, and return the meat to the sauce.
- Serve over your favorite pasta.

5. Instant Pot Cranberry Sauce
Servings: 3 Cups
Total Time: 50 Minutes

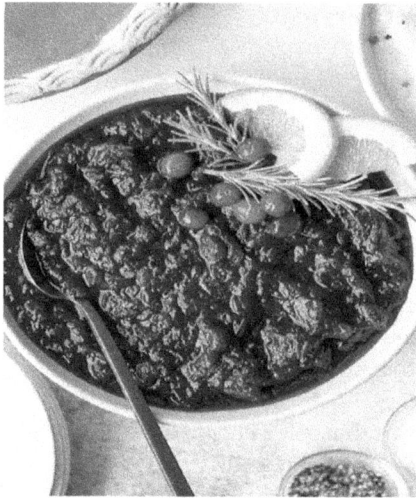

Energy Value Per Serving:
Calories: 86
Protein: 0.1 gram
Total Fat: 0.1 gram
Carbohydrates: 22 grams
Ingredients:
- 2, 12 ounce packages fresh cranberries
- ½ cup brown sugar
- ½ cup freshly squeezed orange juice

- 2 strips orange zest
- 1 cinnamon stick
- ¼ teaspoon ground cloves
- ½ teaspoon vanilla extract

Instructions:

- Place the cranberries, sugar, orange juice, orange zest, cinnamon, and cloves into your instant pot. Stir well.
- Select manual high pressure and set a timer for 4 minutes. Allow the natural release of pressure, 20 minutes.
- Remove the orange zest and cinnamon using a wooden spoon. Mash cranberry mixture until you reach desired consistency. Stir in vanilla and let cool completely.

6. Instant Pot Applesauce
Servings: 4
Total Time: 20 Minutes

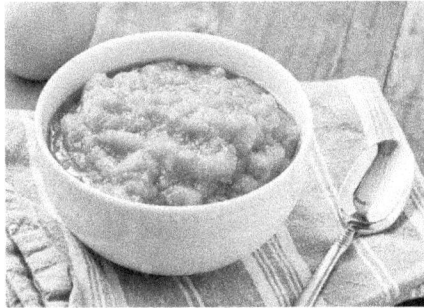

Energy Value Per Serving:
Calories: 90
Protein: 0.4 grams
Total Fat: 0.2 grams
Carbohydrates: 24.1

Ingredients:
- 3 pounds apples
- juice from 1 lemon
- ½ cup of water
- 1 cinnamon stick

Instructions:
- Peel the apples, core, and cut into 8 slices
- Place the apples at the bottom of the instant pot, add lemon juice, water and cinnamon.

- Attach the lid and put on sealing position. Set on manual high pressure for 6 minutes.
- When done, let the pressure release naturally for 6 minutes. Quick release the remainder of pressure. Remove lid carefully, let it cool and remove cinnamon stick.
- Mash with a potato masher. It is now ready to serve.

7. Instant Pot Spicy Curry Hummus
Servings: 12
Total Time: 30 minutes

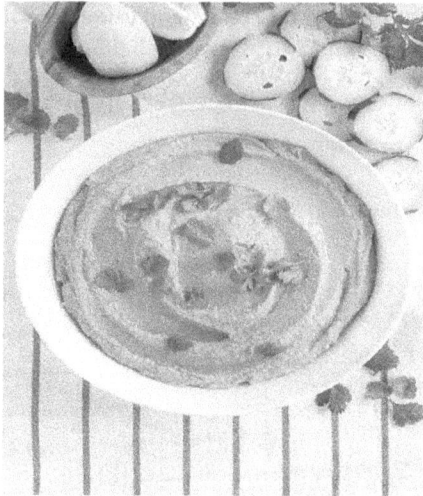

Energy Value Per Serving:
Calories: 372
Protein: 16.7 grams
Total Fat: 12.9 grams
Carbohydrates: 50.9 grams

Ingredients:
- 1 ½ cups garbanzo beans, dry
- 4 cups of water
- ⅓ cup tahini
- ¼ cup extra-virgin olive oil
- 2 cloves garlic, peeled
- 1 tablespoon curry powder
- 1 teaspoon turmeric
- ¼ teaspoon cayenne
- 1 lemon, juiced
- salt and pepper

Instructions:

- Soak garbanzo beans overnight.
- Add garbanzo beans along with 4 cups of water to your instant pot. Set instant post to high pressure for 25 minutes.
- When cooking complete, allow pressure to release naturally. Then quick release to relieve any remaining pressure.
- Let the garbanzo beans cool a bit. In a food processor, add the garbanzo beans, tahini, olive oil, garlic, curry, turmeric, cayenne, lemon juice, salt and pepper. Blend until creamy.
- Hummus ready for serving.

8. Instant Pot Tahini Cashew Curry Recipe
Servings: 2
Total Time: 15 Minutes

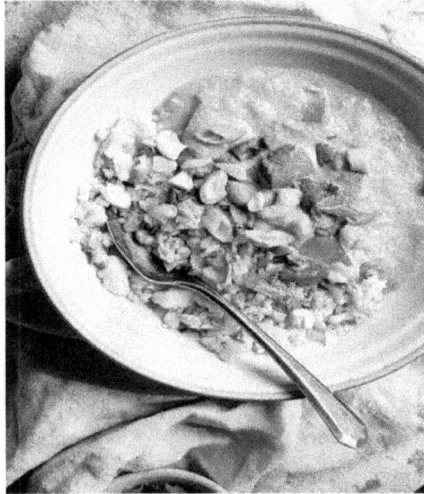

Energy Value Per Serving:
Calories: 232
Protein: 5 grams
Total Fat: 15 grams
Carbohydrates: 20 grams
Ingredients:
- 2 cups unsweetened cashew milk
- 2 tablespoons tahini paste
- 2 teaspoons curry paste
- 2 teaspoons fresh minced ginger
- ½ teaspoon sea salt
- 1 tablespoon turmeric
- 1 tablespoon tapioca starch

- 1 cup cauliflower florets
- ½ cup onion, chopped
- ½ red bell pepper, chopped

Instructions:

- Whisk the cashew milk, tahini paste, curry paste, ginger, sea salt, turmeric together into the instant pot. Set on saute mode and bring to a boil.
- Whisk the tapioca starch with 2 tablespoons of the hot liquid in a separate bowl until smooth. Stir this mixture back into the instant pot until well combined. Boil the curry until it begins to thicken, stirring frequently.
- Stir in cauliflower, onions and pepper into the instant pot. Set it to sealing and cook on manual high pressure for 1 minute. Let pressure release naturally.
- Serve over rice or with pita bread.

9. Instant Pot Mediterranean Pizza Dip

Servings: 8
Total Time: 35 Minutes

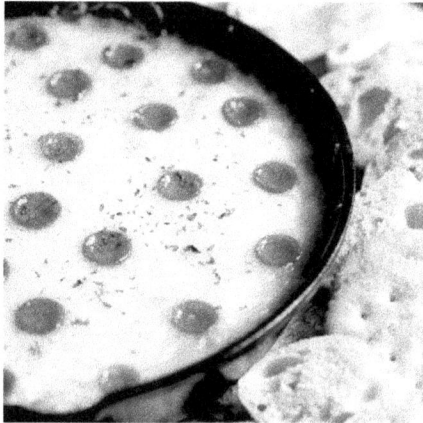

Energy Value Per Serving:
Calories: 285
Protein: 14.1 grams
Total Fat: 23.9 grams
Carbohydrates: 4.3 grams

Ingredients:

- 8 ounce package of cream cheese, cubed and softened
- 8 ounces Monterey Jack cheese, shredded

- 1 cup cherry tomatoes, chopped
- ¾ cup boneless ham steak, chopped
- ½ sliced black olives
- ½ cup marinated artichoke hearts, chopped
- 3 ounces crumbled feta cheese
- 3 cloves garlic, pressed
- ½ tablespoon chopped fresh basil
- 1 teaspoon Italian seasoning

Instructions:

- Combine the cream cheese, Monterey Jack, cherry tomatoes, ham steak, olives, artichoke hearts, feta cheese, garlic, basil, and Italian seasoning in a bowl and mix well. Pour into a rounding glass baking dish and cover with aluminum foil. Make sure the dish will fit inside instant pot.
- Pour 1 cup of water into the insert of your instant pot. Set the metal trivet inside and place baking dish on top. Lock the lid and press manual high pressure for 10 minutes.
- Release the pressure using quick release. Carefully unlock and remove lid. Stir and serve.

10. Instant Pot Marinara Sauce With Fresh Tomatoes

Servings: Two 16 Ounce Jars
Total Time: 30 minutes

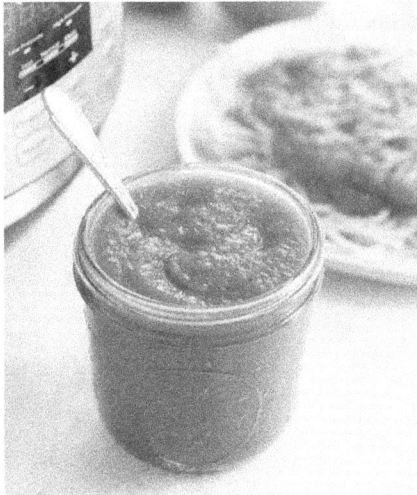

Energy Value Per Serving:
Calories: 65

Protein: 1.8 grams
Total Fat: 1.9 grams
Carbohydrates: 10 grams

Ingredients:

- 1 pound tomatoes, diced
- 1 large onion, diced
- 8 garlic cloves, minced
- 1 tablespoon dried basil
- 1 tablespoon dried oregano
- 1 diced carrot
- 2 tablespoons fresh basil, chopped
- 2 tablespoons fresh parsley, chopped
- 4 ounces vegetable broth
- 2 tablespoon olive oil
- salt to taste

Instructions:

- Press saute on the instant pot and add olive oil to heat. Add garlic, and cook for a minute, then add the dried herbs and onions. Saute for a couple of minutes until you smell the garlic.
- Throw in the tomatoes, carrots, fresh herbs and broth.
- close the lid and seal the vent. Pressure cook on high for 15 minutes. Allow the pressure to naturally release for 10 minutes and then quick release the remaining pressure.
- Place all ingredients in a blender and process until you reach your desired consistency. It is now ready to serve.

11. Instant Pot Chickpeas Curry

Servings: 5
Total Time: 11 Hours

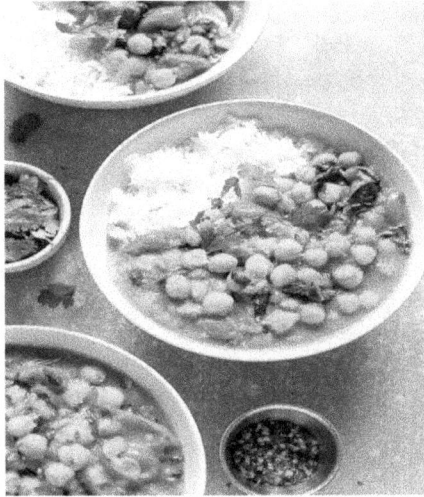

Energy Value Per Serving:
Calories: 205
Protein: 9 grams
Total Fat: 6 grams
Carbohydrates: 31 grams
Ingredients:
- 1 cup dried chickpeas
- 1 tablespoon olive oil
- 1 tablespoon cumin seeds
- 1 tablespoon crushed ginger
- 4 cloves garlic, crushed
- 1 chopped onion
- 2 green chillies, deseeded
- 2 roma tomatoes, finely chopped
- 1 teaspoon salt
- 1 tablespoon coriander powder
- 1 tablespoon garam masala
- 1 teaspoon cumin powder
- ¼ teaspoon cayenne
- 1 teaspoon red chili powder
- ½ teaspoon fennel powder
- 2 cups water

Instructions:

- First, rinse and soak the chickpeas overnight in 4 cups of water. Strain them and rinse thoroughly.
- Turn instant pot to saute setting and add cumin seeds after 30

seconds. When cumin begins to sputter, add onions, garlic, ginger, green chillies, Tomato and saute for a minute.
- Add the spices, chickpeas and water. Close the lid, set to sealing and pressure cook for 35 minutes at bean setting.
- After cooking, naturally release the pressure for 10 minutes, and then quick release the remainder of the pressure. Open the lid and remove contents. Use a wooden spoon to mash a few beans to make the curry more creamy. May garnish with cumin powder and squeeze some fresh lemon juice. It is now ready to serve

12. Instant Pot Sweet Chili Sauce
Servings: 16
Total Time: 25 minutes

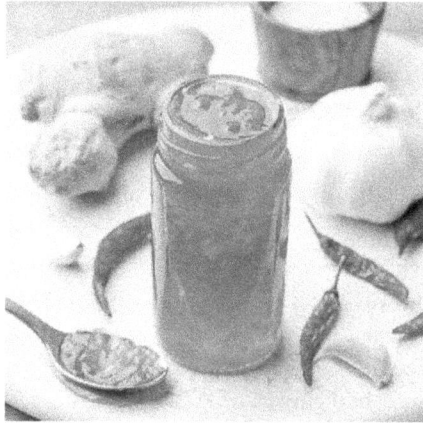

Energy Value Per Serving:
Calories: 37
Protein: 0.2 grams
Total Fat: 0
Carbohydrates: 9.6 grams
Ingredients:
- 2 fresh long chili peppers, halved
- 2 garlic cloves, peeled
- 1-inch peeled ginger
- ½ cup of water
- ½ cup apple cider vinegar
- ½ cup mild honey
- salt to taste
Ingredients:

- Place the chili peppers, garlic, and ginger in a food processor and process until finely chopped.
- Press the saute button on instant pot and let sit until heated, add the chili mixture, water, vinegar, and honey and mix thoroughly.
- Cook and occasionally stir until the sauce thickness is to your liking for 15-20 minutes.
- Add salt to taste.
- Transfer sauce to a jar.

13. Instant Pot Roasted Red Pepper Sauce
Servings: 4
Total Time: 45 Minutes

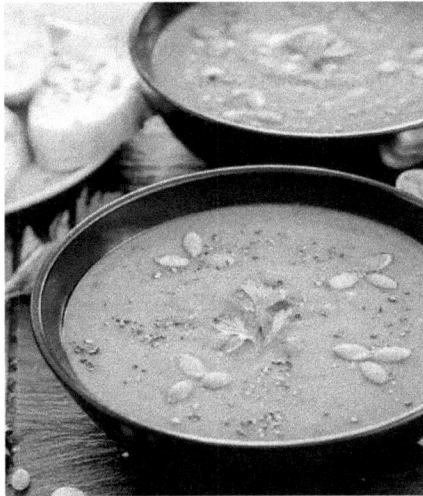

Energy Value Per Serving:
Calories: 336
Protein: 1.9 grams
Total Fat: 31 grams
Carbohydrates: 12 grams
Ingredients:
- 1 teaspoon coconut oil
- 1 onion
- 3 cloves garlic
- ½ teaspoon coriander
- ½ teaspoon cumin
- ½ teaspoon black pepper
- ⅛ teaspoon Ceylon cinnamon
- 1 can diced tomatoes

- 3 roasted red bell peppers, chopped
- 2 teaspoons of apple cider vinegar
- 1 teaspoon chili garlic paste
- ½ teaspoon paprika powder
- ¼ teaspoons Ancho chili powder
- 1 teaspoon salt

Instructions:

- Set your instant pot to saute mode and melt the coconut oil. Fry the onions for 7 minutes until translucent, then add garlic and fry for another minute.
- Add some more coconut oil to one corner of the pot and sprinkle the coriander, cumin, black pepper, and Ceylon cinnamon into the same corner. Fry for 30 seconds and stir well.
- Add diced tomatoes, bell peppers, vinegar, chili garlic paste, paprika, salt, and chili. Let the mixture come to a boil, and then turn off saute mode.
- Close the lid, turn to sealing and set instant pot into pressure cooking mode for 10 minutes.
- Quick release the pressure and transfer sauce into a blender. Blend until smooth.

14. Instant Pot Ace Blender Beef Marinade

Servings: 2.5 cups
Total time: 9 Minutes

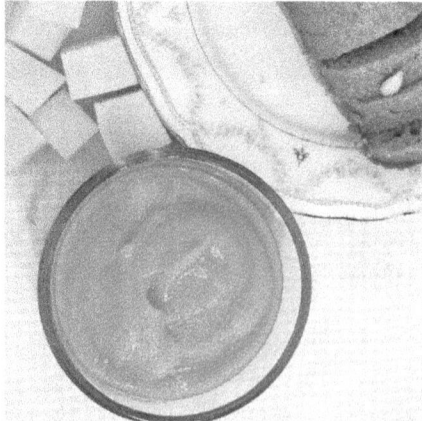

Energy Values Per Serving:
Calories: 9.9
Protein: 0

Total Fat: 0
Carbohydrates: 2 grams
Ingredients:
- ¾ cup tomato juice
- 1 ½ cups balsamic vinegar
- 2 tablespoon Worcestershire sauce
- 2 tablespoons olive oil
- 1 ½ teaspoon ground black pepper
- 1 ½ kosher salt
- ½ teaspoon dried thyme
- 3 cloves of garlic
- ½ yellow onion

Instructions:

- Add all of the ingredients to an Ace blender, by instant pot. Secure and lid and select pulse.
- Blend until smooth

15. Ace Blender Tuscan White Bean Dip
Provides For 6-8 Servings
Total Time: 3 Minutes

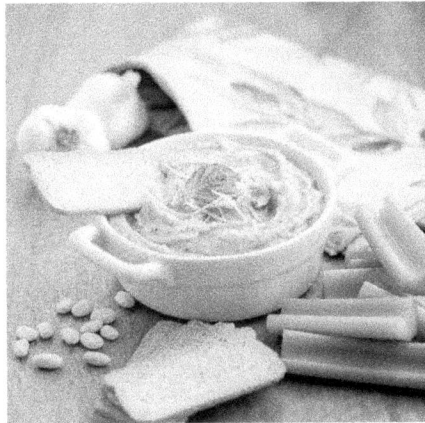

Energy Value Per Serving:
Calories: 34.5
Protein: 2.4 grams
Total Fat: 0.2 grams
Carbohydrates. 6.3 grams
Ingredients:
- 3 teaspoons fresh basil

- 30 ounces cannellini beans
- 2 cloves garlic
- ¼ yellow onion, diced
- ¼ cup vegetable stock
- 1 teaspoon Italian seasoning
- ½ teaspoon black pepper
- ½ teaspoon salt
- ¼ cup extra-virgin olive oil
- ⅓ cup grated Parmesan cheese

Instructions:

- Place all ingredients in an Ace blender, by instant pot. Pulse until smooth.
- Pour into bowl and it is ready to serve. Drizzle a little extra olive oil on top to taste.

MEDITERRANEAN SNACKS

1. Instant Pot Greek Yogurt Cheesecake
Servings: 8
Total Time: 60 Minutes

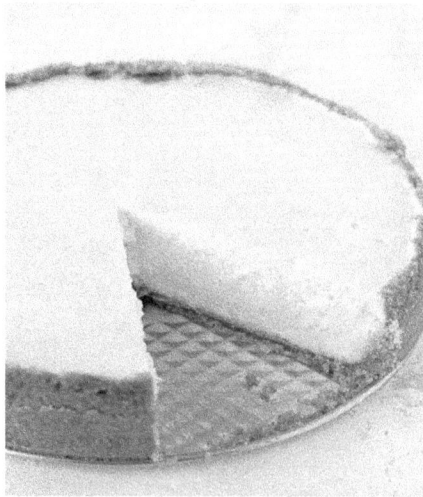

Energy Value Per Serving:
Calories: 280
Protein: 6 grams
Total Fat: 17 grams
Carbohydrates: 26 grams

Ingredients:
- 6 ounce graham crackers
- 4 tablespoons unsalted butter, melted
- 4 ounces regular cream cheese
- 1 ½ cups of whole milk Greek yogurt
- ¼ cup sugar
- 1 teaspoon vanilla
- 2 large eggs

Instructions:

- For the crust, crush the graham crackers into crumbs, then mix in melted butter. Press the mixture onto a 7-inch springform pan, pressing firmly and push the crust firmly halfway up the wall.
- Combine the softened cream cheese, greek yogurt, sugar, and vanilla into a large bowl and whip together smoothly. Add the eggs and mix until combined.
- Pour the filling into the pan, making sure to cover the crust base completely.
- Place the trivet rack into the instant pot and pour 1 cup of water. Place the cheesecake on the trivet and close the lid. Set the value to sealing position and cook on manual high pressure for 30 minutes.
- Release the pressure naturally after cooking, open the lid carefully, and use trivet handles to lift the pan using mitts. Gently blot away any excess water. Allow the cheesecake to sit at room temperature for 1-2 hours, then transfer it to the fridge for at least 4 hours to chill.

2. Instant Pot Creme Brulee
Servings: 3
Total Time: 12 Minutes

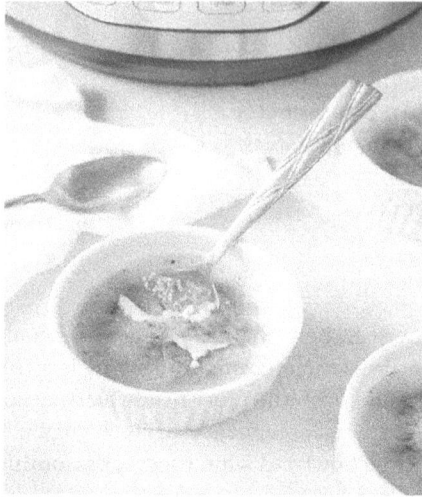

Energy Value Per Serving:

Calories: 335

Protein: 3 grams

Total Fat: 32 grams

Carbohydrates: 8 grams

Ingredients:

- 1 cup whipping cream
- 2 egg yolks
- ¼ fresh vanilla bean pod
- 1 ½ tablespoons of sugar
- 1 teaspoon of caramelized sugar
- 1 cup of cold water

Instructions:

- Prepare your instant pot by placing the trivet inside and pour water at the bottom of the cooker.
- Heat whipping cream for 45 seconds in the microwave, do not let boil.
- Whisk together the egg yolk, vanilla, sugar, and salt into mixing bowl.
- Quickly whisk in 1-2 tablespoons warm cream and then slowly add in the remaining cream, stirring well.
- Divide the cream mixture between 6-ounce heat-safe ramekins and cover with foil.
- Place the custard cups on the trivet and close lid.
- Cook on high for 7 minutes, let the pressure naturally release for 5

minutes and then do a quick release. Open lid, and carefully remove custard cups.

- Refrigerate at least 4 hours before serving.
- Right before serving, top each cup with 1 teaspoon of sugar and then use a kitchen torch and place the flame about 2 inches from the custard. Move in a circular motion and melt the sugar to a caramelized form.

3. Clean Eating Instant Pot Chocolate Cake
Servings: 8
Total Time: 42 Minutes

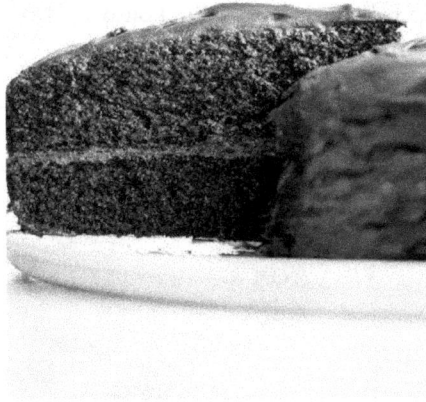

Energy Value Per Serving:
Calories: 168
Protein: 2 gram
Total Fat: 8 grams
Carbohydrates: 24 grams
Ingredients:
- ¾ cup of white whole wheat flour
- ½ cup unprocessed sugar
- ½ cup unsweetened cocoa powder
- 2 teaspoons baking powder
- ⅓ teaspoon salt
- ½ cup unsweetened almond milk
- ¼ cup olive oil
- 2 teaspoons vanilla extract
- 2 teaspoons of apple cider vinegar

Instructions:

- Combine all dry ingredients and whisk well to work out any clumps in the cocoa powder.
- Add in wet ingredients and stir with a wooden spoon until well combined. The batter will be on the thicker side.
- Pour the batter into a greased 6-inch cake pan.
- Place the trivet in your instant pot and add two cups of water
- Place the cake pan on the trivet. Close the lid and the vent.
- Press the manual button and adjust time to 12 minutes. Afterward, allow natural release for 10 minutes and then quick release for the remaining steam.
- Carefully remove the lid.
- Lift the cake pan out and allow to cool.
- Gently lift the cake from the pan and onto a platter.
- Cut and serve.

4. Healthy Instant Pot Chocolate Pudding
Servings: 6
Total Time: 15 Minutes

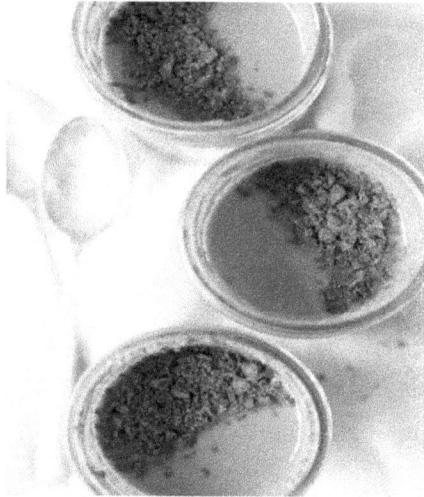

Energy Values Per Serving:
Calories: 208
Protein: 15 grams
Total Fat: 12 grams
Carbohydrates: 31 grams
Ingredients:

- 3-¼ cups of low-fat milk
- 3 organic eggs
- ⅓ cup honey
- 1 ½ tablespoons of vanilla extract
- 1 tablespoon melted ghee butter
- 3-4 tablespoons cocoa powder
- ¼ cup grass-fed collagen
- 3 tablespoons of grass-fed gelatin
- 1 cup of water

Instructions:

- Add milk, eggs, honey, vanilla, ghee, and cocoa powder to a blender. Blend on low for about 30 seconds until fully combined. Remove the vent lid while blender is still blending and add collagen and gelatin. Blend for another 30 seconds.
- Evenly distribute and pour the chocolate pudding mixture into six, ½ pint glass jars, leaving about ½ inch space at the top. Cover the jars with lids.
- Add water into instant pot and place the trivet inside.
- Set all 6 jars on top of trivet.
- Secure the instant pot lid and lock it. Seal the vent. Press the manual high pressure setting and set for 5 minutes.
- When the instant pot is done, it will beep. Turn off the pot, manually release the pressure. Carefully remove the lid after all pressure is released. Using oven mitts, carefully remove the jars and allow them to cool at room temperature. Shake the jars a few times while cooling to prevent separation. Once they have cooled, place them in the fridge.
- While in the fridge, shake a couple of times to prevent separation. Chill at least 6 hours before serving.

5. Instant Pot Baked Apples
Servings: 4
Total Time: 17 Minutes

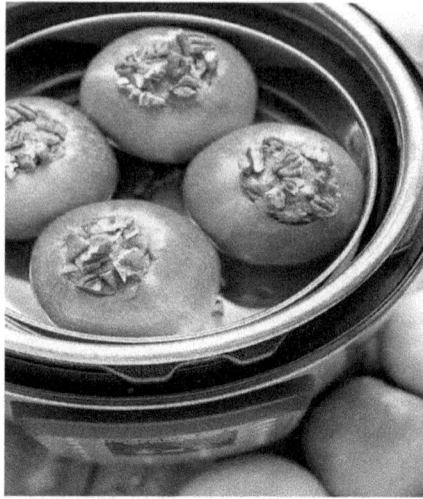

Energy Values Per Serving:

Calories: 406

Protein: 1 gram

Total Fat: 23 grams

Carbohydrates: 53 grams

Ingredients:

- 4 medium apples
- 1 ½ cups of water
- ½ cup unsalted butter
- 1 teaspoon vanilla
- ½ teaspoon nutmeg
- 1 tablespoon cinnamon
- 4 tablespoons brown sugar
- ½ cup walnuts, chopped
- ½ cup raisins

Instructions:

- Pour water into instant pot and add trivet.
- Wash and core the apples, leaving the bottom intact. Make a well that will hold the filling later.
- In a small bowl, mix the butter, vanilla, cinnamon, nutmeg, brown sugar, walnuts, and raisins together. Fill the apples with mixture.
- Arrange the apples on the trivet in the instant pot.
- Lock the lid and move the steam release knob to sealing.
- Press the high pressure for 7 minutes, followed by 5 minute natural release, then quick release for any remaining pressure.
- Open the lid and use tongs to transfer apples to a serving plate.

6. Instant Pot Flourless Brownies

Servings: 16
Total Time: 45 Minutes

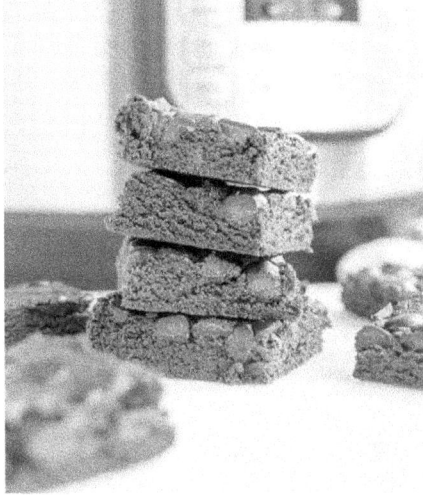

Energy Value Per Serving:

Calories: 125
Protein: 3 grams
Total Fat: 2 grams
Carbohydrates: 12 grams

Ingredients:

- ¾ cup almond butter
- ¾ cup coconut sugar
- ⅓ cup raw cacao powder
- 1 egg
- ¼ teaspoon fine sea salt
- ½ teaspoon baking soda
- ½ teaspoon pure vanilla extract
- ½ cup of dairy free dark chocolate chips
- 1 cup of water

Instructions:

- Use parchment paper to line a 7-inch round pan. For the batter, in a large bowl, combine the egg, salt, baking soda, almond butter, coconut sugar, cacao powder, and vanilla. Stir well.
- Add the batter to the pan and use your hands to press in evenly. Sprinkle with chocolate chips and press them into the batter. Pour

water into instant pot and insert the trivet. Place the pan on the trivet and cover with an upside-down plate.

- Secure the lid and set the steam release valve to sealing. Select the manual pressure to cook on high pressure for 15 minutes. When the cooking is complete, allow natural release of pressure for 10 minutes, then quick release the remaining pressure.
- Carefully remove the lid, lift the trivet and pan out. Let the brownies cool before cutting and serving.

7. Instant Pot Rice Pudding
Servings: 4
Total Time: 30 Minutes

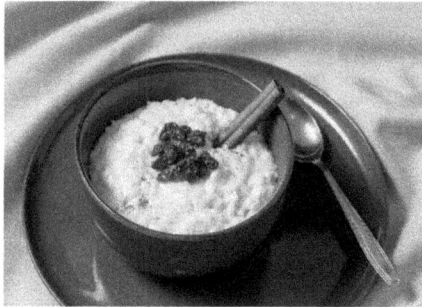

Energy Value Per Serving:
Calories: 151
Protein: 2 grams
Total Fat: 4 gram
Carbohydrates: 26 grams
Ingredients:
- ½ cup rice of your choice
- 1 cup of water
- 400 ml cup full-fat coconut milk
- 10 pitted dates
- 1 medium-sized apple
- ½ teaspoon real vanilla extract
- ¼ teaspoon ground nutmeg
- ½ teaspoon of cinnamon
- pinch of salt
Instructions:

- Wash the rice under cold water.
- Put all ingredients in the instant pot and secure the lid with knob on sealing.

- Press the porage mode, which should be preset to 20 minutes.
- When the pot beeps, naturally release the pressure. This will take about 15 minutes. You may quick release the remaining pressure.
- Open the lid carefully and stir the rice pudding.
- Remove from the pot and then serve.

8. Guilt-Free Instant Pot Chocolate Pudding Cake
Servings: 6
Total Time: 27 Minutes

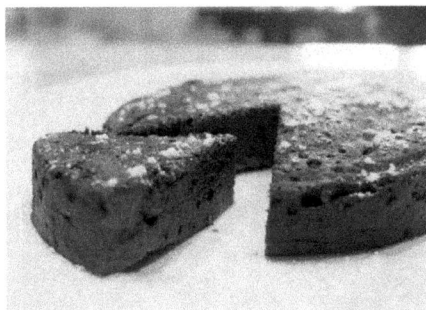

Energy Values Per Serving:
Calories: 155
Protein: 3.6 grams
Total Fat: 8.3 grams
Carbohydrates: 17.5 grams
Ingredients:
- ⅔ cup chopped dark chocolate
- ½ cup applesauce
- 2 eggs
- 1 teaspoon vanilla
- pinch salt
- ¼ cup arrowroot starch
- 3 tablespoons cocoa powder

Instructions:

- Place the trivet inside of the instant pot and pour in 2 cups of water. Measure the chocolate into a heatproof ramekin and set on the trivet. Turn the instant pot on to saute and melt the chocolate over the heated water. Remove ramekin from instant pot when melted.
- Combine applesauce, eggs, and vanilla in a small mixing bowl and whisk well. Add dry ingredients and slowly mix in until no dry streaks are there. Stir in the melted chocolate.

- Grease a 6-inch grease pan with coconut oil and then dust the sides and bottom of pan with cocoa butter. Pour in the cake batter and set the pan on top of the trivet in instant pot.
- Cook on high pressure for 4 minutes. Quick release the pressure when the timer goes off.
- Remove the cake carefully and let it cool for 10 minutes before serving.

9. Instant Pot Greek Yogurt
Servings: 14
Total Time: 45 minutes

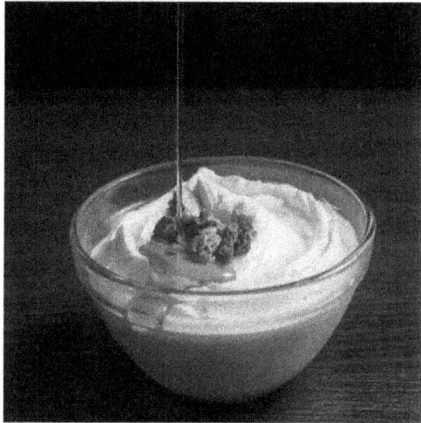

Energy Values Per Serving:
Calories: 166
Protein: 8 grams
Total Fat: 8 grams
Carbohydrates: 13 grams
Ingredients:
- 1 gallon whole milk
- 2 tablespoons yogurt starter
Instructions:

- Pour the milk into the instant pot. Cover the lid and close the pressure valve. Push the yogurt button and then adjust until it says boil. Whisk milk occasionally during boiling cycle.
- When it beeps, open lid, whisk and take temperature. It should be at least 180 F. If not, repeat step.
- Remove cooking pot and place it in kitchen sink full of cold water. Cool the milk, whisking often.

- Temper started-scoop out some milk and whisk in the starter. Pour milk back into the cooking pot and whisk.
- Place cooking pot back in instant pot and cover with lid. Press the yogurt button.
- When the cycle ends, remove the cooking pot to fridge, until cool.
- To make greek yogurt, use a yogurt strainer, and strain the yogurt in refrigerator for at least 2 hours. Using a yogurt strainer provides the easiest method. The whey, or watery part, should be translucent. At this time, you have greek yogurt.

10. Instant Pot Chickpeas With Salsa Verde

Servings: 4
Total Time: 1 hour

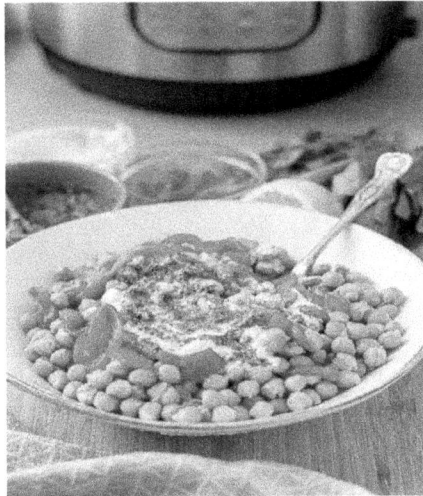

Energy Values Per Serving:

Calories: 367
Protein: 14.6 grams
Total Fat: 16.3 grams
Carbohydrates: 43.7 grams

Ingredients:

- 1 ½ cups of dried chickpeas
- 4 cups of water
- 1 cube of vegetable stock

Ingredients For Salsa Verde:

- A handful of parsley leaves
- A handful of fresh basil
- 2 tablespoons of marinated capers

- 2 cloves of garlic
- 2 ½ tablespoons lemon juice
- ¼ teaspoon of salt
- ¼ cup of olive oil
- ¼ teaspoon of honey
- 2 roasted peppers, thinly sliced
- ¼ cup plant-based yogurt
- 1 teaspoon tahini

Ingredients:

- Add the dried chickpeas to instant pot and cover with water. Add a cube of vegetable stock. Set to high pressure for 45 minutes.
- The instant pot will take about 10 minutes to come to pressure. Once cooked, allow the pressure to release naturally for about 10 minutes, and then do quick release.
- Prepare the salsa verde by adding all of the ingredients to food processor and blend until smooth. Transfer to a bowl.
- Mix yogurt with tahini. Slice the red peppers and place everything on top of the cooked chickpeas.

11. Instant Pot Falafel
Servings: 6
Total Time: 10 Minutes

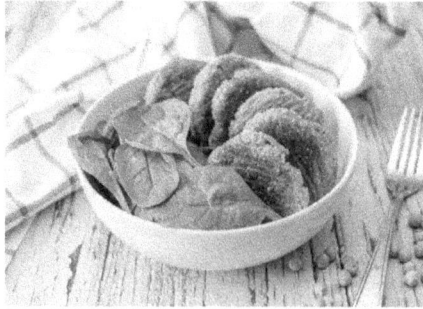

Energy Value Per Serving:
Calories: 57
Protein: 2.3 grams
Total Fat: 3 grams
Carbohydrates: 5 grams
Ingredients:
- 1 cup chickpeas precooked
- 2 cloves garlic, minced
- ½ onion, finely chopped

- 2 tablespoon tahini paste
- 2 teaspoons cumin powder
- 2 tablespoons fresh cilantro, minced
- 1 tablespoon fresh parsley, minced
- 1 tablespoon fresh dill
- 2 tablespoons lemon juice
- ¼ cup flour
- 2 tablespoons sesame oil
- salt to taste

Instructions:

- Blend the chickpeas, garlic, onion, cilantro, parsley, dill, tahini, cumin, lemon juice, and salt in the mixer to obtain a thick paste.
- Add the chickpea flour and stir well.
- Shape some small patties with your hands.
- Pour sesame oil into your instant pot.
- Press saute and add your patties.
- Cook them for 10 minutes until they are roasted and brown on each side.

12. Instant Pot Broccoli

Servings: 2
Total Time: 3 Minutes

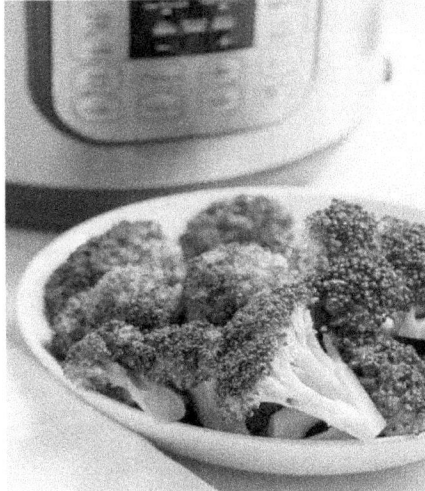

Energy Value Per Serving:
Calories: 30.9
Protein: 2.6 grams

Total Fat: 0.3 grams
Carbohydrates: 6 grams
Ingredients:
- 1 head of broccoli
- ½ cup of water
- salt and pepper to taste

Instructions:

- Wash and cut the broccoli florets.
- Place the steaming basket in the instant pot and add ½ cup of water.
- Add the broccoli to the basket.
- Press manual high pressure for 1 minute.
- Release the pressure immediately and carefully remove broccoli from instant pot
- Add salt and pepper to taste. Light and easy snack.

13. Instant Pot Baby Potatoes
Servings: 6
Total Time: 11 minutes

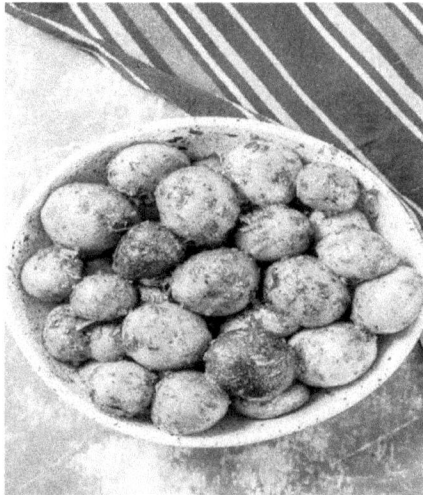

Energy Value Per Serving:
Calories: 170
Protein: 3 grams
Total Fat: 6 grams
Carbohydrates: 25 grams
Ingredients:

- 1 pound baby potatoes
- 1 ½ cups of water
- salt and black pepper to taste
- olive oil to taste

Instructions:

- Press saute mode on instant pot. Add olive oil and potatoes, and saute for 5 minutes.
- Pour water into your instant pot and correctly place the trivet.
- Cook at high pressure for 5 minutes.
- Quick release steam immediately.
- Season your potatoes with salt, pepper, and serve.

14. Instant Pot Mango Sticky Rice

Servings: 6
Total Time: 27 Minutes

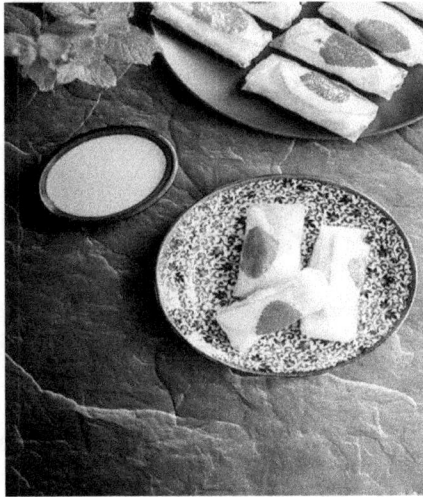

Energy Value Per Serving:

Calories: 493
Protein: 4.9 grams
Total Fat: 25 grams
Carbohydrates: 69 grams

Ingredients:

- 1/2 cup cooked rice
- ⅓ cup cold water
- ⅓ cup coconut milk
- ⅛ cup + ½ tablespoon sugar

- ½ mango, sliced and peeled
- ¼ cup coconut milk
- 1 tablespoon sugar
- 1 pinch of salt
- ½ tablespoon starch

Instructions:

- Add all of the ingredients in the instant pot except mango.
- Close the lid of the instant pot and set the manual at high pressure for 12 minutes. Quick release the pressure when done.
- Open the lid carefully and serve the rice with mango on top.

15. Instant Pot Spicy Boiled Peanuts
Servings: 8
Total Time: 1 Hour and 20 minutes

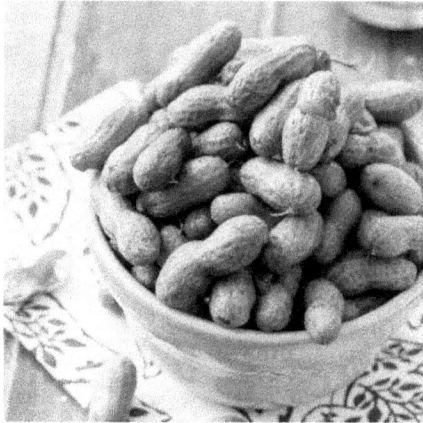

Energy Value Per Serving:
Calories: 120
Protein: 5 grams
Total Fat: 8 grams
Carbohydrates: 5 grams

Ingredients:
- 1 ½ pounds of green peanuts
- ⅓ cup salt
- 1 tablespoon red pepper flakes
- 1 tablespoon Cajun seasoning

Instructions:

- Place the peanuts in the instant pot, and add salt, red pepper flakes, and seasoning.
- Add water to cover the peanuts.
- Place steamer rack for the pot on top of the peanuts to help weight them down.
- Place lid on instant pot, and make sure valve is in sealing position.
- Set to Pressure cook for 75 minutes.
- Do a natural pressure release for 30 minutes and then quick release.

MEDITERRANEAN DRINKS

1. Raspberry Vanilla Smoothie
Servings: over 2 cups
Total time: 5 minutes

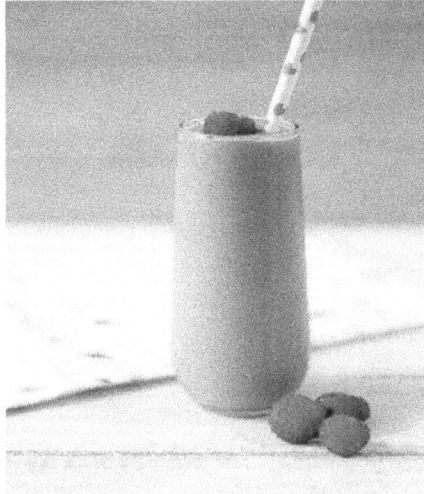

Energy Value Per Serving:
Calories: 155
Protein: 7 grams
Total Fat: 2 grams
Carbohydrates: 30 grams
Ingredients:
- 1 cup frozen raspberries
- 6-ounce container of vanilla Greek yogurt
- ½ cup of unsweetened vanilla almond milk
Instructions:

- Take all of your ingredients and place them in an instant pot Ace blender.
- Process until smooth and liquified.

2. Blueberry Banana Protein Smoothie
Servings: 1
Total time: 5 minutes

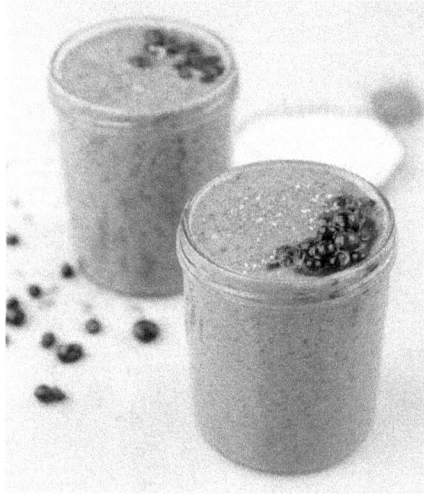

Energy Value Per Serving:
Calories: 230
Protein: 19.1 grams
Total Fat: 2.6 grams
Carbohydrates: 32.9 grams
Ingredients:
- ½ cup frozen and unsweetened blueberries
- ½ banana slices up
- ¾ cup plain nonfat Greek yogurt
- ¾ cup unsweetened vanilla almond milk
- 2 cups of ice cubes
Instructions:

- Add all of the ingredients into an instant pot ace blender.
- Blend until smooth.

3. Honey And Wild Blueberry Smoothie
Servings: 2
Total time: 10 minutes

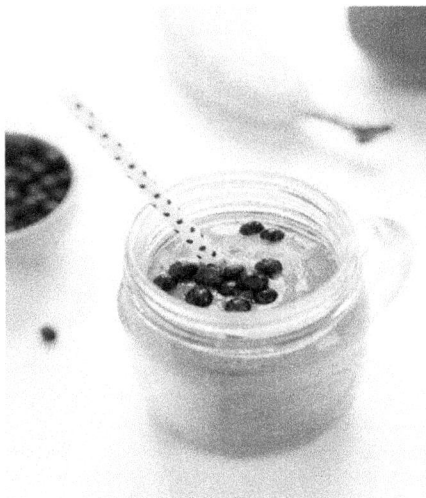

Energy Value Per Serving:
Calories: 223
Protein: 9.4 grams
Total Fat: 1.4 grams
Carbohydrates: 46.8 grams
Ingredients:
- 1 whole banana
- 1 cup of mango chunks
- ½ cup wild blueberries
- ½ plain, nonfat Greek yogurt
- ½ cup milk (for blending)
- 1 tablespoon raw honey
- ½ cup of kale

Instructions:

- Add all of the above ingredients into an instant pot Ace blender. Add extra ice cubes if needed.
- Process until smooth.

4. Oats Berry Smoothie
Servings: 2
Total Time: 10 Minutes

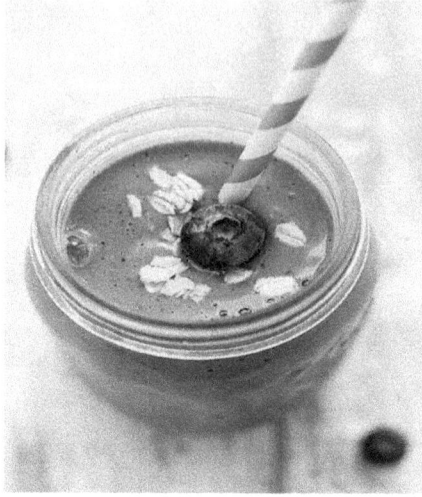

Energy Value Per Serving:
Calories: 295
Protein: 18 grams
Total Fat: 5 grams
Carbohydrates: 44 grams
Ingredients:
- 1 cup of frozen berries
- 1 cup Greek yogurt
- ¼ cup of milk
- ¼ cup of oats
- 2 teaspoon honey

Instructions:

- Place all ingredients in an instant pot Ace blender and blend until smooth.

5. Kale-Pineapple Smoothie
Servings: 2
Total Time: 5 Minutes

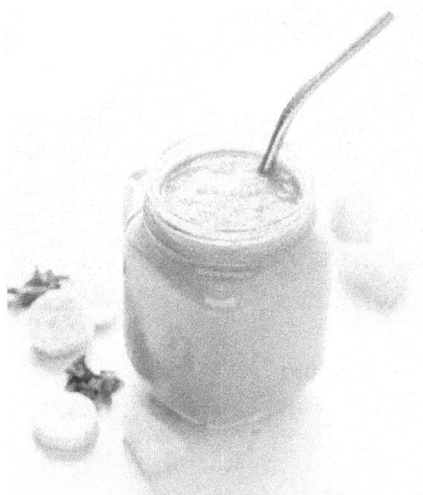

Energy Value Per Serving:
Calories: 140
Protein: 4 grams
Total Fat: 2.5 grams
Carbohydrates: 30 grams

Ingredients:
- 1 Persian cucumber
- fresh mint
- 1 cup of coconut milk
- 1 tablespoon honey
- 1 ½ cups of pineapple pieces
- ¼ pound baby kale

Instructions:

- Cut the ends off of the cucumbers and then cut the whole cucumber into small cubes. Strip the mint leaves from the stems.
- Add all of the ingredients to your instant pot Ace blender and blend until smooth.

6. Moroccan Avocado Smoothie
Servings: 4
Total Time: 5 Minutes

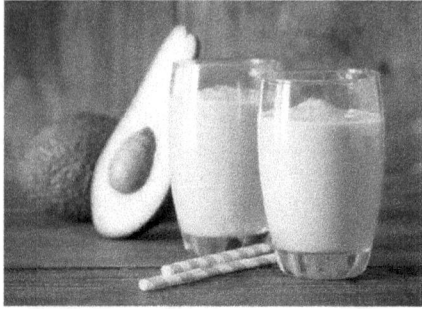

Energy Value Per Serving:
Calories: 100
Protein: 1 gram
Total Fat: 6 grams
Carbohydrates: 11 grams
Ingredients:
- 1 ripe avocado, peeled and pitted
- 1 overripe banana
- 1 cup almond milk, unsweetened
- 1 cup of ice

Instructions:

- Place the avocado, banana, milk, and ice into your instant pot Ace blender.
- Blend until smooth with no pieces of avocado remaining.

7. Mediterranean Smoothie
Servings: 2
Total Time: 5 Minutes

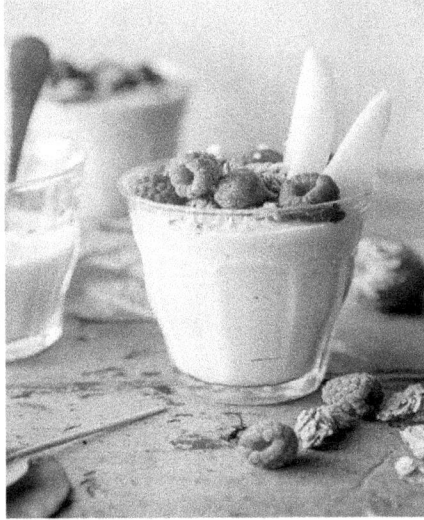

Energy Value Per Serving:
Calories: 168
Protein: 4 grams
Total Fat: 1 gram
Carbohydrates: 39 grams
Ingredients:
- 2 cups of baby spinach
- 1 teaspoon fresh ginger root
- 1 frozen banana, pre-sliced
- 1 small mango
- ½ cup beet juice
- ½ cup of skim milk
- 4-6 ice cubes

Instructions:

- Take all ingredients and place them in your instant pot Ace blender.

8. Mango Strawberry Smoothie With Greek Yogurt
Servings:2
Total Time: 10 Minutes

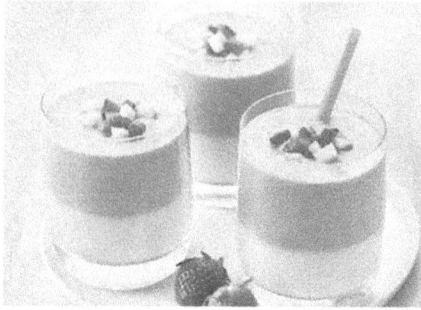

Energy Value Per Serving:
Calories: 184.9
Protein: 18.9 grams
Total Fat: 1 grams
Carbohydrates: 27.5 grams
Ingredients:
- 1 banana
- ½ cup frozen strawberries
- ½ cup frozen mango
- ½ cup Greek yogurt
- ¼ cup almond milk
- ¼ teaspoon turmeric
- ¼ teaspoon ginger
- 1 tablespoon honey

Instructions:

- Place all of these ingredients into your instant pot ace blender and blend until smooth.
- Pour in a glass and serve.

9. Anti-Inflammatory Blueberry Smoothie
Servings: 1
Total Time: 5 Minutes

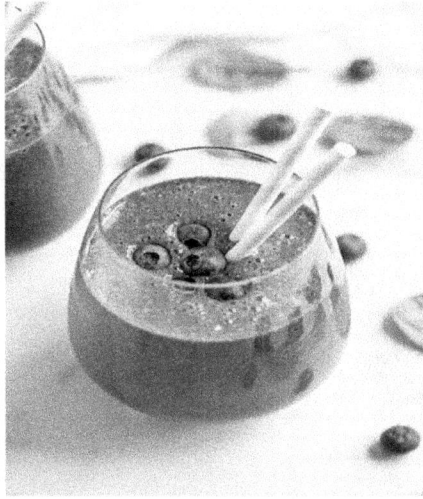

Energy Value Per Serving:
Calories: 340
Protein: 9 grams
Total Fat: 13 grams
Carbohydrates: 55 grams
Ingredients:
- 1 cup of almond milk
- 1 frozen banana
- 1 cup frozen blueberries
- 2 handfuls of spinach
- 1 tablespoon almond butter
- ¼ teaspoon cinnamon
- ¼ teaspoon cayenne
- 1 teaspoon maca powder

Instructions:

- Combine all of these ingredients into your instant pot Ace blender and blend until smooth.

10. Healthy Breakfast Smoothie
Servings: 1
Total Time: 3 Minutes

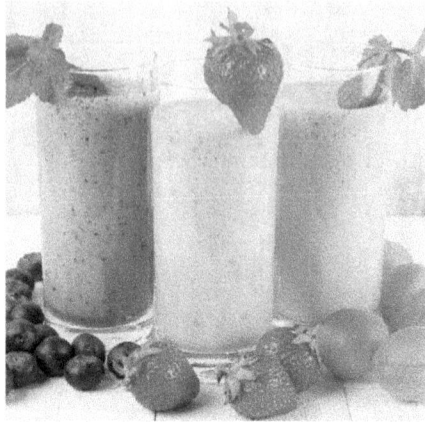

Energy Value Per Serving:
Calories: 300
Protein: 12.5 grams
Total Fat: 11 grams
Carbohydrates: 40 grams
Ingredients:
- 1 medium banana
- ½ cup sliced strawberries
- ¼ cup 2% Greek yogurt
- 1 tablespoon of almond butter
- ½ cup baby spinach
- ½ cup of unsweetened almond milk

Instructions:

- Place all of the ingredients into your instant pot ace blender and blend until smooth.

11. Super Nutrient Smoothie
Servings: 1
Total Time: 5 Minutes

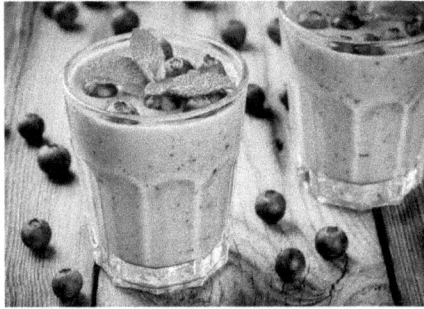

Energy Value Per Serving:

Calories: 214

Protein: 6 grams

Total Fat: 4 grams

Carbohydrates: 41 grams

Ingredients:

- ½ cup of frozen blueberries
- ½ cup of frozen pineapple
- ¼ cup of spinach
- 1 tablespoon of honey
- ½ cup of water

Instructions:

- Combine all of the ingredients into your instant pot Ace blender and blend until smooth.

AFTERWORD

The Mediterranean way of eating is one of the most popular and beloved eating patterns that is known for its health benefits and healthy slimming. This is a diet that is based on fresh, plant-based foods that are rich in healthy fats and whole foods that grow from the ground.

This diet (or eating pattern) is one that has no strict rules. All it suggests is that you get the right ingredients such as fruits, vegetables, olive oil, fish, and seafood, and do what works the best for you.

People who live in the Mediterranean region (Italy, Balkans, Spain, Portugal, France) are known to have fit figures, live longer, and in general, are healthy people. So, if your main goal is to lose weight while eating Mediterranean meals, then you will have made a wonderful choice. Slimming with this diet goes steadily and in a healthy way. There is no restriction or starvation, but rather eating foods that are not processed. Switching to fresh and whole foods might be challenging if you are used to eating fast food, red and processed meats, sweets, white flour, sugar, and alcohol, but it is not impossible.

The risk of cancer, heart failure, high blood pressure, cholesterol, depression, inflammations, poor immunity, and other health issues is significantly higher when your menu consists mostly of unhealthy food. Thus, this diet is a sure way to purge your blood, improve your general mood and health, boost your immunity, and lower the risk of diseases such as Type 2 diabetes, breast and colon cancer, or Alzheimer's disease. Studies have shown that even depression and anxiety are directly connected with the type of food you eat, so it is best to know that foods that grow naturally and under the sun have a far bigger chance to improve your mood and boost your body with serotonin.

One of the greatest things about the Mediterranean way of eating is that you do not have to be an extraordinary cook to prepare your meals. With the right ingredients, you can always make simple and delicious meals that don't require hours in the kitchen.

Prepare your weekly meal plan, buy the groceries, and simply stick to eating the suitable foods. Your energy will be higher, your brain's cognitive functions and memory will improve, and you will never feel bloated. Digestion will become easier, and you will feel happier.

The most important thing for people who want to slim down with this diet is to keep a positive mindset. This is a healthy lifestyle that requires you to pay attention to the food you are eating, spend more time with your loved ones, and do more physical activity.

Once you lose weight, you will keep maintaining your figure by simply eating your favorite meals. Since this diet does not feel like a diet, it is super easy to follow. There is no yo-yo effect because you will remain true to your Mediterranean menu. This diet is also a wonderful way for you to get rid of your unhealthy eating habits and kill all your cravings for junk food.

At the end of the day, nothing is forbidden in this diet. Some foods are recommended to be consumed frequently, while there are other foods that should only be eaten occasionally. When you see that you have lost a couple of pounds within the first week, you will know that you made the right decision.

Finally, what matters most is you feeling content, happy, and good in your own skin. I hope this book answered most of your questions and helped you decide how to start your new lifestyle.

www.ingramcontent.com/pod-product-compliance
Lightning Source LLC
Chambersburg PA
CBHW070857030426
42336CB00014BA/2243